国家卫生健康委员会"十四五"规划教材
全国高等学校药学类专业第九轮规划教材
供药学类专业用

药学英语（上册）

第 6 版

主　编　史志祥　龚长华

副主编　唐　漫　张予阳　付爱玲

编　者（按姓氏笔画排序）

王　炜（湖南中医药大学）　　　　陈　芸（南京医科大学）

亢小辉（大连医科大学）　　　　　陈　菁（中国药科大学）

史志祥（中国药科大学）　　　　　欧田苗（中山大学药学院）

付爱玲（西南大学药学院）　　　　易　玲（苏州大学药学院）

乔玉玲（北京大学医学人文学院）　赵　岩（内蒙古医科大学）

庄　婕（上海健康医学院）　　　　郭　昊（徐州医科大学）

杜伟杰（哈尔滨医科大学）　　　　唐　漫（中国医科大学）

李晨睿（西北工业大学生命学院）　龚长华（广东药科大学）

张予阳（沈阳药科大学）　　　　　符　垚（四川大学华西药学院）

张维芬（潍坊医学院）　　　　　　翟兴英（江西中医药大学）

张朝慧（首都医科大学）

人民卫生出版社
·北　京·

版权所有，侵权必究！

图书在版编目（CIP）数据

药学英语．上册 / 史志祥，龚长华主编．—6 版
．—北京：人民卫生出版社，2023.12（2025.4重印）
ISBN 978-7-117-35771-5

Ⅰ．①药…　Ⅱ．①史…　②龚…　Ⅲ．①药物学–英语
–教材　Ⅳ．①R9

中国国家版本馆 CIP 数据核字（2024）第 004477 号

药学英语（上册）
Yaoxue Yingyu (Shangce)
第 6 版

主　　编：史志祥　龚长华
出版发行：人民卫生出版社（中继线 010-59780011）
地　　址：北京市朝阳区潘家园南里 19 号
邮　　编：100021
E - mail：pmph @ pmph.com
购书热线：010-59787592　010-59787584　010-65264830
印　　刷：天津市银博印刷集团有限公司
经　　销：新华书店
开　　本：850×1168　1/16　印张：17
字　　数：491 千字
版　　次：1986 年 6 月第 1 版　2023 年 12 月第 6 版
印　　次：2025 年 4 月第 3 次印刷
标准书号：ISBN 978-7-117-35771-5
定　　价：68.00 元
打击盗版举报电话：010-59787491　E-mail：WQ @ pmph.com
质量问题联系电话：010-59787234　E-mail：zhiliang @ pmph.com
数字融合服务电话：4001118166　E-mail：zengzhi @ pmph.com

出 版 说 明

全国高等学校药学类专业规划教材是我国历史最悠久、影响力最广、发行量最大的药学类专业高等教育教材。本套教材于1979年出版第1版,至今已有43年的历史,历经八轮修订,通过几代药学专家的辛勤劳动和智慧创新,得以不断传承和发展,为我国药学类专业的人才培养作出了重要贡献。

目前,高等药学教育正面临着新的要求和任务。一方面,随着我国高等教育改革的不断深入,课程思政建设工作的不断推进,药学类专业的办学形式、专业种类、教学方式呈多样化发展,我国高等药学教育进入了一个新的时期。另一方面,在全面实施健康中国战略的背景下,药学领域正由仿制药为主向原创新药为主转变,药学服务模式正由“以药品为中心”向“以患者为中心”转变。这对新形势下的高等药学教育提出了新的挑战。

为助力高等药学教育高质量发展,推动“新医科”背景下“新药科”建设,适应新形势下高等学校药学类专业教育教学、学科建设和人才培养的需要,进一步做好药学类专业本科教材的组织规划和质量保障工作,人民卫生出版社经广泛、深入的调研和论证,全面启动了全国高等学校药学类专业第九轮规划教材的修订编写工作。

本次修订出版的全国高等学校药学类专业第九轮规划教材共35种,其中在第八轮规划教材的基础上修订33种,为满足生物制药专业的教学需求新编教材2种,分别为《生物药物分析》和《生物技术药物学》。全套教材均为国家卫生健康委员会“十四五”规划教材。

本轮教材具有如下特点:

1. 坚持传承创新,体现时代特色　本轮教材继承和巩固了前八轮教材建设的工作成果,根据近几年新出台的国家政策法规、《中华人民共和国药典》(2020年版)等进行更新,同时删减老旧内容,以保证教材内容的先进性。继续坚持“三基”“五性”“三特定”的原则,做到前后知识衔接有序,避免不同课程之间内容的交叉重复。

2. 深化思政教育,坚定理想信念　本轮教材以习近平新时代中国特色社会主义思想为指导,将“立德树人”放在突出地位,使教材体现的教育思想和理念、人才培养的目标和内容,服务于中国特色社会主义事业。各门教材根据自身特点,融入思想政治教育,激发学生的爱国主义情怀以及敢于创新、勇攀高峰的科学精神。

3. 完善教材体系,优化编写模式　根据高等药学教育改革与发展趋势,本轮教材以主干教材为主体,辅以配套教材与数字化资源。同时,强化“案例教学”的编写方式,并多配图表,让知识更加形象直观,便于教师讲授与学生理解。

4. 注重技能培养,对接岗位需求　本轮教材紧密联系药物研发、生产、质控、应用及药学服务等方面的工作实际,在做到理论知识深入浅出、难度适宜的基础上,注重理论与实践的结合。部分实操性强的课程配有实验指导类配套教材,强化实践技能的培养,提升学生的实践能力。

5. 顺应“互联网+教育”,推进纸数融合　本次修订在完善纸质教材内容的同时,同步建设了以纸质教材内容为核心的多样化的数字化教学资源,通过在纸质教材中添加二维码的方式,“无缝隙”地链接视频、动画、图片、PPT、音频、文档等富媒体资源,将“线上”“线下”教学有机融合,以满足学生个性化、自主性的学习要求。

众多学术水平一流和教学经验丰富的专家教授以高度负责、严谨认真的态度参与了本套教材的编写工作,付出了诸多心血,各参编院校对编写工作的顺利开展给予了大力支持,在此对相关单位和各位专家表示诚挚的感谢!教材出版后,各位教师、学生在使用过程中,如发现问题请反馈给我们(renweiyaoxue@163.com),以便及时更正和修订完善。

人民卫生出版社
2022年3月

主 编 简 介

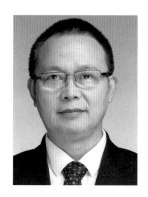

史志祥

　　中国药科大学教授,硕士生导师,外国语学院副院长。《药学英语》(上、下册)第4版、第5版主编,《中国药科大学学报》编委兼英文主审,《药学进展》英文主审。中国中医药研究促进会中医药翻译与国际传播专业委员会常务理事,江苏省翻译协会理事。近年主持"药学英语"省级一流课程,主讲"中国文化"省级全英文精品课程、"英语口译"校级精品课程、"博士药学国际学术交流英语"等。多次荣获校优秀教学成果一、二等奖,主持多项省部级科研及教改课题,主编医药英语相关教材十余部。

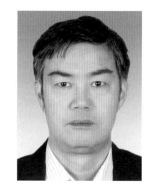

龚长华

　　广东药科大学教授,博士,外国语学院院长。广东省外国语言学会常务理事,广东省普通高校大学英语课程教学指导委员会委员,中华中医药学会翻译分会副主委,世界中医药学会联合会翻译专业委员会常务理事。主持医药英语研究与教学类省级课题6项,发表科研、教学文章十余篇,主编、副主编医药英语类教材8部。

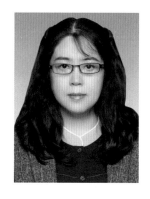

唐　漫

　　临床医学学士,病理生理学硕士,美国得克萨斯州大学药学院药理学博士,莱斯康制药公司神经科学部博士后。留美学习工作十三年,曾任莱斯康制药公司科学家,美国得克萨斯脊椎指压疗法学院副教授,通过美国执业医师考试(USMLE)。2010 年回国,任中国医科大学临床药理学教授。近十年主持省级教改课题,发表多篇医学教育论文,主编或参编人民卫生出版社等多家出版社本科生及研究生规划教材十余部。科研以抑郁症发病机制为主线,主持国家、教育部、省市级课题,发表多篇 SCI 论文。

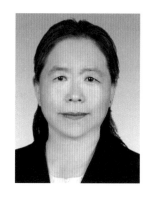

张予阳

　　沈阳药科大学教授、博士;2009—2010 年美国南佛罗里达大学医学院脑修复研究中心访问学者;辽宁省药学会药理专业委员会委员、辽宁省细胞生物学学会中药化学专业委员会理事、辽宁省医疗机构制剂审评专家、沈阳市高层次(领军)人才、国家自然科学基金委评议专家、教育部学位中心评审专家、辽宁省科技奖励评审专家;主持辽宁省教育厅项目 2 项、承担"重大新药创制"科技重大专项课题 1 项、承担国家自然科学基金面上项目 2 项;发表论文百余篇;主编或参编教材及专著 20 余部。

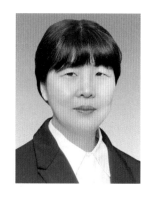

付爱玲

　　教授,博士生导师。从事一线教学工作 20 余年,主要承担本科生和研究生的药学专业英语课程,以及生物化学、药理学的中英文教学工作,提倡学以致用的教学方法。先后主持国家自然科学基金、教育部新世纪优秀人才支持计划、重庆市科技重点项目等多项科研任务。科研方向为药物合成与线粒体治疗的工作。分别在 *J Med Chem, Bioeng Transl Med* 和 *Asian J Pharm Sci* 等国内外学术期刊上发表论文 90 余篇,其中 SCI 论文 60 余篇。出版著作 2 部,教材 3 部。

前　言

《药学英语》（上、下册）第 5 版于 2016 年面世以来，在设有药学类及医药英语相关专业的全国医药院校和综合性大学药学院（系）得到了较好的使用，收到了很好的效果。

为了确保本教材能更好地适应新医药背景下药学教育的新形势和新任务以及国际化背景下医药行业的新发展和新需要，真正将药学英语教材和药学相关专业人才知识获取、能力训练和素质提高结合起来，做到立德树人，本套教材编委会全体成员认真学习国家相关文件精神以及人民卫生出版社相关要求，充分考虑药学学科的发展变化和高校药学英语教学的实际情况，推出第 6 版教材。

《药学英语》（第 6 版）包括上、下两册：上册为基础药学英语部分，选课文 28 篇（按专业题材分成 14 个单元，每个单元 2 篇文章），每个单元包括单元导入（Lead-in）、课文 A（Text A）、习题（Exercises）、思政短文（Value-Oriented Reflective Reading）、课文 B（Text B）、医药英语词汇学习（Medical and Pharmaceutical Terminology）以及英汉翻译技巧（English-Chinese Medical Translation Strategy）；下册为专业药学英语部分，选课文 20 篇（按专业学科领域分成 10 个单元，每个单元 2 篇文章），每个单元包括学科导入（Lead-in）、课文 A（Text A）、习题（Exercises）、思政短文（Value-Oriented Reflective Reading）、课文 B（Text B）、学术英语写作（Academic Writing）以及汉英翻译技巧（Chinese-English Medical Translation Strategy）。

为了便于学生及药学英语爱好者自学，本教材上、下册在每篇课文之后均配有词汇表（Word Study）和注释（Notes）。同时，教材还首次利用数字平台提供每个单元第一篇单元导入及课文 A 的录音、习题参考答案、课文 A 参考译文、医药分类词汇拓展等，广大读者只需扫描教材中的二维码即可随时进入数字内容的学习或参考。为了方便各院校老师使用，本教材在提供以上录音、主要练习参考答案和参考译文的基础上，还通过数字平台专区提供了其他补充材料和线上课程共享等数字增值服务。

为了体现药学学科的完整性以及教材内容的适用性，《药学英语》（第 6 版）上、下册涵盖了药学基础、药学科学、临床药学、制药工程、药物监管等方面。与第 5 版相比，上册增加了"药品国际注册"单元，下册增加了"药物发现及评价"单元。

《药学英语》（第 6 版）上册可供全国各高校药学类各专业及医药英语类专业本、专科生"药学英语"教学用，在注重学生药学英语阅读及词汇能力提高的同时强调学生药学英语听、说、读、译等综合能力的提升；下册可供开设两个学期药学英语课的高校药学类各专业本科生第二学期用，也可以供药学类本科各专业学生"专业外语"或研究生"专业药学英语"教学用，在注重学生药学专业英语水平提高的同时强调学生汉英药学英语翻译能力和药学学术英语写作能力的提升，为他们未来在医药行业从业及用英语进行药学国际学术英语交流打下扎实的基础。

本套教材编写队伍阵容强大，全套教材由本人及广东药科大学龚长华教授担任主编，中国医科大学唐漫教授、沈阳药科大学张予阳教授及西南大学付爱玲教授担任副主编。编委单位包括中国药科大学、沈阳药科大学、广东药科大学三所一流药学专业性院校，包括北京大学、中山大学、四川大学、西北工业大学、苏州大学、西南大学、南京医科大学、中国医科大学、大连医科大学、哈尔滨医科大学等知名医药院校；编委中既有博通医药的复合型英语专家，也有长期从事相关药学领域教学及研究且精通英语的药学各领域专家。所有编者除了完成自己分工的内容之外，还协助其他编者完成相关编写及审校工作，多次进行线下、线上交流，不辞辛劳。

　　南京医科大学药学院的杨静老师、中国药科大学外国语学院药学英语系张宇辉老师、美国纽约州立大学布法罗分校药学院在读 PharmD（药学博士）史博诚等提供了不同形式的帮助，在此一并表示感谢。

　　由于编者水平有限，不足之处在所难免，敬请各位专家及读者指正。

中国药科大学　史志祥

shizhixiang@cpu.edu.cn

2023 年 3 月

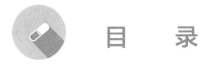

目　录

Unit One

Physiology and Pathology

Stated most simply and broadly, physiology is the study of how living organisms work. As applied to human beings, its scope is extremely broad. At one end of the spectrum, it includes the study of individual molecules—for example, how a particular protein's shape and electrical properties allow it to function as a channel for sodium ions to move into or out of a cell. At the other end, it is concerned with complex processes that depend on the interplay of many widely separated organs in the body—for example, how the brain, heart, and several glands all work together to cause the excretion of more sodium in the urine when a person has eaten salty food.

Pathology is the science of diseases, which deals with the studies of etiology, pathogenesis, morphologic structures, changes in functions and metabolism in the living organisms by means of natural science. It illustrates the discipline of the development and the evolution of diseases and the essence of diseases to provide a theoretical basis for the treatment and prevention of varied types of diseases.

Pathophysiology is the study of functional changes in the body which occur in response to diseases or injuries. The field of pathophysiology is designed to help people study the progress of diseases so that they can quickly identify diseases and consider various treatments. One of the major issues in pathophysiology is that every human body is different. What may be normal in one person could be abnormal in another, and diseases will not always behave in the same way. For this reason, it is critical for the researchers in this field to be exposed to a diversity of patients and disease manifestations, so that they see real-world examples of physiological and pathological differences.

非常简明而广义地讲,生理学就是研究生物体是如何工作的。就人体生理学而言,其研究范畴极为广泛。一方面,生理学研究的是单个分子,例如某个特定蛋白质的形状和带电生理特性如何发挥传运通道作用,允许钠离子进出细胞。另一方面,生理学关注散布于人体各处的器官相互作用所产生的复杂过程,例如人体摄入咸的食物后,脑、心脏和数种腺体如何彼此协调,通过尿液将多余的钠排出体外。

病理学是研究疾病的科学,通过自然科学的方法研究生物体的发病原因、发病机制、形态结构、功能和代谢变化。病理学阐述了疾病发生和演化的规律,揭示了疾病的本质,为各种疾病的防治提供理论基础。

病理生理学研究机体应对疾病或损伤所产生的功能性改变。该领域的研究旨在帮助人们研究疾病的进展,以便快速识别疾病,斟酌不同治疗方案。病理生理学主要关注点之一就是个体之间是有差异的。对于某一个体正常的状况对另一个体可能就是不正常,而且疾病的表现并非一成不变。因此,该领域的研究人员有必要接触各种患者,了解疾病的表现,这样才能观察到真实世界中不同个体的生理和病理差异。

Text A
Introduction to Physiology

Introduction

Physiology is the study of the functions of living matter. It is concerned with how an organism performs its varied activities: how it feeds, how it moves, how it adapts to changing circumstances, and how it **spawns** new generations. The subject is vast and embraces the whole of life. The success of physiology in explaining how organisms perform their daily tasks is based on the notion that they are intricate and **exquisite** machines whose operation is governed by the laws of physics and chemistry.

Although some processes are similar across the whole spectrum of biology–the replication of the genetic code for example–many are specific to particular groups of organisms. For this reason, it is necessary to divide the subject into various parts such as bacterial physiology, plant physiology, and animal physiology.

To study how an animal works it is first necessary to know how it is built. A full appreciation of the physiology of an organism must, therefore, be based on a sound knowledge of its anatomy. Experiments can then be carried out to establish how particular parts perform their functions. Although there have been many important physiological investigations on human volunteers, the need for precise control over the experimental conditions has meant that much of our present physiological knowledge has been derived from studies on other animals such as frogs, rabbits, cats, and dogs. When it is clear that a specific physiological process has a common basis in a wide variety of animal species, it is reasonable to assume that the same principles will apply to humans. The knowledge gained from this approach has given us an insight into human physiology and **endowed** us with a solid foundation for the effective treatment of many diseases.

The building blocks of the body are the cells, which are grouped together to form tissues. The principal types of tissue are **epithelial**, connective, nervous, and muscular, each with its own characteristics.[1] Many connective tissues have relatively few cells, but have an extensive **extracellular matrix**. In contrast, smooth muscle consists of densely packed layers of muscle cells linked together via specific cell junctions. Organs such as the brain, heart, lungs, intestines and liver are formed by the aggregation of different kinds of tissues. The organs themselves are parts of distinct physiological systems. The heart and blood vessels form the cardiovascular system; the lungs, trachea, and bronchi together with the chest wall and diaphragm form the respiratory system; the skeleton and skeletal muscles form the musculoskeletal system; the brain, spinal cord, autonomic nerves and ganglia, and peripheral somatic nerves form the nervous system, and so on.[2]

Cells differ widely in form and function but they all have certain common characteristics. First, they are bounded by a limiting membrane, the **plasma membrane**. Second, they have the ability to break down large molecules to smaller ones to liberate energy for their activities. Third, they possess a nucleus which contains genetic information in the form of **deoxyribonucleic acid** (DNA) at some point in their life history.

Living cells continually transform materials. They break down **glucose** and fats to provide energy for other activities such as motility and the synthesis of proteins for growth and repair. These chemical changes are collectively called **metabolism**. The breakdown of large molecules to smaller ones is called **catabolism** and the synthesis of large molecules from smaller ones is called **anabolism**.

In the course of evolution, cells began to differentiate to serve different functions. Some developed the ability to contract (muscle cells), others to conduct electrical signals (nerve cells). A further group developed the ability to secrete different substances such as **hormones** (endocrine cells) or **enzymes**. During embryological development, this process of differentiation is re-enacted as many different types of cells are formed from the **fertilized egg**.

Most tissues contain a mixture of cell types. For example, blood consists of red cells, white cells, and **platelets**. The red cells transport oxygen around the body. The white cells play an important role in defending against infection and the platelets are vital components in the process of blood clotting. There are a number of different types of connective tissue but all are characterized by having cells distributed within an extensive noncellular matrix. Nerve tissue contains nerve cells and **glial cells**.

The Principal Organ Systems

The cardiovascular system

The cells of large multicellular animals cannot derive the oxygen and nutrients they need directly from the external environment. The oxygen and nutrients must be transported to the cells. This is one of the principal functions of the blood, which circulates within blood vessels by virtue of the pumping action of the heart. The heart, blood vessels and associated tissues form the cardiovascular system.

The heart consists of four chambers, including two atria and two ventricles, which form a pair of pumps arranged side by side.[3] The right ventricle pumps deoxygenated blood to the lungs where it absorbs oxygen from the air, while the left ventricle pumps oxygenated blood returning from the lungs to the rest of body to supply the tissues. Physiologists are concerned with establishing the factors responsible for the heartbeat, how the heart pumps the blood around the circulation, and how it is distributed to perfuse the tissues according to their needs. Fluid exchanged between the blood plasma and the tissues passes into the lymphatic system, which eventually drains back into the blood.

The respiratory system

The energy required for performing the various activities of the body is ultimately derived from respiration. This process involves the oxidation of foodstuffs to release the energy they contain. The oxygen needed for this process is absorbed from the air in the lungs and carried to the tissues by the blood. The carbon dioxide produced by the respiratory activity of the tissues is carried to the lungs by the blood in the pulmonary artery, where it is excreted in the expired air. The basic questions to be answered include the following: How is the air moved in and out of the lungs? How is the volume of air breathed adjusted to meet the requirements of the body? What limits the rate of oxygen uptake in the lungs?

The digestive system

The nutrients needed by the body are derived from the diet. Food is taken in by the mouth and broken down into its component parts by enzymes in the **gastrointestinal tract**. The digestive products are then absorbed into the blood across the wall of the intestine and pass to the liver via the portal vein. The liver makes nutrients available to the tissues for their growth and repair and for the production of energy. In the case of the digestive system, key physiological questions are: How is food ingested? How is it broken down and digested? How are the individual nutrients absorbed? How is the food moved through the gut? How are the indigestible remains eliminated from the body?

The kidneys and urinary tract

The chief function of the kidneys is to control the composition of the extracellular fluid. In the course of this process, they also eliminate **non-volatile** waste products from the blood. To perform these functions, the kidneys produce **urine** of variable composition which is temporarily stored in the **bladder** before voiding. The key physiological questions in this case are: how do the kidneys regulate the composition of the blood? How do they eliminate toxic waste? How do they respond to stresses such as dehydration? What mechanisms allow the storage and elimination of the urine?

The reproductive system

Reproduction is one of the fundamental characteristics of living organisms. The **gonads** produce specialized sex cells known as **gametes**. At the core of sexual reproduction is the creation and fusion of the male and female gametes, the sperm and ova (eggs), with the result that the genetic characteristics of two separate individuals are mixed to produce offspring that differ genetically from their parents.[4]

The musculoskeletal system

This consists of the bones of the skeleton, skeletal muscles, joints, and their associated tissues. Its primary function is to provide a means of movement, which is required for **locomotion**, for the maintenance of posture, and for breathing. It also provides physical support for the internal organs. Here, the mechanism of muscle contraction is a central issue.

The endocrine and nervous systems

The activities of the different organ systems need to be coordinated and regulated so that they act together to meet the needs of the body. Two coordinating systems have evolved: the nervous system and the endocrine system. The nervous system uses electrical signals to transmit information very rapidly to specific cells. Thus, the nerves pass electrical signals to the skeletal muscles to control their contraction. The endocrine system secretes chemical agents, hormones, which travel in the bloodstream to the cells upon which they exert a regulatory effect. Hormones play a major role in the regulation of many different organs and are particularly important in the regulation of the **menstrual cycle** and other aspects of reproduction.

The immune system

The immune system provides the body's defenses against infection both by killing invading organisms and by eliminating diseased or damaged cells.

Although it is helpful to study how each organ performs its functions, it is essential to recognize that the activity of the body as a whole is dependent on the intricate interactions between the various organ systems. If one part fails, the consequences are found in other organ systems throughout the whole body. For example, if the kidneys begin to fail, the regulation of the internal environment is impaired, which in turn leads to disorders of function elsewhere.

Homeostasis

Complex mechanisms are at work to regulate the composition of the **extracellular fluid** and individual cells have their own mechanisms for regulating their internal composition. The regulatory mechanisms stabilize the internal environment despite variations in both the external world and the activity of the animal. The process of stabilization of the internal environment is called homeostasis, which is essential if the cells of the body are to function normally.

Taking one example, the beating of the heart depends on the rhythmical contractions of cardiac muscle cells. This activity depends on electrical signals which, in turn, depend on the concentration of **sodium**

and **potassium** ions in the extracellular and intracellular fluids. If there is an excess of potassium in the extracellular fluid, the cardiac muscle cells become too excitable and may contract at inappropriate times rather than in a coordinated manner. Consequently, the concentration of potassium in the extracellular fluid must be kept within a narrow range if the heart is to beat normally.

How Does the Body Regulate Its Own Composition?

The concept of balance

In the course of a day, an adult consumes approximately 1 kg of food and drinks 2–3 liters of fluid. In a month, this is equivalent to around 30 kg of food and 60–90 liters of fluid. Yet, in general, body weight remains remarkably constant. Such individuals are said to be in balance; the intake of food and drink matches the amounts used to generate energy for normal bodily activities plus the losses in urine and **feces**. In some circumstances, such as starvation, intake does not match the needs of the body and muscle tissue is broken down to provide glucose for the generation of energy. Here, the intake of protein is less than the rate of breakdown and the individual is said to have a negative **nitrogen** balance. Equally, if the body tissues are being built up, as is the case for growing children, pregnant women and athletes in the early stages of training, the daily intake of protein is greater than the normal body turnover and the individual is in positive nitrogen balance.

This concept of balance can be applied to any of the body constituents including water and salt and is important in considering how the body regulates its own composition. Intake must match requirements and any excess must be excreted for balance to be maintained. Additionally, for each chemical constituent of the body there is a desirable concentration range, which the control mechanisms are adapted to maintain. For example, the concentration of glucose in the plasma is about 4–5 mmol/L between meals. Shortly after a meal, plasma glucose rises above this level and this stimulates the secretion of the hormone **insulin** by the **pancreas**, which acts to bring the concentration down. As the concentration of glucose falls, so does the secretion of insulin. In each case, the changes in the circulating level of insulin act to maintain the plasma glucose at an appropriate level. This type of regulation is known as negative feedback. During the period of insulin secretion, the glucose is being stored as either **glycogen** or fat.

A negative feedback loop is a control system that acts to maintain the level of some variables within a given range following a disturbance. Although the example given above refers to plasma glucose, the basic principle can be applied to other physiological variables such as body temperature, blood pressure, and the **osmolality** of the plasma. A negative feedback loop requires a sensor of some kind that responds to the variable in question but not to other physiological variables.[5] Thus, an **osmoreceptor** should respond to changes in osmolality of the body fluids but not to changes in body temperature or blood pressure. The information from the sensor must be compared in some way with the desired level by some form of comparator. If the two do not match, an error signal is transmitted to an **effector**, a system that can act to restore the variable to its desired level. These features of negative feedback can be appreciated by examining a simple heating system. The controlled variable is room temperature, which is sensed by a **thermostat**. The effector is a heater of some kind. When the room temperature falls below the set point, the temperature difference is detected by the thermostat which switches on the heater. This heats the room until the temperature reaches the pre-set level whereupon the heater is switched off.

To summarize, the body is actually a social order of about 100 trillion cells organized into different functional structures, some of which are called organs. Each functional structure contributes its share to the maintenance of homeostatic conditions in the extracellular fluid, which is called the internal environment. As long as normal conditions are maintained in this internal environment, the cells of the body continue to live and function properly. Each cell benefits from homeostasis, and in turn, each cell contributes its share toward the maintenance of homeostasis. This **reciprocal** interplay provides continuous automaticity of the body until one or more functional systems lose their ability to contribute their share of function. When this happens, all the cells of the body suffer. Extreme dysfunction leads to death; moderate dysfunction leads to sickness.

Word Study

1. anabolism [əˈnæbəˌlɪzəm] *n.* 合成代谢，同化，同化作用
2. bladder [ˈblædə(r)] *n.* 膀胱，囊状物
3. catabolism [kəˈtæbəlɪzəm] *n.* 分解代谢，异化，异化作用
4. deoxyribonucleic acid [diːˌɒksiːraɪbəʊnuˈkliːɪk ˈæsɪd] *n.* 脱氧核糖核酸
5. effector [ɪˈfektə(r)] *n.* 效应器
6. endow [ɪnˈdaʊ] *vt.* 捐助，赋予，使具有某种品质
7. enzyme [ˈenzaɪm] *n.* 酶
8. epithelial [ˌepɪˈθiːlɪəl] *adj.* 上皮的
9. exquisite [ɪkˈskwɪzɪt] *adj.* 精挑细选的，精致的，细腻的，强烈的
10. extracellular fluid [ˌekstrəˈseljʊlə ˈfluːɪd] 细胞外液
11. extracellular matrix [ˌekstrəˈseljʊlə ˈmeɪtrɪks] 细胞外基质
12. feces [ˈfiːsiːz] *n.* 粪便，排泄物
13. fertilized egg [ˈfɜːrtɪlaɪzd eg] 受精卵
14. gamete [ˈgæmiːt] *n.* 配子，接合体
15. gastrointestinal tract [ˌgæstrəʊɪnˈtestɪnl trækt] 胃肠道
16. glial cell [ˈglaɪəl sel] 神经胶质细胞
17. glucose [ˈgluːkəʊs] *n.* 葡萄糖
18. glycogen [ˈglaɪkəʊdʒen] *n.* 糖原
19. gonad [ˈgəʊnæd] *n.* 性腺
20. homeostasis [ˌhəʊmiəˈsteɪsɪs] *n.* 稳态，体内平衡
21. hormone [ˈhɔːməʊn] *n.* 激素
22. insulin [ˈɪnsjəlɪn] *n.* 胰岛素
23. locomotion [ˌləʊkəˈməʊʃn] *n.* 运动，移动，转位
24. menstrual cycle [ˈmenstruəl ˈsaɪkl] 月经周期
25. metabolism [məˈtæbəlɪzəm] *n.* 新陈代谢
26. nitrogen [ˈnaɪtrədʒən] *n.* 氮
27. non-volatile [ˈnʌnˌvɒlətaɪl] *adj.* 不易挥发的
28. osmolality [ɒsməˈlælɪtɪ] *n.* 渗透浓度
29. osmoreceptor [ɒzməʊrɪˈseptə] *n.* 渗透压感受器
30. pancreas [ˈpæŋkriəs] *n.* 胰腺
31. plasma membrane [ˈplæzmə ˈmembreɪn] 质膜，细胞膜
32. platelet [ˈpleɪtlət] *n.* 血小板
33. potassium [pəˈtæsiəm] *n.* 钾

34. reciprocal [rɪ'sɪprəkl] *adj.* 互补的，相互的，相反的

35. sodium ['səʊdiəm] *n.* 钠

36. spawn [spɔːn] *v.* 产卵，种菌丝，产生，造成

37. thermostat ['θɜːməstæt] *n.* 恒温器，自动调温器，温度调节装置

38. urine ['jʊərɪn] *n.* 尿

Notes

1. The principal types of tissue are epithelial, connective, nervous, and muscular, each with its own characteristics. 译为：组织的基本类型包括上皮组织、结缔组织、神经组织和肌肉组织，每种组织都有各自的特征。此处，each + with 为代词 + 介词短语构成的独立主格结构，在句子中作状语。

2. The heart and blood vessels form the cardiovascular system; the lungs, trachea, and bronchi together with the chest wall and diaphragm form the respiratory system; the skeleton and skeletal muscles form the musculoskeletal system; the brain, spinal cord, autonomic nerves and ganglia, and peripheral somatic nerves form the nervous system, and so on. 译为：心脏和血管组成心血管系统；肺、气管、支气管以及胸壁和膈肌一起组成呼吸系统；骨骼和骨骼肌组成骨骼肌肉系统；脑、脊髓、自主神经、神经节以及周围躯体神经组成神经系统；等等。此句的难点是医学术语的翻译。

3. The heart consists of four chambers, including two atria and two ventricles, which form a pair of pumps arranged side by side. 译为：心脏有四个腔，包括两个心房和两个心室，它们构成了一对并排存在的泵。此处，consist of 意为"由……构成"，使用时应当避免与 be composed of 混淆。

4. At the core of sexual reproduction is the creation and fusion of the male and female gametes, the sperm and ova (eggs), with the result that the genetic characteristics of two separate individuals are mixed to produce offspring that differ genetically from their parents. 译为：性生殖核心是雌雄配子（即精子和卵子）的产生和融合，其结果就是两个单独个体的遗传特征融合在一起，产生不同于双亲基因的后代。此句是倒装句，介词短语放在句首充当主语成分，翻译成中文时应适当调整语序，增强中文译文的可读性。

5. A negative feedback loop requires a sensor of some kind that responds to the variable in question but not to other physiological variables. 译为：负反馈环要求某种感受器对所待测的变量产生应答，然而对其他生理变量不产生应答。句中"that"引导定语从句；"in question"在这里表示"讨论的、关注的、待测的"。

Exercises

1. **Decide whether the following statements are true (T) or false (F) according to the text.**

(1) Much of our present physiological knowledge has been accumulated through the experiments and studies on human beings.

(2) Living cells break down glucose and fats to provide energy for other activities, which is called catabolism.

(3) The right atrial pumps deoxygenated blood to the lungs where it absorbs oxygen from the air.

(4) The nervous system uses electrical signals to transmit information very rapidly to specific cells.

(5) With the level of sodium increasing in the extracellular fluid, the cardiac muscle cells become too excitable and may contract.

(6) A negative feedback loop is a control system that acts to maintain the level of some variables within a given range following a disturbance.

2. Questions for oral discussion.

(1) What is physiology mainly concerned with?

(2) What are the common characteristics of different forms of cells?

(3) How do you understand the concept of balance in the human body?

(4) How do the endocrine and nervous systems coordinate body organs to perform their functions?

3. Choose the best answer to each of the following questions.

(1) Which of the following descriptions about physiology is wrong?

    A. It is the study of how living organisms work.

    B. It illustrates the discipline of the development and the evolution of disease and the essence of disease.

    C. It is to study the living phenomena and the function activities of living organs.

    D. It is to explain how organ systems are regulated and integrated.

(2) Which of the following are specialized in producing force and movement?

    A. Muscle cells.   B. Connective tissues.

    C. Nerve cells.   D. Epithelial cells.

(3) The fluid environment surrounding each cell is called the _____.

    A. intracellular fluid   B. extracellular fluid

    C. internal environment   D. external environment

(4) Which of the following is not the fundamental characteristic of living organisms?

    A. Metabolism.   B. Adaption.

    C. Reproduction.   D. Massive diffusion.

(5) Which of the following is a physiological process with negative feedback?

    A. Blood coagulation.   B. Process of passing urine.

    C. Aortic baroreflex.   D. Process of parturition.

(6) Which of the following is not the characteristic of regulation by hormone?

    A. Diffuse in nature.   B. Longer in duration.

    C. Accurate in action.   D. Active in overcorrection.

(7) Which of the following is not the characteristic of cells?

    A. They are bound by the plasma membrane.

    B. They have the ability to break down large molecules to smaller ones to liberate energy for their activities.

    C. They possess a nucleus which contains genetic information in the form of deoxyribonucleic acid (DNA).

    D. Living cells cannot transform materials.

(8) The breakdown of large molecules to smaller ones is called _____.

    A. respiration   B. anabolism

    C. catabolism   D. absorption

(9) Which of the following descriptions about the characteristics of nervous regulation is wrong?

    A. It responds fast.   B. It acts exactly.

    C. It responds slowly.   D. Duration is short.

(10) Which of the following descriptions about the control of body function is wrong?

    A. Homeostasis is kept by feedback control.

B. Negative feedback minimizes the changes, leading to stability.

C. Positive feedback is not useful.

D. Feed-forward makes human body foresee and adapt itself to the environment promptly.

4. Write down each word in the box before its corresponding description.

> anabolism, excitability, homeostasis, hormones, internal environment, kidney, metabolism, pathology, physiology, right ventricle

(1) _____ The study of how living organisms work. The goal is to study the normal functions and their regular patterns of organs or organ systems of living organism.

(2) _____ It illustrates the discipline of the development and the evolution of disease.

(3) _____ It means all the chemical reactions in all the cells of the body, and includes all material and energy transformations that occur in the body.

(4) _____ The synthesis of large molecules from smaller ones.

(5) _____ It is the environment that all cells of the body live.

(6) _____ It pumps deoxygenated blood to the lungs where it absorbs oxygen from the air.

(7) _____ Its chief function is to control the composition of the extracellular fluid.

(8) _____ They play a major role in the regulation of many different organs and are particularly important in the regulation of the menstrual cycle and other aspects of reproduction.

(9) _____ The state maintenance of constancy and balance in one's internal environment.

(10) _____ It is the ability of certain kinds of cells (excitable cells) to make response to the stimulus. Essentially, it is the ability of cells to generate action potential.

5. Translate the following sentences and paragraphs into Chinese.

(1) The success of physiology in explaining how organisms perform their daily tasks is based on the notion that they are intricate and exquisite machines whose operation is governed by the laws of physics and chemistry.

(2) Metabolism, excitability, adaptability and reproduction are the basic characteristics of life activity.

(3) If there is an excess of potassium in the extracellular fluid, the cardiac muscle cells become too excitable and may contract at inappropriate times rather than in a coordinated manner.

(4) Signal transduction refers to the processes by which intercellular messengers (such as neurotransmitters, hormones and cytokines) which bind to specific receptors on or in the target cell, and are converted into biochemical and/or electrical signals within that cell.

(5) All cells of the body are surrounded by extracellular fluid and so extracellular fluid forms the internal environment of the body. A stable internal environment is necessary for normal cell function and survival of the living organs. Homeostasis is the maintenance of a steady state in the body by coordinated physiological mechanism.

(6) Usually, a constancy of physiological variable requires a feedback mechanism that feeds the output information back to the control system so as to modify the nature of control. Negative feedback system works to restore the normal value of a variable and thus exert a stabilizing influence; while positive feedback amplifies the changes in order to finish the certain physiological process. Feed-forward control mechanisms often sense a disturbance and can therefore take corrective action that anticipates changes.

Value-Oriented Reflective Reading

Ivan Petrovich Pavlov

Inspired by I. M. Sechenov, the father of Russian physiology, Ivan Petrovich Pavlov decided to devote his life to science. In 1870 he entered the faculty of physics and mathematics to study natural science.

Pavlov became keenly interested in physiology, which in fact remained its fundamental importance to him throughout his life. It was during this first course that he, together with another student, produced his first learned treatise, a work on the physiology of pancreatic nerves, which was widely acclaimed and won him a gold medal.

In 1875, Pavlov finished his course and received the degree of Candidate of Natural Sciences. Due to his strong interest in physiology, he decided to continue his study at the Academy of Medical Surgery. He completed this in 1879 and was again awarded a gold medal. After a competitive examination, Pavlov won a fellowship at the Academy, and this together with his position as Director of the Physiological Laboratory at the clinic of the famous Russian clinician, S. P. Botkin, enabled him to continue his research work. In 1883 he presented his doctoral dissertation on the subject of *The centrifugal nerves of the heart*, in which he developed his idea of nervism, using as example the intensifying nerve of the heart he had discovered, and furthermore laid down the basic principles on the trophic function of the nervous system. In this as well as other works, resulting mainly from his research in the laboratory at the Botkin clinic, Pavlov showed that there existed a basic pattern in the reflex regulation of the activity of the circulatory organs.

In 1890, Pavlov was invited to organize and direct the Department of Physiology at the Institute of Experimental Medicine. With his 45-year efforts till the end of his life, this Institute became one of the most important centers of physiological research. He was appointed in the same year professor of pharmacology at the Military Medical Academy and was appointed 5 years later to the then vacant chair of physiology, which he held till 1925.

Pavlov did most of his research on the physiology of digestion at the Institute of Experimental Medicine from 1891 to 1900. It was here that he developed the surgical method of the "chronic" experiment with extensive use of fistulas, which enabled the functions of various organs to be observed continuously under relatively normal conditions. This discovery opened a new era in the development of physiology. Until then the principal method used had been "acute" vivisection, and the function of an organism had only been approached by a process of analysis. This meant that research into the functioning of any organ necessitated disruption of the normal interrelation between the organ and its environment. Such a method was inadequate as a means of determining how the functions of an organ were regulated or of discovering the laws governing the organism as a whole under normal conditions-problems which had hindered the development of the whole medical science. With his research, Pavlov opened the way for new advances in theoretical and practical medicine. He showed with extreme clarity that the nervous system played the dominant role in regulating the digestive process, which in fact has been the basis of modern physiology of digestion. Pavlov made known the results of his research in this field in lectures which he delivered in 1895 and published on the function of the principal digestive glands in 1897. His research is of great importance in practical medicine.

Pavlov's research into the physiology of digestion led to his logical creation of a science of conditioned reflexes. His discovery of the function of conditioned reflexes made it possible to study all "psychic" activity objectively, instead of resorting to subjective methods as had hitherto been necessary; it was possible to investigate by experimental means the most complex interrelations between an organism and its external environment. According to Pavlov, a conditioned reflex should be regarded as an elementary psychological phenomenon, which at the same time is a physiological one. It followed from this that the conditioned reflex was a clue to the mechanism of the most highly developed forms of reaction in animals and humans to their environment and it made an objective study of their psychic activity possible.

Even in the early stages of his research Pavlov received world acclaim and recognition. In 1901, he was elected a corresponding member of the Russian Academy of Sciences. In 1904 he was awarded a Nobel Prize, and in 1907 he was elected Academician of the Russian Academy of Sciences. In 1912, he was given an honorary doctorate at Cambridge University and in the following years honorary membership of various scientific societies abroad. Finally, upon the recommendation of the Medical Academy of Paris, he was awarded in 1915 the Order of the Legion of Honour.

Pavlov directed all his indefatigable energy towards scientific reforms. He devoted much effort to transforming the physiological institutions headed by him into world centers of scientific knowledge, and it is generally acknowledged that he succeeded in this endeavour.

Questions for oral discussion:

1. What are the major contributions Pavlov made to the study of physiology?
2. What is conditioned reflex?
3. What do you think can be the major reason(s) for the great success of Pavlov?

Text B
General Pathology

Pathology is the science or study of diseases. In its broadest sense, pathology is literally abnormal biology, the study of individuals who are ill or disordered. As a basic biologic science, pathology includes fields such as plant pathology, insect pathology, comparative pathology, as well as human pathology.

Pathology, in the context of human medicine, is not only a basic or theoretical science, but also a clinical medical specialty. Pathologists specialize in laboratory medicine; they consult with other physicians, thereby assisting in the diagnosis and treatment of disease. The scope of laboratory medicine includes all of the studies performed on patient samples, including samples of tissues, blood and other body fluids. Laboratory studies involve **anatomic pathology** study and assess morphologic alterations in cells and tissues. Surgical pathology, **cytopathology**, and **autopsy pathology** are included in this category. Many studies are performed using other means. These areas of clinical pathology include clinical chemistry, microbiology, **hematology**, immunology and immunohematology. Pathophysiology deals with the dynamic aspects of the disease process. It is the study of disordered or altered functions, for example, the physiologic changes caused by disease in a living organism.

Concept of Normalcy

Most people have some notion of normal and would define disease or illness as a deviation from or an absence of that normal state. However, on closer scrutiny, the concept of normalcy turns out to be complex and cannot be defined simply; correspondingly, the concept of disease is far from simple.

Any parameter of measurement applied to an individual or group of individuals has some sort of average value that is considered normal. Average values for height, weight, and blood pressure are derived from observations on many individuals and include a certain amount of variation.

Variations in normal values occur for several reasons. First, individuals differ from one another in their genetic makeup. Thus, no two individuals in the world, except those derived from the same fertilized ovum, have exactly the same genes. Second, individuals differ in their life experiences and in their interaction with the environment. Third, in every individual there are variations in physiologic parameters because of the way in which the control mechanisms of the body function. For instance, blood glucose concentrations in a healthy person vary significantly at different times during the day, depending on food intake, activities of the individual, and so forth. These variations generally occur within a certain range. The situation is somewhat analogous to a thermostatically controlled room. The temperature may dip slightly below the desired level before such a drop is sensed by the thermostat. The corrective action triggered by the thermostat may, in turn, overshoot the ideal slightly before the heat input is halted. Indeed, such variations in body temperature, even in the normal state, occur in all individuals. Finally, for physiologic parameters measured by fairly intricate means, a significant amount of variation in observed values may result from error or imprecision inherent in the measurement process itself.

Because of these considerations, determining a normal range of variation from an average value is a complex matter. This complexity includes knowing the degree of physiologic oscillation of a particular measurement, accounting for the degree of variation among normal individuals even under baseline conditions, and figuring the precision of the measurement method.[1] Finally, the biologic significance of the measurement must be estimated. Single measurements, observations or laboratory results that seem to indicate abnormality must always be judged in the context of the entire individual. A single reading of elevated blood pressure does not make an individual hypertensive; a single slightly elevated blood glucose level does not mean that the individual is diabetic; and a single hemoglobin value lower than average does not necessarily indicate anemia.

To place the above considerations in perspective, concepts of normalcy and even of disease are, to an extent, arbitrary and influenced by cultural values as well as by biologic realities. For example, in our culture a defect of a central nervous system function may produce a significant reading disability and would be an abnormality, whereas the same defect might never be noted in a primitive culture. Furthermore, a trait that might be average and thus normal in one population might be considered distinctly abnormal in another. Consider, for instance, how a "normal" person from our population would be viewed by a group of central African pygmies; or conversely, how an infant from a primitive culture, with the "normal" chronic diarrhea and poor weight gain, might be viewed in one of our well-baby clinics.

Concept of Disease

Disease can be defined as changes in individuals that cause their health parameters to fall outside the normal range. The most useful biologic yardstick for normalcy relates to the individual's ability to meet the demands placed on the body and to adapt to these demands or changes in the external environment so as to maintain reasonable constancy of the internal environment.[2] All cells in the body need a certain amount of oxygen and nutrients for their continuing survival and function, and they also require an environment that provides narrow ranges of temperature, water content, acidity and salt concentration. Thus, the maintenance of internal conditions within fairly narrow limits is an essential feature of the normal body. When some of the structures and functions of the body deviate from the norm to the point where the ability to maintain homeostasis is destroyed or threatened or where the individual can no longer meet environmental challenges, disease is said to exist.[3] A person's subjective perception of disease is related to impairment of the ability to carry on daily activities comfortably.

Disease does not involve the development of a completely new form of life but rather is an extension or distortion of the normal life processes presented in the individual. Even in the case of an obviously infectious disease, where the body is literally invaded, the infectious agent itself does not constitute the disease but only evokes the changes that ultimately are manifested as disease.

Thus, disease is actually the sum of the physiologic processes that have been distorted. To understand and adequately treat the disease, the identity of the normal processes interfered with, the character of the disturbances and the secondary effects of such disturbances on other vital processes must be taken into account.

A theme that will recur, with variations, is that disease above all is part and parcel of the patient.[4] Normal and abnormal processes represent different points on the same continuous spectrum. In fact, the seeds of disease often lie within the adaptive mechanisms of the body itself, mechanisms that constitute a potential two-edged sword. For instance, the very same mechanism that allows us to become immune to certain infections evokes reactions such as **hay fever** and asthma when some of us are challenged by particular environmental agents. Similarly, the mechanism of cellular proliferation that allows us to repair wounds and constantly renew cell populations in various tissues may run amok, giving rise to cancer.[5]

Development of Disease

Etiology

Etiology, in its most general definition, is the assignment of causes or reasons for phenomena. A description of the cause of a disease includes the identification of those factors that provoke the particular disease. Thus, the tubercle bacillus is designated as the etiologic agent of **tuberculosis**. Other etiologic factors in the development of tuberculosis include age, nutritional status, and even the occupation of the individual. Even in the case of an infectious disease, such as tuberculosis, the agent itself does not constitute the disease. Instead, all of the resulting responses to that agent, all the **perversions** of biologic processes taken together, constitute the disease.

Pathogenesis

Pathogenesis of a disease refers to the development or evolution of the disease. To continue with the above example, the pathogenesis of tuberculosis would include the mechanisms whereby the invasion of the body by the tubercle bacillus ultimately leads to the observed abnormalities.

Such an analysis would relate the proliferation and spread of tubercle bacilli to the evolving inflammatory responses, to the immunologic defenses of the body, and to the destruction of cells and tissues. The pattern and extent of the tissue damage would be ultimately related to the **overt** manifestations of disease. Pathogenesis also takes into account the sequential occurrence of certain phenomena and the temporal aspects of the evolving disease. A given disease is not static, but it is a dynamic phenomenon with a rhythm and natural history of its own. In the diagnostic evaluation of patients and the assessment of therapy, it is essential to keep in mind this concept of natural history and the range of variation among different diseases with respect to their natural history. Some diseases characteristically have a rapid **onset**, whereas others have a long **prodrome**. Some diseases are self-limited, that is, they clear up spontaneously in a brief time. Others become chronic, and still others are subject to frequent **remissions** and exacerbations.

When considering the totality of human disease, the number of etiologic factors and the number of separately named diseases seem to be endless. However, the situation is not as difficult as indicated by sheer numbers. The response mechanisms of the body are finite. Therefore, disease A differs from disease B because it varies somewhat in terms of this or that pathogenetic mechanism being exaggerated. Thus, understanding a manageable number of pathogenetic mechanisms and their evolution permits understanding of a large number of seemingly different diseases.

Manifestations

Early in the development of a disease, the etiologic agent or agents may provoke a number of changes in biologic processes that can be detected by laboratory analysis even though there are no subjective symptoms. Thus, many diseases have a subclinical stage, during which the patient functions normally even though the disease processes are well established. The structure and function of many organs provide a large reserve or safety margin, and functional impairment may become evident only when the disease has become quite advanced. For example, chronic renal disease could completely destroy one kidney and partly destroy the other before any symptoms related to decreased renal function would be perceived. However, some diseases seem to begin as functional derangements and actually become clinically evident although no anatomic abnormalities can be detected at the time. Such functional illnesses may lead to secondary structural abnormalities.

As certain biologic processes are encroached on, the patient begins to feel subjectively that something is wrong. These subjective feelings are called symptoms of disease. By definition, symptoms are subjective and can be reported only by the patient to an observer. However, when manifestations of the disease can be objectively identified by an observer, these are termed signs of the disease. Nausea, malaise, and pain are symptoms, whereas fever, reddening of the skin, and a palpable mass are signs of disease.[6] A demonstrable structural change produced in the course of a disease is referred to as a lesion. Lesions may be evident at a gross and/or a microscopic level. The outcome of a disease is sometimes referred to as a **sequela**. For example, the sequela to an inflammatory process in a given tissue might be a scar in that tissue. The sequela to acute rheumatic inflammation of the heart might be scarred, deformed cardiac valves. A **complication** of a disease is a new or separate process that may arise secondarily because of sonic change produced by the original entity. For example, bacterial pneumonia may be a complication of viral infection of the respiratory tract. Fortunately, many diseases can also undergo what is termed resolution, and the host returns to a completely normal state, without sequelae or complications. Resolution can occur spontaneously, that is, owing to body defenses, or it can result from successful therapy.

Finally, it is essential to reemphasize that disease is dynamic rather than static. The manifestations of disease in a given patient may change from day to day as biologic equilibria shift or as compensatory mechanisms are brought into play. Environmental influences brought to bear on the patient will also affect the disease. Therefore, every disease has a range of manifestations and a spectrum of expressions that may vary from patient to patient.

Word Study

1. anatomic pathology [ˌænəˈtɒmɪk pəˈθɒlədʒi] 解剖病理学

2. anemia [ə'ni:mɪə] *n.* 贫血

3. autopsy pathology ['ɔ:tɒpsi pə'θɒlədʒi] 尸检病理学

4. complication [,kɒmplɪ'keɪʃn] *n.* 并发症

5. cytopathology [,saɪtəʊpə'θɒlədʒɪ] *n.* 细胞病理学

6. etiology [,i:tɪ'ɒlədʒɪ] *n.* 病因学

7. hay fever [heɪ 'fi:və(r)] *n.* 花粉症，枯草热

8. hematology [,hi:mə'tɒlədʒi] *n.* 血液学

9. hemoglobin [,hi:məʊ'gləʊbɪn] *n.* 血红蛋白

10. onset ['ɒnset] *n.* 发作，发病，开始

11. overt [əʊ'vɜ:t] *adj.* 显性的，公开的

12. pathogenesis [,pæθə'dʒenɪsɪs] *n.* 发病机制

13. perversion [pə'vɜ:ʃn] *n.* 变态，倒错，反常

14. prodrome ['prəʊdrəʊm] *n.* 前驱症状，先兆

15. remission [rɪ'mɪʃn] *n.* 缓解，减轻

16. sequela [si:'kwɪlə] *n.* 后遗症

17. tuberculosis [tju:,bɜ:kju'ləʊsɪs] *n.* 结核病

Notes

1. This complexity includes knowing the degree of physiologic oscillation of a particular measurement, accounting for the degree of variation among normal individuals even under baseline conditions, and figuring the precision of the measurement method. 译为：这种复杂性包括了解某一特定测量值的生理振荡程度，解释正常个体在基线条件下的变化程度，并且计算测量方法的精度。该句的结构是"主＋谓＋宾"，宾语部分由三个动名词短语"knowing, accounting for, figuring"构成并列结构。

2. The most useful biologic yardstick for normalcy relates to the individual's ability to meet the demands placed on the body and to adapt to these demands or changes in the external environment so as to maintain reasonable constancy of the internal environment. 译为：评估正常状态最有用的生物学标尺是个体有能力满足机体的需求，有能力适应这些需求或外部环境的变化，以便将内环境维持在可以接受的稳定状态。此处，to meet the demands 与 to adapt to these demands or changes in the external environment 并列，共同做 ability 的定语。

3. When some of the structures and functions of the body deviate from the norm to the point where the ability to maintain homeostasis is destroyed or threatened or where the individual can no longer meet environmental challenges, disease is said to exist. 译为：机体的某些结构和功能偏离正常范围，以至于维持体内平衡的能力受到破坏或威胁，或者个人不能应对环境挑战时，疾病就出现了。此处，to the point 中的 point 表示某一程度，其后 where 引导定语从句。

4. A theme that will recur, with variations, is that disease above all is part and parcel of the patient. 译为：一个主题反复出现，尽管略有变化，即疾病首先是病人的一部分。part and parcel 为必不可少、必要部分，part 与 parcel 彼此押头韵（首字母发音相同），用以加强语气。

5. Similarly, the mechanism of cellular proliferation that allows us to repair wounds and constantly renew cell populations in various tissues may run amok, giving rise to cancer. 译为：同样，细胞增殖机制可使伤口得到修复，各种组织的细胞数量不断增加，这种机制也会失控，导致癌症。此句的主干是 the mechanism of cellular proliferation ... may run amok，其中 run amok 意为失控。

6. Nausea, malaise, and pain are symptoms, whereas fever, reddening of the skin, and a palpable mass are

signs of disease. 译为：恶心、不适和疼痛是疾病的症状，而发热、皮肤变红和可触及的肿块是疾病的体征。此句的难点是医学术语的翻译和辨析，例如 malaise 和 reddening of the skin 的翻译、symptom 和 sign 的差别。

Supplementary Parts

1. Medical and Pharmaceutical Terminology (1)

(1) How to Build your Medical and Pharmaceutical English Vocabulary

1) 英语词汇构成基础知识：英语和其他语言一样，其词汇是由词素（morpheme）结合而构成的，词素是语言中最小的包含有意义的单位，是不能再分的最小的语言结构单位。

英语词素按其功能可分为变词词素和构词词素，前者指那些语法范畴中表示语法作用的构形词缀，后者根据其在构词过程中的作用可分为词根词素和附加词素，词根词素是词汇意义的基本组成部分，附加词素是指那些依附于词根（或词干）的词素，词根（root）是构词的主要部分，是词的核心部分，附加成分是词的辅助部分，叫作构词词缀（affix）。

词素按其构词性质可以分为自由词素（free morpheme）及黏着词素（bound morpheme），前者指那些可以作为有独特意义的词来使用的词素，如 act、quick 等，它们可以单词形式单独出现，也可以和各种构词词素自由结合，而后者指那些不能作为一个有独立意义的词来使用的词素，如 reject 中的"re-"和"-ject"，英语单词中的派生词和合成词是以这两种类型的词素作为构词成分的。

2) 英语词汇的构成方法：在现代英语中，词汇结构主要有四种类型，即：①根词（简单词）；②派生词；③复合词和结合词；④缩略词。

从构词方法上来看有派生法（derivation 或 affixation）、转化法（conversion）、合成法（或合词法）（composition）、缩略法（shortening）、逆生法（back-formation）等。在科技英语中，还经常会见到从人名、地名、星座名等造词的现象。

下面分别介绍几种常见的构词法：

A. 派生法（derivation）：在一个词根或词干上增加构词词缀，从而构成新词。

如：electron（电子）+ -ics → electronics 电子学

infra（外、超出）+ red（红）→ infrared 红外线

pleur（肋膜、胸膜）+ -itis（炎症）→ pleuritis 胸膜炎

总体上讲，构词词缀（前后缀）相对数量较少，因而较易掌握，而能否记住大量的词根便成了词汇识记的关键。尤其是在科技词汇中，涉及大量的学科名词术语，需要记忆大量的相关词根，难易显而易见。然而，"世上无难事，只怕有心人"。只要用心去记去学，在掌握规律性方法的前提之下，记忆大量的专业术语词根，就可以真正提高专业英语词汇的数量及记忆效果。

B. 转化法（conversion）：这主要是指词类的转化，而且一般涉及比较简单的词，因此掌握起来比较容易，但切记不要创造性地使用词汇，否则会闹出一些笑话，比如将 instead 错用作动词等。

C. 合成法（composition）：把两个或两个以上的单词（词干或词根）组合起来构成新词，在英语词汇构成中是一种很常见的方法，如 weekend、workload、spaceship 等，这种方法可以构成不同词类的合成词。

D. 缩略法（shortening）：随着现代英语词汇的不断发展，缩略法被广泛用来构成一些含义丰富的词和略语，科技英语中尤其如此。缩略词就结构而言可以分为紧缩词（或拼缀词）(blends)、音节缩略词（clipping）及字母缩略词（acronyms）三大类，举例如下：

①紧缩词（blends）

brunch = breakfast + lunch

motel = motor + hotel

smog = smoke + fog

heliport = helicopter + airport

newscast = news + broadcast

travelog = travel + catalog

②音节缩略词（clipping）

advertisement → ad 或 advert

examination → exam

laboratory → lab

memorandum → memo

microphone → mike

photograph → photo

public house → pub

telephone → phone

aeroplane → plane

influenza → flu

refrigerator → fridge

③字母缩略词（acronyms)

AIDS → acquired immune deficiency syndrome

laser → light amplification by stimulated emission of radiation

radar → radio detecting and ranging

UFO → unidentified flying objects

CNS → central nervous system

HSLC → high speed liquid chromatography

UVL → ultraviolet light

E.　逆生法（back-formation）：这是指删除派生词词缀的构词法。

television → televise　　*v.* 播放电视

laser → lase　　*v.* 放射激光

diagnosis → diagnose　　*v.* 诊断

burglar → burgle　　*v.* 撬门而入

editor → edit　　*v.* 编辑

以上介绍了几种常见的构词法，结合医药英语词汇的特点以及中高级英语学习的特点，建议大家重点关注如何通过识记一定量的词素来达到识记并牢记大量词汇而展开。

3）如何学习医药科技英语词汇：在医药英语词汇课程的教学中特别重视培养学生医药英语的词汇能力，而不仅仅是向学生介绍大量的科技词汇。在现代英语中，词汇结构主要有四种类型，即根词（简单词）、派生词、复合词和结合词以及缩略词，因此整个课程的教学往往从英语构词法入手，介绍派生法（derivation 或 affixation)、转化法（conversion)、合成法（或合词法）（composition)、缩略法（shortening）以及逆生法（back-formation）等。

分析医药英语词汇的特点之后不难发现，它们主要有四种形式。

A.　基础词汇型：指基础英语词汇在科技英语中被赋予新的含义，如 addition 加成、lead 铅等。

B.　科技缩略型：指用首字母将由两个以上词汇或词根组成的术语用缩略字母来代表，如 AIDS 代表 acquired immune deficiency syndrome 艾滋病、HPLC 代表 high performance liquid chromatography 高效液相色谱、DNA 代表 deoxyribonucleic acid 脱氧核糖核酸等。

  C. 专业术语型：指一般不用缩略，在某些专业领域使用的词汇，如 leukocyte 白细胞、hypercalcemia 高血钙／高钙血症。

  D. 专有名词型：指由人名、地名、星座名等造词的现象来表达的术语，如 volt 伏特是由意大利物理学家 Alessandro Volt（1745—1827）的姓氏而来，polonium 钋是由居里夫人的祖国波兰（Poland）得名的。

  除了以上四种类型词汇之外，大多数科技英语词汇均可用现代英语构词法来进行解释，所以现代英语构词法对医药英语词汇的学习同样具有实际指导意义。

(2) Common Morphemes in Terms of English for Physiology and Pathology

Morpheme	Meaning	Example
acus	听觉	paracusis 听觉倒错，错听
alg	疼痛	analgia 痛觉缺乏，无痛
anaphyl	过敏	anaphylatoxin 过敏毒素
ancyl, ankyl	弯曲	ankylosis 关节强硬，关节强直
anomal	异常	anomalous 异常的
asthen	无力，衰弱	asthenia 无力，虚弱
atel	发育不全	atelectasis 肺不张
carcin	癌	carcinoma 癌
choler	霍乱	cholera 霍乱
copr	粪	coprology 粪便学
crin	分泌	endocrine 内分泌
crypt	隐	cryptitis 隐窝炎
dacry	泪	dacryagogue 催泪剂
diabet	糖尿病	diabetes 糖尿病，多尿症
digest	消化	digestion 消化
diphther	白喉	diphtheria 白喉
ectas	扩张	ectasia 扩张，膨胀
edem	水肿	edema 水肿
emes, emet	呕吐	emesis 呕吐
emia	血症	anoxemia 缺氧血症
epidem	流行病	epidemic 流行性的，流行病
esthes, esthet	感觉	esthesia 感觉，知觉
fert	生育	fertility 生育力；多产，肥沃
galact	乳	galactagogue 催乳剂
gen	原	antigen 抗原
genit	生殖	generation 生殖，世代
gest	妊娠	progesterone 孕酮，黄体酮
gon	生殖；精液；淋病	gonosome 性染色体；gonococcus 淋球菌
gravid	妊娠	unigravida 初孕妇
hallucin	幻觉	hallucinogen 致幻剂
helc	溃疡	helcoid 溃疡状的
hemat	血	hematology 血液学
hered	遗传	heredity 遗传
hidr	汗	hidrosis 多汗
hormon	激素	parahormone 副激素
hypn	睡眠	hypnagogic 催眠的

续表

Morpheme	Meaning	Example
hyster	癔症	hysteria　癔症,歇斯底里
immun	免疫	immunology　免疫学
kines	运动	kinematics　运动学
lacrim	泪	lacrimator　催泪剂
lact	乳	lacteal　乳状的; lactate 乳酸
lymph	淋巴	lymphadenitis　淋巴结炎
malac	软	malacia　软化症
man	疯狂	monomania　偏狂
meno	月经	menopause　绝经
menstru	月经	menstruation　月经
ment	精神	amentia　智力缺陷
morb	病	morbid　病态的,疾病的
muc	黏液	mucoid　黏液样的
narc	睡眠 , 麻醉	narcolepsy　发作性睡病; narcotic analgesic　麻醉性镇痛药
nat	分娩、生产	neonatal　新生的
nos	病	nosology　疾病分类学
nutr	营养	nutrient　营养的,营养物
odyn	疼痛	odynophagia　吞咽疼痛
onc	肿瘤	oncology　肿瘤学
osm	嗅觉	osmoreceptor　渗透压感受器,嗅觉感受器
oz	臭	ozena　臭鼻症
par	分娩	primipara　初产妇
part	分娩	parturifacient　催产的,催产剂
path	情感	empathy　移情
path	病	pathology　病理学
pector	痰	expectoration　痰,咳痰
pept, peps	消化	dyspepsia　消化不良
phag	吞噬	phagosome　吞噬体
phor	隐斜	heterophoria　隐斜
phren	精神	phrenic　精神的,膈的
physi	生理	physiology　生理学
phyt	生长	exophytic　外部生长的
plas	发育	metaplasia　（组织）化生
pleg	麻痹	diplegia　双侧瘫痪
pnea	呼吸	eupnea　正常呼吸（平静呼吸）
prax	运动	apraxia　失用症,失用[症]
pregn	妊娠	pregnancy　妊娠,怀孕
psych	精神	psychiatry　精神病学
pyo-	脓	pyemia　脓血症
rheumat	风湿	rheumatic　风湿性的
rig	硬	rigid　刚硬的,刚性的
saliv	唾液	salivation　流涎,多涎
sanguin	血	exsanguinate　放血,使无血
schist, schiz	裂	diaschisis　神经功能联系不能

续表

Morpheme	Meaning	Example
scler	硬	sclerema 硬化病
secret	分泌	secretory 分泌的
semin	精液	semen 精液,种子
sens	情感	sensation 感觉,知觉
seps, sept	腐烂	septic 腐败性的,败血病的
sequestr	死骨	sequestrum 死骨,死骨片
ser	血清	serology 血清学
skat	粪	skatology 粪便学
somn	睡眠	somnambulism 梦游症
sorb, sorpt	吸收	absorption 吸收
spasm	痉挛	spasmolysis 解痉作用
sphygm	脉搏	sphygmomanometer 血压计
spir	呼吸	spirograph 呼吸描记器
sten	狭窄	stenosis 狭窄
steril	不育	sterilization 绝育,灭菌
stimul	刺激	stimulation 刺激,兴奋
stip	便秘	constipation 便秘
syphil	梅毒	syphilis 梅毒
terat	畸形,畸胎	teratology 畸形学,畸胎学
tetan	破伤风	tetanus 破伤风;强直收缩
thromb	血栓,血小板	thrombus 血栓;thrombocyte 血小板
traumat	外伤,创伤	trauma 外伤,创伤
trop	斜视	esotropia 内斜视
trophy	营养	amyotrophy 肌萎缩
tubercul	结核,结节	tuberculin 结核菌素
tum	肿,瘤	tumefaction 肿胀,肿大
typh	伤寒	typhoid 伤寒
typhl	盲	typhlosis 盲,视觉缺乏
ulcer	溃疡	ulceration 溃疡形成
urin	尿	urination 排尿
varic	曲张	varicocele 精索静脉曲张
varicell	水痘	varicelloid 水痘样的
venere	性	venereology 性病学

(3) Fill in the blanks with the missing word root, prefix or suffix.

1) an_____ia   痛觉缺乏

2) _____ectasis   肺不张

3) _____atoxin   过敏毒素

4) endo_____   内分泌

5) _____osis   关节强硬

6) _____ambulism   梦游症

7) pro_____erone   孕酮,黄体酮

8) _____agogue   催乳剂

9) _____oid   溃疡状的

10) _____ology　血液学

11) _____ema　硬化病

12) _____olepsy　发作性睡病

(4) Word-matching.

1) ectasia		A.	副激素
2) anoxemia		B.	正常呼吸
3) parahormone		C.	感觉,知觉
4) menopause		D.	缺氧血症
5) dyspepsia		E.	血小板
6) eupnea		F.	解痉作用
7) thrombocyte		G.	消化不良
8) exsanguinate		H.	扩张,膨胀
9) sensation		I.	外部生长的
10) spasmolysis		J.	血栓
11) thrombus		K.	绝经
12) exophytic		L.	放血,使无血

2. English-Chinese Translation Skills: 药学英语词汇特点与翻译

　　药学英语属于科技英语,具有科技英语的特点。药学英语词汇一般主要有四个特点:专业术语多、两栖词汇多、有隐喻性词汇、首字母缩略词汇多。

(1) 专业术语多:药学英语涉及范围广,关联学科多,不仅含有药学领域专业词汇,还有很多相关领域词汇,包括生理学、病理学、微生物学等。药学英语专业词汇数量虽多,但是语义固定,绝大多数可以通过专业词典找到汉语完全对等词,直译即可。如果词典中找不到对应词,可以采用以下三种办法。

1) 分析原词的组成结构,拆分词根,造出对应的汉语表达。如 glycerol phenylbutyrate 可以译为"苯丁酸甘油酯",因为 glycerol 意思是"甘油",而 phenylbutyrate 是"丁酸苯酯",再根据汉语表达习惯将化合物的译名顺序稍加调整就可以了。

2) 如果在语义上难以造出对应的新词,可以考虑音译法。例如: Viagra(伟哥、万艾可)。

3) 意译与音译相结合。例如: carbidopa-levodopa 中的 levo 有"左旋的"的意思,该词可译为"卡比多巴 - 左旋多巴"(一种延迟释放制剂)。同理, hydrocodone 可译为"氢可酮"。

(2) 两栖词汇多:两栖词汇是指那些既可以用于普通领域,又可以用于专业领域的词汇。药学英语中很多普通英语词汇被赋予了专业含义。翻译这类词汇,要结合上下文语境,参考专业词典或查阅相关资料。例如, administration 在普通英语中表示"行政管理""管理层"等意思,但在医药领域则是"给药""用药"的意思。其动词形式是 administer。有些两栖词汇在医药学不同学科内的意思也有差别,如 develop 在普通英语中意思是"发展",在薄层色谱法中表示"显色",而在描述微生物概念时则表示"生长"; formulation 在普通英语中意思是"规划,制定",表示药物配方时可译为"处方",表示药物制品时则应译为"制剂"。

(3) 有隐喻性词汇:药学英语中也有一些词汇存在隐喻现象,在翻译中应该采用直译还是意译要根据具体情况具体分析。如 orphan drugs 可以直接翻译成"孤儿药",这种药物是指用于治疗罕见病的药物,适用人群少,销量有限,大部分医药公司不愿意投资研发,就好像"孤儿"一样无人照管,这种直译可保留原词的隐喻义,也为业界普遍接受。但是,隐喻性药学专业名词也不都采用直译法翻译,如 sandwich ELISA(夹心 ELISA)是用于测量抗原量的酶联免疫吸附法,在该测定法中被测量的抗原需要与上下两层抗体相结合,恰如三明治的结构,由此得名。但如果直译为"三明治

ELISA"则感觉缺乏科学的严谨性,因此意译为"夹心 ELISA"。同样,sandwiched osmotic tablet system 可译为"三层渗透泵片"。

(4) 首字母缩略词汇多:首字母缩略词是指把构成术语的多个单词用它们各自开头字母大写缩略而成的特殊单词,医药英语中大量使用首字母缩略词。例如:BPC(bulk pharmaceutical chemical,原料药)、CFU(colony forming unit,菌落形成单位)、USP(United States Pharmacopoeia,美国药典)、OTC(over-the-counter drug,非处方药)、BBB (blood brain barrier,血脑屏障)、QSAR(quantitative structure-activity relationship,定量结构 - 活性关系,简称定量构效关系)等。这些缩略词都有规范译法,直接采用即可。有些缩略词可以分别表示不同术语意思,例如,TDDS 既可以表示为 transdermal drug delivery system(透皮给药系统),又可以表示为 targeting drug delivery system(靶向给药系统),要根据具体语境选择正确词义进行翻译。

（郭　昊　杜伟杰　史志祥　龚长华）

Unit Two

Microbiology

Unit Two
数字内容

Life on earth is impossible without microorganisms, which are the ancestors of all living systems. Microbiology encompasses the whole of studying microscopic organisms, such as bacteria, protozoa, fungi, some types of algae and viruses. The need to study these minute organisms started when scientists discovered the association of microbes to specific diseases. The roles of microbiology in the advances in pharmaceutical and medical industry have led to great discoveries from vaccines to devices.

Pharmaceutical microbiology is one of the many facets of applied microbiology, having a special bearing on pharmacy in all its aspects. It can be defined as the study of microorganisms that are pertinent to the production of antibiotics, enzymes, vitamins, vaccines, and other pharmaceutical products; it also incorporates the study of microorganisms that cause pharmaceutical contamination, and degradation and deterioration of pharmaceutical raw materials and finished products.

Over the years, pharmaceutical microbiology has evolved and expanded significantly to encompass various other aspects, e.g., research and development of new anti-infective agents, the use of microorganisms to detect mutagenic and carcinogenic potential in drugs, and the use of microorganisms in the manufacture of insulin and human growth hormone.

地球上的生命不可能离开微生物而存在，它们是所有生物系统的祖先。微生物学涉及所有的微生物研究，如细菌、原生动物、真菌、某些类型的藻类和病毒。当科学家发现微生物与特定疾病相关时，就有了对这些微小生物体的研究需求。微生物学促进了制药和医疗行业的发展，带来了从疫苗到医疗器械领域的许多重大发现。

药物微生物学是应用微生物学的众多分支之一，对药学的各个领域都有特殊的影响。可以说它既研究与生产抗生素、酶、维生素、疫苗和其他药品相关的微生物，也包括导致药物污染、原料药及成品的降解和变质的微生物的研究。

多年来，药物微生物学已得到显著发展和延伸，涵盖了许多其他方面，例如新抗感染药物的研发，使用微生物检测药物的致突变性和致癌性，以及使用微生物生产胰岛素和人生长激素。

Text A
The Other Side of Antibiotics

Antibiotics have eliminated or controlled so many infectious diseases that virtually everyone has benefited from their use at one time or another. Even without such personal experience, however, one would have to be isolated indeed to be unaware of the virtues, real and **speculative**, of these "miracle" drugs.[1] The American press, radio, and television have done a good job of reporting the truly remarkable story of successes in the chemical war on germs. What's more, any shortcomings on their part have been more than made up for by the aggressive public relations activity of the pharmaceutical companies which manufacture and sell antibiotics.

In comparison, the inadequacies and potential dangers of these remarkable drugs are much less widely known. And the lack of such knowledge can be bad, especially if it leads patients to pressure their doctors into prescribing antibiotics when such medication isn't really needed, or leads them to switch doctors until they find one who is, so to speak, antibiotics-minded.[2]

Because the good side of the antibiotics story is well-known, there seems more point here to a review of some of the immediate and long-range problems that can come from today's casual use of these drugs. It should be made clear in advance that calamities from the use of antibiotics are rare in relation to the enormous amounts of the drugs administered. But the potential hazards, so little touched on generally, do need a clear statement. The antibiotics are not, strictly speaking, exclusively prescription drugs. A number of them are permitted in such over-the-counter products as nasal sprays, creams and **ointments**. Even if these products do no harm, there is no point whatsoever in using them. If you have an infection serious enough to warrant the launching of chemical **warfare**, you need much bigger doses of the antibiotics than any of the non-prescription products are allowed to contain.

Over-the-counter products, however, account for only a small percentage of total antibiotics production. It is the prescription dosages that give people trouble. These drugs—even allowing for the diverse abilities of the many narrow-spectrum ones and the versatility of the broad-spectrum ones—are not the cure-alls, they often are billed as being. There are wide gaps in their ability to master contagious diseases. Such important infections as **mumps**, **measles**, common colds, influenza, and infectious **hepatitis** still await conquest. All are virus infections and despite intense efforts, very little progress has been made in chemotherapy against viruses. Only small progress has been achieved against fungi. Many strains of bacteria and fungi are naturally resistant to all currently available antibiotics and other chemotherapeutic drugs. Some microorganisms originally sensitive to the action of antibiotics, especially **staphylococcus**, have developed resistant strains. This acquired resistance imposes on the long range value of the drugs a very important limitation, which is not adequately met by the frequent introduction of new **antimicrobial** agents to combat the problem.[3]

It has been pretty well established that the increase in strains of bacteria resistant to an antibiotic correlates directly with the duration and extent of use of that antibiotic in a given location. In one hospital a survey showed that, before **erythromycin** had been widely used there, all strains of staphylococci taken from patients and personnel were sensitive to its action. When the hospital started extensive use of erythromycin, however, resistant staphylococcus strains began to appear.

The development of bacterial resistance can be minimized by a more discriminating use of antibiotics,[4] and the person taking the drug can help here. When an antibiotic must be used, the best way to prevent the development of resistance is to wipe out the infection as rapidly and thoroughly as possible. Ideally, this requires a **bactericidal** drug, which destroys, rather than a **bacteriostatic** drug, which inhibits. And the drug must be taken in adequate dosage for as long as it is necessary to **eradicate** the infection completely. The doctor, of course, must choose the drug, but patients can help by being sure to take the full course of treatment recommended by the doctor, even though symptoms seem to disappear before all the pills are gone. In rare instances the emergence of resistance can be delayed or reduced by combinations of antibiotics. Treatment of tuberculosis with streptomycin alone results in a high degree of resistance, but if

para-aminosalicylic acid or **isoniazid** is used with streptomycin the possibility that this complication will arise is greatly reduced.

In hospital treatment of severe infections, the sensitivity of the infecting organism to appropriate antibiotics is determined in the laboratory before treatment is started. This enables the doctor to select the most effective drug or drugs; it determines whether the antibiotic is bactericidal or bacteriostatic for the germs at hand; and it suggests the amount needed to destroy the growth of the bacteria completely.[5] In either hospital or home, **aseptic** measures can help to reduce the **prevalence** of resistant strains of germs by preventing cross infection and the resultant spreading of organisms.

Every one of the antibiotics is potentially dangerous for some people. Several serious reactions may result from their use. One is a severe, sometimes fatal, shock-like **anaphylactic** action, which may strike people who have become **sensitized** to penicillin. Anaphylactic reaction happens less frequently and is less severe when the antibiotic is given by mouth. It is most apt to occur in people with a history of allergy, or a record of sensitivity to penicillin. Very small amounts of penicillin, even the traces which get into the milk of cows for a few days after they are treated with the antibiotic for **mastitis,** may be sufficient to sensitize; hence, the strong campaign by food and drug officials keeps such milk off the market.[6]

To minimize the risk of anaphylactic shock in illnesses where injections of penicillin are the preferred treatment, a careful doctor will question the patient carefully about allergies and previous reactions. In case of doubt, another antibiotic will be substituted if feasible[7], or other **precautionary** measures will be taken before the injection is given.

Other **untoward** reactions to antibiotics are gastrointestinal disorders—such as sore mouth, cramps, diarrhea, or **anal itch**—which occur most frequently after use of the tetracycline group but have also been encountered after use of penicillin and streptomycin. These reactions may result from **suppression** by the antibiotic of bacteria normally found in the gastrointestinal tract. With their competition removed, antibiotic-resistant staphylococci or fungi, which are also normally present, are free to flourish and cause what is called a **super-infection**. Such infections can be extremely difficult to cure.

A few antibiotics have such toxic effects that their usefulness is strictly limited. They include streptomycin and **dihydro-streptomycin**, which sometimes cause deafness, and chloramphenicol, which may injure the bone marrow. Drugs with such serious potential dangers as these should be used only if life is threatened and nothing else will work. All the possible troubles that can result from antibiotic treatment should not keep anyone from using one of these drugs when it is clearly indicated. Nor should they discourage certain preventive uses of antibiotics which have proved extremely valuable.

Word Study

1. anal ['eɪnl] *adj.* 肛门的
2. anaphylactic [ˌænəfɪ'læktɪk] *adj.* 过敏的
3. antimicrobial [ˌæntɪmaɪ'krəubɪəl] *adj.* 抗菌的, 杀菌的
4. aseptic [ˌeɪ'septɪk] *adj.* 无(病)菌的, 防腐的
5. bactericidal [bæk,tɪərɪ'saɪdl] *adj.* 杀菌的
6. bacteriostatic [bæk,tɪrɪəs'tætɪk] *adj.* 抑菌的; *n.* 抑菌剂
7. dihydro-streptomycin [diː'haɪdrəu 'streptə'maɪsɪn] *n.* 双氢链霉素
8. eradicate [ɪ'rædɪkeɪt] *vt.* 根除, 消灭
9. erythromycin [ɪˌrɪθrə'maɪsɪn] *n.* 红霉素

10. hepatitis [ˌhepə'taɪtɪs] *n.* 肝炎

11. isoniazid [ˌaɪsəʊ'naɪəzɪd] *n.* 异烟肼（一种抗结核药）

12. itch [ɪtʃ] *n.* 痒; *v.* 发痒

13. mastitis [mæ'staɪtɪs] *n.* 乳腺炎

14. measles ['miːzlz] *n.* 麻疹

15. mumps [mʌmps] *n.* 流行性腮腺炎

16. ointment ['ɔɪntmənt] *n.* 油膏, 软膏, 药膏

17. para-aminosalicylic acid ['pærə ə,miːnəʊ,sælɪ,sɪlɪk 'æsɪd] *n.* 对氨基水杨酸

18. precautionary [prɪ'kɔːʃənəri] *adj.* 预先警告的

19. prevalence ['prevələns] *n.* 传播, 流行

20. sensitize ['sensətaɪz] *v.* (使) 敏感

21. speculative ['spekjələtɪv] *adj.* 纯理论的, 推测的

22. staphylococcus [ˌstæfɪlə'kɒkəs] ([复]cocci ['kɒksaɪ]) *n.* 葡萄球菌

23. super-infection [suːpər ɪn'fekʃn] *n.* 双重感染, 继发感染

24. suppression [sə'preʃn] *n.* 抑制

25. untoward [ˌʌntə'wɔːd] *adj.* 不利的, 不适当的

26. warfare ['wɔːfeə(r)] *n.* 战争

Notes

1. Even without such personal experience, however, one would have to be isolated indeed to be unaware of the virtues, real and speculative, of these "miracle" drugs. 译为：然而，即使没有这样的亲身体验，一个人也只有完全离群索居才不知道这些"神奇"药物的或真实或推测的优点。在本句中，one would have to be isolated indeed 在功能上相当于一个条件句与 to be unaware of 构成意义衔接。"real and speculative" 作为后置定语对 "virtue" 进行补充说明。

2. ...especially if it leads patients to pressure their doctors into prescribing antibiotics when such medication isn't really needed, or leads them to switch doctors until they find one who is, so to speak, antibiotics-minded. 译为：……特别是如果这导致患者向医生施压，要求他们在并不真正需要抗生素的情况下开抗生素，或者导致他们更换医生，直到找到一个可以说有抗生素意识的医生。在 "if" 引导的条件状语从句中包括两个由 "or" 连接的并列句，两个并列句的主语均是 "it"，指代主句中的 "the lack of such knowledge"。"antibiotics-minded" 的意思是 "脑子里想着抗生素的"。

3. This acquired resistance imposes on the long range value of the drugs a very important limitation, which is not adequately met by the frequent introduction of new antimicrobial agents to combat the problem. 译为：这种获得耐药性极大地限制了抗生素的长期价值，即使频繁引入新的抗菌剂也不能完全解决这一问题。"impose...on..." 的意思是 "将……强加于……"。定语从句 "which is not adequately met by..." 中，"met" 可以理解为 "解决"。

4. The development of bacterial resistance can be minimized by a more discriminating use of antibiotics... 译为：更有区别地使用抗生素可以最大限度地减少细菌耐药性的产生。本句中的 "discriminating" 应解释为 "having or demonstrating the ability to recognize or draw fine distinctions"，即 "有识别力的、加以区分的"。

5. In hospital treatment of severe infections, the sensitivity of the infecting organism to appropriate antibiotics is determined in the laboratory before treatment is started. This enables the doctor to select the most effective drug or drugs; it determines whether the antibiotic is bactericidal or bacteriostatic for

the germs at hand; and it suggests the amount needed to destroy the growth of the bacteria completely. 译为：在医院治疗严重感染时，开始治疗前在化验室确定感染微生物对合适抗生素的敏感性。这使医生能够选择最有效的一个或多个药物，决定抗生素对眼下的细菌起到杀灭还是抑制作用，提出完全破坏细菌生长所需（药物）的量。在这段话中，"infecting organism"、"the germs" 和 "the bacteria" 均指引起严重感染的致病菌，作者使用这些意思相近的词是为了避免表达上的重复；第二句中三个分句的主语 "this"、"it" 和 "it" 均指第一句表达的内容。

6. Very small amounts of penicillin, even the traces which get into the milk of cows for a few days after they are treated with the antibiotics for mastitis, may be sufficient to sensitize; hence, the strong campaign by food and drug officials keeps such milk off the market. 译为：极少量的青霉素，甚至是在奶牛用抗生素治疗乳腺炎几天后进入牛奶中的微量青霉素，都可能足以引起过敏；因此，食品和药品监管官员采取了强有力的行动，阻止这种牛奶进入市场。本句中 "even the traces" 指 "even the traces of penicillin"，指用青霉素治疗奶牛乳腺炎后残留在牛奶中的极少量的青霉素。

7. In case of doubt, another antibiotic will be substituted if feasible. 译为：如有疑问，在可行的情况下将用另外一种抗生素代替。In case of + 名词，表示条件。

Exercises

1. Decide whether each of the following statements is true (T) or false (F) according to the text.

(1) Pharmaceutical companies which manufacture and sell antibiotics have made out a clear list of the shortcomings of their manufactured drugs.

(2) The serious harms caused by the use of antibiotics are comparatively rare in proportion to the amount of the drugs administered.

(3) It is the over-the-counter antibiotic products that cause the potential hazards of using the drugs.

(4) Scientists have barely achieved progress in the development of chemotherapeutic drugs against viruses and fungi.

(5) The combination of antibiotics proves to accelerate the emergence of resistance.

(6) People may possibly develop anaphylactic reaction if they drink milk of the cows treated with penicillin.

(7) In spite of the potential dangers of antibiotics, their use in treatment and prevention should be recommended if the indication is clear.

2. Questions for oral discussion.

(1) What is the difference between narrow-spectrum and broad-spectrum antibiotics? Could you give some examples of the two types of antibiotics, and then describe their respective advantages and disadvantages?

(2) What factors correlate with the increase of bacteria resistance to antibiotics? Please illustrate your viewpoints based on relevant research literature.

(3) What are the possible ways to minimize the development of antibiotic resistance?

(4) What would be your suggestions to our society regarding the control of antibiotic abuse?

3. Choose the best answer to each of the following questions.

(1) What is an antibiotics-minded doctor?

A. A doctor with a good knowledge of antibiotics.

B. A doctor who tends to prescribe antibiotics without considering if the drug is really needed.

C. A doctor who often denies patients' requests for antibiotics.

D. A doctor who is very careful in the prescription of antibiotics.

(2) As to "OTC antibiotics" and "prescription antibiotics", which of the following statements is false?

A. It is of great significance for patients to use OTC antibiotics.

B. Prescription drugs contain bigger doses of antibiotics than OTC products.

C. The troubles brought by antibiotics are usually from the use of prescription dosages.

D. Dosage forms like spray, ointment and lozenges usually contain OTC dosages.

(3) For viral infections, _____.

A. antibiotics do not work at all

B. many successful chemotherapeutic drugs have been developed

C. the use of prescription antibiotics is warranted

D. most of them have been tackled

(4) Determination of the sensitivity of the infecting bacteria to appropriate antibiotics before treatment is started can help doctors do the following things except _____.

A. select the most effective drug or drugs

B. determine whether the antibiotic is bactericidal or bacteriostatic

C. determine the amount needed to destroy the growth of bacteria completely

D. prevent cross-infection among patients

(5) The development of antibiotic resistance can be minimized by the following strategies except _____.

A. taking the full course of treatment

B. combination of antibiotics

C. using broad-spectrum antibiotics to kill as many types of bacteria as possible

D. taking aseptic measures in hospitals

(6) As to allergic reaction to antibiotics, which of the following statements is false?

A. Some of them can be serious and even fatal.

B. It happens less frequently and is less severe when the antibiotic is given orally.

C. A big dose is needed to elucidate an allergic reaction.

D. It is more likely to happen in people with a history of allergy.

(7) Which of the following is not a reasonable use of antibiotics?

A. Antibiotics with severe potential dangers should be used only if life is threatened and nothing else will work.

B. Preventive use of antibiotics should always be prohibited.

C. Antibiotic should not be prescribed when the drug is not really needed by the patient.

D. The doctor should question the patient carefully about allergic history before prescription.

(8) A super-infection is caused by _____.

A. suppression of resistant microorganisms in the gastrointestinal tract by antibiotics

B. suppression of resistant microorganisms in the gastrointestinal tract by normal microbiota

C. overgrowth of normal microbiota in the gastrointestinal tract

D. overgrowth of sensitive microorganisms in the gastrointestinal tract

(9) Which of the following does not belong to "the other side of antibiotics"?

A. Antibiotics are not cure-alls.

B. The development of resistance caused by the use of antibiotics is inevitable.

C. Only a few antibiotics are available as OTC products.

D. Some antibiotics can cause severe adverse reactions.

(10) Which of the following underlined words has a completely different meaning from the others?

    A. Approximately 10% of patients report an <u>allergy</u> to penicillin.

    B. <u>Hypersensitivity</u> reactions related to nonsteroidal anti-inflammatory drugs (NSAIDs) may be due to immunological or non-immunological mechanisms.

    C. Drug-induced <u>anaphylaxis</u> (DIA) is also associated with more severe outcomes than other triggers.

    D. The goal of antimicrobial <u>sensitivity</u> testing is to predict the *in vivo* success or failure of antibiotic therapy.

(11) Some microorganisms originally sensitive to the action of antibiotics, especially staphylococcus, have _____ resistant strains.

    A. developed   B. occurred

    C. emerged   D. formed

(12) Many drugs can be _____ orally as liquids, capsules, tablets, or chewable tablets.

    A. eaten   B. swallowed

    C. applied   D. administered

(13) In order to wipe out the infection as rapidly and thoroughly as possible, a _____ antibiotic which _____ the bacteria is required.

    A. bactericidal, inhibits   B. bactericidal, destroys

    C. bacteriostatic, inhibits   D. bacteriostatic, destroys

4. Fill in the blanks with the words or phrases given below in their proper forms.

> anaphylactic, apt, warrant, untoward, eradicate, speculative, substitute, be billed as, suppression, precautionary

(1) It is necessary to closely monitor the therapeutic and _____ response of children when the antibiotic medication is initially administered.

(2) The _____ cure-all antibiotics are supposed to have the ability to combat all contagious diseases.

(3) Those with a mind to "live for today" are _____ to be indifferent to health risks that have a very long incubation period.

(4) Although these substances would not _____ the AIDS virus, but can effectively control their reproduction.

(5) Most allergies are mild, but very allergic individuals may develop serious _____ shock within a few minutes of exposure.

(6) Certain conditions of invasive aspergillosis (曲霉病) _____ consideration for surgical resection of the infected focus.

(7) The virus destroys a subgroup of lymphocytes, resulting in _____ of the body's immune response.

(8) Food supplements are intended to supplement the diet and should not be regarded as a _____ for a varied diet and a healthy lifestyle.

(9) We employ this approach to stockpile antiviral drugs as a _____ measure against possible influenza pandemic.

(10) The discovery of penicillin _____ a major breakthrough, selected as one of the most important science discoveries in the 20th century.

5. Translate the following sentences and paragraphs into Chinese.

(1) No advance in medical or surgical practice would remain successful if patients developing infections

could not be treated reliably. Developments in chemotherapy for malignancy and organ transplantation make patients more vulnerable to infection, due to immunosuppression. These medical advances would be less meaningful if a patient survived the initial therapy, only to succumb to infection later.

(2) Microorganisms can be either intrinsically resistant to an antibiotic or develop resistance following exposure to that antibiotic (acquired resistance). Resistance can develop as a result of mutation or direct transfer of genes encoding a resistance mechanism.

(3) Not only does antibiotic resistance have a huge financial impact, but more worryingly, there is a major concern about the lack of development of new antibiotics. Between 1940 and 1962, more than 20 new classes of antibiotics were marketed. Since then, only two new classes have reached the market. Many of the other newer antibiotics are modifications of older drugs rather than new classes of agents.

(4) All antibiotics that are currently used in modern medicine have their origins as by-products of bacterial secondary metabolism. Today, technology has allowed advances in areas of antibiotic research and development that have led to alterations and the production of semi-synthetic derivatives of antibiotics first isolated from bacterial cultures. The importance of these antibiotic products cannot be understated in the treatment of infectious diseases, and as multidrug resistance rises in emerging pathogens, the continued discovery and isolation of new antibiotics from bacteria is ever important.

(5) Penicillin-binding proteins (PBPs) are a group of proteins that are characterized by their affinity for and binding to penicillin. They are a normal constituent of many bacteria and involved in the final stages of the synthesis of peptidoglycan, which is the major component of bacterial cell walls. Bacterial cell wall synthesis is essential to growth, cell division (thus reproduction) and maintaining the cellular structure in bacteria. All β-lactam antibiotics bind to PBPs, causing defects in cell wall structure, irregularities in cell shape and eventual cell death and lysis.

(6) Since the resistance to the first commercial antimicrobial agent (penicillin) was identified in 1948, almost every known bacterial pathogen has developed resistance to one or more antibiotics in clinical use. Bacteria have a remarkable genetic plasticity that allows them to respond to a wide array of environmental threats, including the presence of antibiotic molecules that may jeopardize their existence. From an evolutionary perspective, bacteria use two major genetic strategies to adapt to the antibiotic "attack": i) mutations in gene(s) often associated with the mechanism of action of the compound, and ii) acquisition of foreign DNA coding for resistance determinants through horizontal gene transfer (HGT).

Value-Oriented Reflective Reading

Penicillin: An Accidental Discovery Changed the Course of Medicine

Sir Alexander Fleming, a Scottish researcher, is credited with the discovery of penicillin. In 1928, he started to research common staphylococcal bacteria (葡萄球菌). Before Fleming left for a two-week vacation, a petri dish (培养皿) containing a staphylococcus culture was left on a lab bench and never placed in the incubator as intended. Somehow, in preparing the culture, a *Penicillium* (青霉菌, 青霉菌属) mold spore had been accidentally introduced into the medium—perhaps coming in through a window, or more likely floating up a stairwell from the lab below where various molds were being cultured. After returning from the vacation, Fleming noticed that many of the microbial cultures were infected with a fungus and threw them into a detergent container. But then he had to show to a visitor what he was looking for, so he took some of the tablets (培养皿) that were not submerged in the detergent. Then he noticed a zone around the mold that was free of bacteria. This should have happened if the mold produced some bactericidal substance.

Fleming managed to isolate a specimen of mold, he correctly identified it as a *Penicillium* fungus, and for that reason the new substance took the name of penicillin. He found that it affected generally all Gram positive pathogens which cause diseases like diphtheria, gonorrhea, meningitis, pneumonia, and scarlet fever. Fleming published his findings in 1929. However, his efforts to purify the unstable compound from the extract proved beyond his capabilities. For a decade, no progress was made in isolating penicillin as a therapeutic compound. During that time, Fleming sent his *Penicillium* mold to anyone who requested it in hopes that they might isolate penicillin for clinical use.

Then in 1938, Ernst Chain, a biochemist working with pathologist Howard Florey at Oxford University, came across Fleming's paper while he was researching antibacterial compounds. Scientists in Florey's lab started working with penicillin, which they eventually injected into mice to test if it could treat bacterial infections. Their experiments were successful and they went on to test it in humans, where they also saw positive results.

In June 1941, Florey decided to take penicillin to the US in hope of finding a way to scale up production. In Peoria, Illinois, a new team was set up in the Department of Agriculture's research laboratory. They utilized their expertise in fermentation and designed new techniques using deep fermentation tanks to make the purification of penicillin as efficient as possible. They also found more productive strains of *Penicillium notatum* which produced six times more penicillin than Fleming's original strain. Penicillin quickly became known as the war's "miracle drug", curing infectious disease and saving millions of lives.

"Chance favors the prepared mind," remarked Louis Pasteur, a founder of microbiology who had made several serendipitous discoveries himself. Fruitful ideas do not come in an intellectual vacuum. They may pop up at a bus stop or a mountain road, but are only caught by a prepared mind. Most accidents that led to discoveries occurred in laboratories, which were themselves designed for explorations. Experiments are not passive experiences but active inquiries. An experiment is a question by which scientists try to wrestle answers from nature. The answers may be unexpected, but in setting up experiments, scientists have already primed their minds to pounce on surprises. Chance unlocks a door and most people just walk pass. A few with prepared mind open the door and look inside the room. However, without an open mind ready to exploit new possibilities and connect the dots, one may not discover that the room hides more doors that lead to even greater treasures. Fleming's discovery was not a mere chance. A person with unprepared mind would wash out the penicillin with the dirty dish. In contrast, Fleming tried various ways to concentrate it, classified it as a slow-acting antiseptic, and promoted it as a laboratory reagent to differentiate and select microbes. A prepared and open mind is also necessary for students during their journey of scientific exploration.

Questions for oral discussion:

1. What are the factors driving the successful discovery and development of penicillin?
2. How to understand "Fruitful ideas do not come in an intellectual vacuum"?
3. Have you ever had any unexpected gains due to careful observation in research?

Text B
Microorganisms-Friend and Foe to Human Health

Microbiology studies microorganisms, or microbes, a diverse group of generally minute simple life-forms that include bacteria, archaea, algae, fungi, protozoa, and viruses. The field is concerned with the structure, function, and classification of such organisms and with ways of both exploiting and controlling their activities. The 17th century discovery of living forms existing invisible to the naked eye was a significant milestone in the history of science, for from the 13th century onward it had been postulated that "invisible" entities were responsible for decay and disease. The word microbe was coined in the last quarter of the 19th century to describe these organisms, all of which were thought to be related. As microbiology eventually developed into a specialized science, it was found that microbes are a very large group of extremely diverse organisms.

Daily life is interwoven inextricably with microorganisms. In addition to populating both the inner and outer surfaces of the human body, microbes abound in the soil, in the seas, and in the air. Abundant, although usually unnoticed, microorganisms provide ample evidence of their presence—sometimes unfavorably, as when they cause decay of materials or spread diseases, and sometimes favorably, as when they ferment sugar to wine and beer, cause bread to rise, flavor cheeses, and produce valued products such as antibiotics and insulin. Microorganisms are of incalculable value to Earth's ecology, disintegrating animal and plant remains and converting them to simpler substances that can be recycled into other organisms.

Microbiology Came into Being Largely through Studies of Bacteria

The experiments of Louis Pasteur in France, Robert Koch[1] in Germany, and others in the late 1800s established the importance of microbes to humans. The research of these scientists provided proof for the germ theory of disease[2] and the germ theory of fermentation. It was in their laboratories that techniques were devised for the microscopic examination of specimens, culturing (growing) microbes in the laboratory, isolating pure cultures from mixed-culture populations, and many other laboratory manipulations. These techniques, originally used for studying bacteria, have been modified for the study of all microorganisms— hence the transition from bacteriology to microbiology.

The organisms that constitute the microbial world are characterized as either prokaryotes or eukaryotes; all bacteria are prokaryotic—that is, single-celled organisms without a membrane-bound nucleus. Their DNA (the genetic material of the cell), instead of being contained in the nucleus, exists as a long, folded thread with no specific location within the cell.

Until the late 1970s, it was generally accepted that all bacteria are closely related in evolutionary development. This concept was challenged in 1977 by Carl R. Woese and co-investigators at the University of Illinois, whose research on ribosomal RNA from a broad spectrum of living organisms established that two groups of bacteria evolved by separate pathways from a common and ancient ancestral form. This discovery resulted in the establishment of a new terminology to identify the major distinct groups of microbes—namely, the eubacteria (the traditional or "true" bacteria), the archaea (bacteria that diverged from other bacteria at an early stage of evolution and are distinct from the eubacteria), and the eukarya (the eukaryotes).[3]

Are We More Bacterial than Human?

Humans are born into an environment laden with microorganisms, and colonization of the human body begins at the time of birth. Colonization simply implies the establishment of microorganisms on the body surface which, by extension, continues internally (oral cavity, gastrointestinal tract, ear canals, etc.).[4] Throughout life, the skin and mucous membranes exposed to the outside world harbor a variety of **indigenous** bacteria, the normal flora.

The microorganisms living on and in the body even include species that have not been fully characterized and classified. Some examples of the principal resident bacteria include *Staphylococcus*, *Micrococcus* and *Propionibacterium* found on the skin; *Lactobacillus*, *Streptococcus*, *Neisseria*, *Corynebacterium* and *Bacteroides* in the mouth; and *Bacteroides*, *Clostridium*, *Lactobacillus*, *Streptococcus* and many species of the Family **Enterobacteriaceae** in the intestinal tract. Usually the normal flora cause no disturbances in the health of their host. In fact, they often benefit the host by outcompeting pathogenic bacteria, yeasts and protozoa which are encountered occasionally.

It's often said that the bacteria and other microbes in our body outnumber our own cells by about ten to one. That number was first introduced in 1972 as more of a vague estimate, without much significant factual basis, and has been **perpetuated** ever since. In 2014, a researcher from the National Institutes of Health called this very issue into question, noting that there were very few good estimates for the numbers of human and microbial cells in the body. The new calculation made by researchers from Israel and Canada came down to about 39 trillion bacteria to about 30 trillion human cells, a roughly 1.3 : 1 ratio. It's important to note though, that this ratio is still an estimation, not an undisputed fact. However, it seems to reveal that we're basically just as human as we are microbe.

Culprit in Infectious Diseases

In the mighty but invisible kingdom of microbes present within human body, many of them are useful for the body and perform various useful functions. Some reside in the intestine and release such components which help in the digestion of food. Some regulate the production of vitamins and nutrients essential to keeping our bodies strong and healthy. Some are involved in the defense against infection. However, some are indeed detrimental. Microorganisms that can cause disease are collectively known as pathogens. Some pathogens are from the human **microbiota**, which consists of the microbes that live on and within the human body. Most of these microbes are beneficial or **commensal** (causing no harm) to humans, but some may become pathogenic in the face of disturbances such as dietary changes, stress, and antibiotic use. Other pathogens may come from our surrounding environment-in the air, soil, and surfaces we touch, as well as from other organisms, including livestock, wild animals, and humans.

In order to cause disease, these microorganisms must enter the human body, stick to specific human cells and tissues, and grow and replicate. Many of these microorganisms only invade specific parts of the body. For example, *Vibrio cholerae* specifically affects the digestive tract; it does not infect the skin or the lungs. This is because pathogens will only adhere to the human cells and tissues by which they grow best. To do this, they often use cell surface receptors, which are proteins on the cell surface. This is comparable to gluing puzzle pieces together: specific pathogen cell surface receptors only fit and stick to certain human cell surface receptors. Once bound, these microorganisms will begin growing and replicating. Some pathogens will simply steal nutrients from the surrounding environment. Other pathogens will invade the host cell and **hijack** the host cells' nutrients or cellular machinery. This may cause host cells to die or malfunction, making us sick. Furthermore, some pathogens produce toxins as they grow, which can also make us ill.

Following the establishment of the germ theory of disease in the mid-1880s and the development of laboratory techniques for the isolation of microorganisms (particularly bacteria), the causative agents of many common diseases were discovered in rapid succession. Some common diseases and the date of discovery of their causative agent illustrate this point: **anthrax** (1876), **gonorrhea** (1879), **typhoid fever** (1880), **malaria** (1880), tuberculosis (1882), **diphtheria** (1883), **cholera** (1884), and **tetanus** (1884). Medical microbiology is the study of pathogenic microbes and the role of microbes in human illness, which includes the study of microbial pathogenesis and **epidemiology** and is related to the study of disease pathology and immunology. Some of the most notable successes of medical microbiology include the development of vaccines beginning in the 1790s, antibiotics during the mid-20th century, and the global eradication of smallpox by 1977. Despite such great advances in identifying and controlling agents of disease and in devising methods for their control, the world still faces the threat of diseases such as AIDS and **hantavirus pulmonary syndrome (HPS)**, the reemergence of old **scourges** such as tuberculosis, cholera, and diphtheria, and the increasing resistance of microbes to antibiotics.

Tiny but Powerful Drug—making Machines

Through millions of years of evolution and exchanging genes between one another, these tiny microbes are poised to make unique and complex molecules that can have many useful properties. One important use of natural products from microorganisms is antibiotics. Ever since the **serendipitous** discovery of penicillin in 1928, which was a natural product from fungi that could kill bacteria, the scientific community rushed to explore other natural products that could also be used as antibacterial drugs. Because microbes often pump out molecules that can kill other microorganisms in the environment in an attempt to outcompete one another, such natural products were thought to be especially great resources for finding potential antibiotics.

In addition to antibiotics, many bacterial natural products have other therapeutic uses. For example, rapamycin, also known as sirolimus, is made by the bacteria *Streptomyces hygroscopicus*, and is used clinically as an immunosuppressant, especially during a kidney transplant. Bleomycin, a natural product found from *Streptomyces verticillus*, is a chemotherapy drug used in the treatment for a range of cancers.

It turns out that calling bacteria a molecule-making factory is not too far from the truth: many bacterial natural products are made in a way that is very similar to an assembly line.[5] Bacteria have enzymes: proteins that catalyze, or speed up, chemical reactions. These enzymes work together in a manner similar to factory workers; some enzymes are tasked with putting on a certain building block, thus "building" up the molecule, while others take the resulting chain of building blocks and rearrange them to form the final compound. The genes in the bacteria that encode for each of these enzymes are typically lined up side-by-side, which are called biosynthetic gene cluster (BGC)[6].

For industrial purposes, mass culture of producing strains in the fermenter leads to product formation. Fermentation can be divided into upstream processes and downstream processes. During upstream processes, the right organisms that provide the maximum product yield are selected and their growth conditions in the fermenter are optimized. The organisms must be able to grow rapidly and vigorously, be non-pathogenic, and must have stable characteristics to produce an appreciable amount of the product from a particular raw material. They are also referred to as 'biocatalysts' since the fermentation process is solely dependent on the biochemical reactions conducted by these microorganisms. Recombinant DNA technology is used nowadays for the efficient production of desired products. When using genetically engineered organisms or cells, the first step is the selection of the appropriate expression systems with the purpose of reducing batch to batch variation of the product yield. The downstream process mainly involves product recovery and purification, product concentration and preparing products for commercialization. It usually initiates with the rupture or lysis of cells, especially when the product is not secreted into the medium. Following purification, products may require concentration by techniques such as solvent extraction, crystallization, evaporation, **desiccation** and **lyophilization**.

Word Study

1. ancestral [æn'sestrəl] *adj.* 祖传的, 祖先的
2. anthrax ['ænθræks] *n.* 炭疽
3. archaea [ɑ:'ki:ə] *n.* (单数 archaeon) 古核生物, 古生菌, 古菌
4. *Bacteroides* [ˌbæktə'rɔidi:z] *n.* 拟杆菌属, 拟杆菌
5. cholera ['kɒlərə] *n.* 霍乱
6. *Clostridium* [klɒs'trɪdɪəm] *n.* 梭状芽孢杆菌属, 梭状芽孢杆菌
7. coin [kɔɪn] *vt.* 创造 (新词语)
8. commensal [kə'mensl] *adj.* 共生的, 共栖的 ; *n.* 共食者, [生] 共生体
9. *Corynebacterium* [ˌkɒrɪnɪbæk'tɪərəm] *n.* 棒状杆菌属, 棒状杆菌
10. culprit ['kʌlprɪt] *n.* 罪魁祸首, 引起问题的事物
11. desiccation [ˌdesɪ'keɪʃn] *n.* 干燥, 枯竭
12. diphtheria [dɪf'θɪərɪə] *n.* 白喉
13. diverge [daɪ'vɜ:dʒ] *vi.* 偏离, 分歧
14. Enterobacteriaceae ['entərəuˌbæktəri'eisiˌi:] *n.* 肠杆菌科
15. epidemiology [ˌepɪˌdi:mi'ɒlədʒi] *n.* 流行病学
16. eubacteria [ju:bæk'tɪərɪə] *n.* (单数 eubaterium) [微] 真细菌, 真细菌类
17. eukarya [u:'keərɪə] *n.* 真核域
18. eukaryote [ju'kærɪəut] *n.* 真核生物
19. foe [fəu] *n.* 敌人, 仇敌
20. gonorrhea [ˌɡɒnə'ri:ə] *n.* 淋病
21. hantavirus pulmonary syndrome (HPS) ['hæntəˌvaɪrəs 'pʌlmənerɪ 'sɪndrəum] *n.* 汉坦病毒肺综合征
22. hijack ['haɪdʒæk] *vt.* 劫持 (交通工具, 尤指飞机) ; *n.* 劫持, 敲诈
23. indigenous [ɪn'dɪdʒənəs] *adj.* 本地的, 当地的, 土生土长的
24. inextricably [ˌɪnɪk'strɪkəbli] *adv.* 不可分开地, 密不可分地
25. interweave [ˌɪntə'wi:v] *v.* 交织, 交错编织
26. *Lactobacillus* [ˌlæktəubə'sɪləs] *n.* 乳杆菌属, 乳杆菌
27. lyophilization [laɪˌɒfəlaɪ'zeɪʃən] *n.* 冷冻干燥法
28. malaria [mə'leərɪə] *n.* 疟疾
29. microbiota [maɪkrəubə'ɪɒtə] *n.* 微生物区系
30. *Micrococcus* [maɪkrəu'kɒkəs] *n.* 微球菌属, 微球菌
31. *Neisseria* [nai'siərɪə] *n.* 奈瑟菌属, 奈瑟菌

32. perpetuate [pə'petʃueɪt] *vt.* 延续,使永久化

33. prokaryote [prəʊ'kærɪəʊt] *n.* 原核生物,原核细胞型微生物

34. prokaryotic [prəʊkærɪ'ɒtɪk] *adj.* 原核的

35. *Propionibacterium* [ˌprəʊpiˌɔnibæk'tɪəriəm] *n.* 丙酸杆菌属,丙酸杆菌

36. protozoa [ˌprəʊtəʊ'zəʊə] *n.*（单数 protozoan）原生动物

37. scourge [skɜːdʒ] *n.* 天灾,祸害

38. serendipitous [ˌserən'dɪpətəs] *adj.* 偶然的,偶然发生的,有意外收获的

39. *Staphylococcus* [ˌstæfɪlə'kɒkəs] *n.* 葡萄球菌属,葡萄球菌

40. *Streptococcus* [ˌstreptə'kɒkəs] *n.* 链球菌属,链球菌

41. *Streptomyces hygroscopicus* [streptəʊ'maɪsiːz haɪɡrə(ʊ)ɪskɒpɪkəz] *n.* 吸水链霉菌

42. *Streptomyces verticillus* [ˌstreptəʊ'maisiːz ˌvəːtɪ'sɪləz] *n.* 轮枝链霉菌

43. tetanus ['tetənəs] *n.* 破伤风

44. typhoid fever ['taɪfɔɪd 'fiːvə(r)] *n.* 伤寒

45. Vibrio cholerae ['vɪbrɪəʊ 'kɒlərə] *n.* 霍乱弧菌

Notes

1. Robert Koch (1843—1910): 德国医师兼微生物学家,为细菌学始祖之一,与路易·巴斯德、费迪南德·科恩共享盛名。

2. the germ theory of disease: 疾病的细菌学说,是目前公认的许多疾病的科学理论,它指出被称为病原体或"细菌"的微生物会导致疾病。这些微小的生物体必须通过放大才能看到,它们会侵入人类、其他动物和其他活的宿主。它们在宿主内的生长和繁殖会导致疾病。

3. This discovery resulted in the establishment of a new terminology to identify the major distinct groups of microbes—namely, the eubacteria (the traditional or "true" bacteria), the archaea (bacteria that diverged from other bacteria at an early stage of evolution and are distinct from the eubacteria), and the eukarya (the eukaryotes). 译为：这一发现导致建立新的术语,用来识别微生物主要的不同群组,即真细菌(传统的或"真正的"细菌)、古生菌(在进化的早期阶段与其他细菌分道扬镳,并且不同于真细菌)和真核生物(真核生物)。这就是美国微生物学家和生物物理学家卡尔·乌斯 (Carl Richard Woese, 1928—2012) 等人在 1977 年提出的三域系统 (Three-domain system),其将细胞生命形式分为古菌域 (Domain Archaea)、细菌域 (Domain Bacteria) 和真核域 (Domain Eukarya)。

4. Colonization simply implies the establishment of microorganisms on the body surface which, by extension, continues internally (oral cavity, gastrointestinal tract, ear canals, etc.). 译为：定植仅仅意味着微生物在体表生长,而这一过程会进一步延伸到人体的内部(口腔、胃肠道、耳道等)。"which"引导的对于从句修饰 "the establishment of microorganisms on the body surface"。

5. It turns out that calling bacteria a molecule-making factory is not too far from the truth: many bacterial natural products are made in a way that is very similar to an assembly line. 译为：事实证明,把细菌称为分子制造工厂并不是太离谱,许多细菌的天然产物是以一种非常类似于装配线的方式制造出来的。 本句中，"It turns out that..." 是一个常用固定结构,表示"结果是,被证明是",此表达带有一些对结果感到吃惊意外的感觉,其中 it 是形式主语,真正的主语是 that 引导的从句。从句中 "not too far from the truth" 可译为"并不太离谱"。

6. biosynthetic gene cluster (BGC): 生物合成基因簇,是紧密相连的一组非同源基因,参与共同的、独立的代谢途径。在基因组中,这些基因在物理上彼此相邻,它们的表达常常受到共同的调控。生物合成基因簇是细菌和大多数真菌基因组的共同特征,在其他生物体中很少见。

Supplementary Parts

1. Medical and Pharmaceutical Terminology (2): Common Morphemes in Terms of English for Microbiology

Morpheme	Meaning	Example
acar	螨虫	acaricide 杀螨的,杀螨剂
ameb	阿米巴	ameba 阿米巴,变形虫
aspergill	曲霉	aspergillus 曲霉
bacill	杆菌	bacillus 杆菌,芽孢杆菌
bacteri	细菌	bacteriology 细菌学
brucell	布鲁氏菌	brucella 布鲁氏菌
coccidioid	球孢子菌	coccidioides 球孢子菌
coccus	球菌	coccobacillus 球杆菌
ferment	发酵	ferment 酶,酵素;发酵
fung	真菌	fungus 真菌,霉菌
germ	病菌	germicide 杀菌剂
monil	念珠菌	monilia 念珠菌
myc	霉菌	mycelium 菌丝体
nematod	线虫	nematode 线虫
parasit	寄生虫	parasite 寄生虫,寄生物
penicill	青霉	penicillin 青霉素
spirochaet	螺旋体	spirochaeta 螺旋体
staphyl	葡萄	staphylococcus 葡萄球菌
strept	链	streptobacillus 链球杆菌属
virus	病毒	arbovirus 虫媒病毒
zym	发酵	zymogenic 引起发酵的

(1) Decompose the following words and translate them into Chinese.

1) actinomycetales   _____

   sample: actino-mycetales 放线菌目

2) bacteriology   _____

3) colicin   _____

4) chlamydiosis   _____

5) microbiota   _____

6) mycobacteriology   _____

7) mycoplasmal   _____

8) salmonellosis   _____

9) septicemia   _____

10) sporocyst   _____

11) immunotoxin   _____

12) vibriosis   _____

(2) Word-matching.

1)	fungus	A.	虫媒病毒
2)	monilia	B.	曲霉
3)	penicillin	C.	念珠菌属
4)	arbovirus	D.	引起发酵的
5)	staphylococcus	E.	线虫
6)	zymogenic	F.	酶,酵素;发酵
7)	nematode	G.	真菌,霉菌
8)	coccobacillus	H.	杆菌属,芽孢杆菌属
9)	aspergillus	I.	杀螨的,杀螨剂
10)	acaricide	J.	球杆菌
11)	bacillus	K.	青霉素
12)	ferment	L.	葡萄球菌

2. English-Chinese Translation Skills: 药学英语句式特点与翻译

药学英语在句式上最显著的特点体现在句子主语上,一般有两种情况:①使用无灵主语;②使用名词化动词作主语。

(1) 跟其他科技英语类一样,药学英语经常使用无灵主语,把动作发出者隐退,强调动作和结果本身,表现在整个句子结构上就是被动语态,动作发出者有时候省略,有时候通过介词短语保留。

例 1：Bacteriology, a subdiscipline of microbiology later, was founded in the 19th century by Ferdinand Cohn, a botanist whose studies on algae and photosynthetic bacteria led him to describe several bacteria including bacillus and beggiatoa.

参考译文：19 世纪,费迪南德·科恩创建了细菌学(后来成为微生物学的一个分支学科),这位植物学家对藻类和光合细菌进行了研究,描述了包括杆菌和贝日阿托氏菌在内的一些细菌。

说明：在翻译被动语态句子时,要不要加上动作发出者作主语,要看情况而定,上面这个例句,由于这个动作发出者是专有名词,就必须保留,译文改成了主动句,而且这个主语以不同方式重复了三次:"费迪南德·科恩""这位植物学家"和"他"。而原文主语只有一个 bacteriology,在以 whose 引导的定语从句的主语是 studies。

药学英语通常描述药物、药剂等专业内容或者有关药物性质、作用等客观现象,这些内容或现象经常出现在句子主语位置,这也是药学英语使用无灵主语多的另外一种情况,对于这类句子,直接翻译就可以。如：

例 2：Calcium ion plays a critical role in coupling surface membrane depolarization to muscle contraction.

参考译文：钙离子在耦联表面膜去极化和肌肉收缩方面起到关键作用。

例 3：Vaccines are used to combat infectious diseases, however, the last decade has witnessed a revolution in the approach to vaccine design and development. Sophisticated technologies such as genomics, proteomics, functional genomics, and synthetic chemistry can be used for the rational identification of antigens, the synthesis of complex glycans, and the generation of engineered carrier proteins.

参考译文：疫苗用来抵御传染病,然而过去的十年里彻底改变了疫苗设计和开发方法,高端技术如基因组学、蛋白质组学、功能基因组学和合成化学能用于抗原合理识别、复杂多聚糖合成以及工程载体蛋白质的生成。

说明：在上面例句中，三个主语都是无灵主语：vaccines、the last decade、sophisticated technologies，在翻译时都采取了不同的策略。第一句是被动结构，翻译时没有刻意译成被动结构；第二句是一个隐喻结构，时间 the last decade 作主语，连接动词 witness（见证），如果按照原文结构翻译"过去 10 年见证了……"，这类语言表达结构不太适合汉语科技文章；第三句就是按照原文的结构自然译成，也符合汉语表达结构。

翻译药学英语使用无灵主语的句子时，需要根据不同语境采用不同策略，这些在以后的章节中会分别讲解，这里不过多介绍。

(2) 名词化就是将动词转换成名词，名词化动词可以作主语、宾语等，这种结构可以使行文简洁、内容确切，将动作发出者退出主语位置，把动作本身作为信息点突显出来。药学英语中大量使用名词化动词作主语。

例 4：Absorption of moisture by the core and subsequent swelling leads to the release of drugs.

参考译文：片芯吸收水分后逐渐膨胀，从而使药物释放。

说明：在上面例句中有三个名词性动词：absorption、swelling 和 release，在翻译中三个名词性动词的处理方式不一样：absorption 和 release 都译成了动词形式，swelling 保留了名词形式，这样的表达符合汉语语言习惯。

例 5：While his work on the Tobacco Mosaic Virus established the basic principles of virology, it was his development of enrichment culturing that had the most immediate impact on microbiology by allowing for the cultivation of a wide range of microbes with wildly different physiologies.

参考译文：他研究烟草花叶病病毒的成果确立了病毒学的基本原理，与此同时，他发展的富集培养技术，可以大量培养具有不同生理特征的微生物，对微生物学产生直接影响。

说明：上面例句中主句和从句都是名词化动词作主语，这样的表达结构相对弱化动作发出者而突出动作本身，在翻译名词化动词作主语时，要注意英汉语言差别。汉语中一般都由动作发出者做主语，要适当改变原文结构。在该例句中，his work on... 和 his development of... 分别译成"他研究……的成果"和"他发展的……技术"都对原主语进行了适当的改变，使其符合汉语表达习惯。

翻译名词化结构作主语不能仅停留在表层结构上，要理解深层次的语义，名词化动词可以翻译成动词结构，也可以翻译成名词词组，这取决于具体语境。

（陈　菁　庄　婕　乔玉玲　史志祥　龚长华）

Unit Three

Biochemistry

Biochemistry, sometimes abbreviated as "BioChem", is the study of chemical processes in living organisms. Biochemistry governs all living organisms and living processes. By controlling information flow through biochemical signaling and the flow of chemical energy through metabolism, biochemical processes give rise to the seemingly magical phenomenon of life. Much of biochemistry deals with the structures and functions of cellular components such as proteins, carbohydrates, lipids, nucleic acids, and other biomolecules, although increasingly processes rather than individual molecules are the main focus. Over the last 40 years biochemistry has become so successful at explaining living processes that now almost all areas of the life sciences from botany to medicine are engaged in biochemical research. Today the main focus of pure biochemistry is in understanding how biological molecules give rise to the process that occur within living cells which in turn greatly relates to the study and understanding of whole organisms.

Biochemistry and medicine enjoy a mutually cooperative relationship. Biochemical studies have illuminated many aspects of health and disease, and the study of various aspects of health and disease has opened up new areas of biochemistry. Drug discovery is a long process that covers many different fields of activity. Rising costs in drug discovery, coupled with high attrition rates throughout the pipeline, particularly during clinical trials, have been a major cause for concern within the drug industry in recent years. Skillful application of traditional and modern techniques in biochemistry and molecular biosciences have the capacity to play a pivotal role in reducing attrition by providing better target selection, more suitable chemical choices, and improving success in translational research and clinical development.

生物化学,有时缩写为"BioChem",是研究生命体内化学过程的学科。生物化学掌控所有生命体和生命过程。通过控制生化信号转导通路的信息流和新陈代谢的化学能流动,生物化学过程引发看似神奇的生命现象。尽管生物化学的研究焦点逐渐从单个的分子转移到生命过程,生物化学更多地仍是研究细胞组成成分的结构和功能,例如蛋白质、糖类、脂类、核酸和其他生物分子。在过去的40年中,生物化学非常成功地解释了生命过程,以至于目前从植物学到医药学几乎所有生命科学领域都涉及生物化学研究。当今生物化学的主要研究焦点是解释生物分子如何在活细胞中参与生命过程,而这又与进一步研究和理解整个有机体密切相关。

生物化学与医学是一种相辅相成的关系。生物化学研究阐明了健康与疾病的方方面面,而对健康与疾病各方面的探索又开辟了生物化学的新领域。药物研发是一个漫长的过程,涵盖了许多不同的研究领域。近年来,药物研发成本的不断攀升,加上整个研发过程(尤其是临床试验期间)的高失败率,一直是制药行业担忧的主要问题。生物化学和分子生物科学中传统和现代技术的熟练运用可以通过更好的靶点选择、更合适的化学研究方案来发挥关键作用,降低新药研发失败率,提高转化研究和临床开发的成功率。

Text A
Statins: From Fungus to Pharma

Background

Cardiovascular disease (CVD) is a class of diseases that involve the heart or blood vessels. There are many types, including coronary artery disease, angina, and heart failure. According to the World Health Organization, CVD is the leading cause of death, taking an estimated 17.9 million lives each year and accounting for about 30 percent of global mortality.

The study of cardiovascular diseases and the search for effective therapeutics have a long history. More than 100 years ago the German pathologist Virchow observed that the artery walls of patients dying of occlusive vascular disease, such as myocardial infraction, were often thickened and irregular, and contained a yellowish fatty substance subsequently identified as cholesterol. This pathological condition was termed atheroma, the Greek word for porridge. In 1913, Anitschkow and Chalatow showed that feeding cholesterol to rabbits rapidly produces atheromatous disease similar to that found in man. In the 1950s and 1960s, it became apparent that elevated concentrations of plasma cholesterol were a major risk factor for the development of coronary heart disease, which led to the search for drugs that could reduce plasma cholesterol. One possibility was to reduce cholesterol biosynthesis, and the rate-limiting enzyme in the cholesterol biosynthetic pathway, 3-hydroxy-3-methyl-glutaryl-CoA (HMG-CoA) reductase, was a natural target.

1. Cholesterol in Cardiovascular Disease

The modern understanding of cardiovascular disease started to emerge in 1961, when the first reports from the *Framingham Heart Study* were published. This project examined 5,209 men and women, ages 30–62, who lived in Framingham, Massachusetts, a small, predominantly middle-class town just outside of Boston. The results revealed that high blood pressure, smoking and high levels of blood cholesterol are all bad for your heart. In particular, this study showed that there is a tight correlation between blood-cholesterol levels and the likelihood of later developing cardiovascular disease. Pivotal as these findings were, they were only the prologue to a story that was to prove more complex.

First, cholesterol is not all bad news. This lipid makes up a crucial component of biological membranes and serves as a precursor for other necessary substances, including the sex hormones estrogen and testosterone. Indeed, because of its necessity cholesterol does not come exclusively from dietary sources but is also manufactured by the liver and to a lesser extent by a few other tissues, including the intestine.

Second, it is not cholesterol in general that is the problem, but rather the form it is in that matters. Atherosclerosis ("hardening of the arteries") arises from the low-density lipoprotein (LDL) form of cholesterol. These LDLs—globules of about 20 nanometers or so across—encapsulate cholesterol derivatives called cholesteryl esters.

When the bloodstream contains a surplus of LDLs, they enter the innermost layer of cells of the arterial wall and accumulate. Eventually, these lipids oxidize, which triggers metabolic and structural changes in the arterial wall, not unlike those elicited by infection from a pathogen. The immune system identifies these changes as damage, driving the formation of capped plaques replete with fat-engorged white blood cells. It is when these plaques are disrupted that trouble arises: blood leaks through the fissure into the lipid-rich core of the structure to make contact with proteins that promote **coagulation**, resulting in clots. That is the downside.

The upside of cholesterol comes from the high-density lipoprotein (HDL) form, which, unlike its LDL counterpart, is **cardioprotective**. HDLs—globules only 8–11 nanometers across—pick up cholesterol from the blood and prevent or impede **plaque** progression by retrieving arterial **cholesterol** deposits and limiting the rate and extent of LDL oxidation. Higher levels of HDLs thereby reduce the risk of **cardiovascular** disease. Of course, that is not to say that there can never be too much of a good thing: Some studies indicate that very high levels of HDLs also increase the risk of cardiovascular diseases.

Third, cholesterol tightly regulates its own production. A seminal finding in the science of cholesterol came in 1966 when Marvin D. Siperstein and Violet M. Fagan—both then at the University of Texas Southwestern Medical School—showed how the body controls cholesterol levels. These investigators discovered that the enzyme that converts a substance named HMG-CoA to mevalonic acid, the immediate precursor of cholesterol, is inhibited by cholesterol. By feedback inhibiting the pacemaker enzyme that catalyzes the first committed and rate-limiting step in the pathway, cholesterol downregulates its own synthesis.[1]

A major culprit in heart disease—cholesterol—and a potential therapeutic target—the enzyme HMG-CoA reductase—had been discovered.

2. Blue Cheese's Cousin

A Japanese biochemist, Akira Endo, made a vital contribution to the finding of HMG-CoA reductase **inhibitors**. He set out to explore whether inhibiting HMG-CoA reductase could decrease blood cholesterol levels. Although other researchers had the same thing in mind, Endo took a fungal angle. He speculated that there must be at least a few fungal **species** capable of elaborating compounds—niche-carving[2] **antimetabolites**—that target HMG-CoA reductase to do battle with fungal competitors that require cholesterol-like compounds for survival.

By 1971, Endo and his colleague Masao Kuroda had started their search for fungal compounds that **interfered** with cholesterol production—via HMG-CoA reductase—in rat-liver extracts. After two years of painstakingly screening 6,000 microbial strains, Endo and Kuroda found a hit from *Penicillium citrinum*, which is a relative of the organism responsible for the blue in blue cheese and the fungal mats that grow on old oranges. By purifying active compounds from 2,900 liters of **filtered** liquid drawn from *P. citrinum* cultures, they isolated compound ML-236B, a compound known as mevastatin, signifying a substance that stops mevalonic acid synthesis. Mevastatin is a structural **analogue** of HMG-CoA: It is able to dock[3] onto the enzyme HMG-CoA reductase and obstruct HMG-CoA binding, thus preventing its conversion into **mevalonic acid** for the synthesis of cholesterol.

With such a potentially promising inhibitor in hand, they faced two make-or-break questions: Does mevastatin do what it should *in vivo* and if so, is it free of **deleterious** side effects? Endo started exploring these questions in depth with rats and found that mevastatin was effective only in the short term. Over longer trials, even at relatively high doses, it produced no consistent effect. That was very bad news—news that could have easily brought work on this compound as a cholesterol-lowering drug to an abrupt end.

3. Cholesterol's Complexities

Before further examining the history of the statins, it is instructive to consider a perplexing question, or at least a question that is perplexing with the benefit of hindsight. That is, if statins diminish all types of cholesterol, why do they reduce the risk of cardiovascular diseases? Surely, a block on cholesterol production should decrease both the good and the bad, the HDLs as well as the LDLs. Well, the short answer to this question is: Luckily, these drugs are more **selective** than could have been anticipated when they were first discovered. Treatment with statins does appreciably decrease LDLs, as expected. But, in addition, statins increase HDLs, and by more than 7.5 percent, according to some studies.

The liver is the hub when it comes to LDLs. When the production of cholesterol in liver cells is diminished by the inhibition of HMG-CoA reductase, fewer LDLs enter the circulation. And because the liver cells have fewer LDLs entering to contribute to the cholesterol pool, they generate more LDL **receptors** on their surfaces to grab more of this substance from the blood. The combination of producing less cholesterol in general—including the LDL fraction—and pulling more LDLs from the blood into liver cells serves to deplete circulating levels of LDL cholesterol. All other things being equal, high numbers of LDL receptors in liver cells equate with low levels of LDLs in the blood.

Currently, there is no consensus on just how statins increase blood HDL levels. Some scientists suspect that statins inhibit the transfer protein responsible for unloading the **cholesteryl ester** cargo of HDLs. A variety of experiments on animals and humans show that blocking the cholesteryl ester transfer protein triggers increases in the levels of HDLs. Another possibility is that statins stimulate the expression of HDL transport proteins, which in turn ferry this form of cholesterol from the liver to the blood.

It is intriguing to consider that the mechanisms that nearly stalled Endo's first screens of mevastatin, because they were done on rats, are the very mechanisms that make these drugs so effective **therapeutically** in humans. Rats are an exception because their **steady-state** blood levels of LDLs are low; most of their blood cholesterol is in HDLs. What this means is that even if statins decreased blood LDL levels enough to be noticeable in the short term in rats, any long-term effects at the level of total blood cholesterol would be offset by a subsequent increase in HDLs. As Endo's work with chickens and subsequently other animals (including humans and other primates) was to show, a lowering of total blood cholesterol is typically seen because LDL cholesterol ordinarily represents a sizeable fraction of the total—a much larger fraction than in rats and other rodents.

4. Merck Moves Ahead

From July 1976 to October 1978, Sankyo offered Merck crystals of mevastatin and its **pharmacological** and **toxicological** data under a "Disclosure Agreement". After confirming the findings of Endo and colleagues, Merck initiated fungal-culture screens to find another statin, one that Merck could call its own. In Feb 1979, Merck independently isolated lovastatin from the common soil **fungus** *Aspergillus terreus*, which is structurally identical to mevastatin except for a single methyl group.

By then, Sankyo was running clinical trials on mevastatin. A rumor was circulating that the company discovered intestinal lymphomas in dogs treated with very large doses of mevastatin over a long period of time and terminated all the trials. Knowing that only a **methyl** group distinguished lovastatin from mevastatin, Merck, too, immediately halted its testing on people, recalling all outstanding samples from clinical investigators and notifying the U.S. Food and Drug Administration (FDA).

Instead of pursuing a drug to treat the general population, Merck executives turned to focus their efforts on the small fraction with a condition called <u>heterozygous familial **hypercholesterolemia**[4]</u>, which afflicts approximately 1 in 500 people. In this genetic disease, a person carries two different copies of a gene, hence the term heterozygous. One copy works normally, and one does not. The possession of one aberrant copy of the gene in this **autosomal-dominant** disease is sufficient to cause problems because of a **deficiency** in the cellular receptors responsible for the removal of circulatory LDLs. As a result, people with this disease have a severe elevation of LDLs, and they typically develop cardiovascular disease between the ages of 30 and 40 if left untreated.

Since mevastatin has already been used on similar patients with some favorable results, the case was compelling: After all, people with hypercholesterolemia faced a great and certain danger, whereas the cancer potential of mevastatin remained only speculation. For this reason, many of the clinicians involved in the early trials of lovastatin urged Merck to continue. After extensive testing, the Merck scientists concluded that the effects observed after treatment with lovastatin were due to its **mechanism** of action and not to **off-target** or drug-based **toxicity**. They reasoned that the "**lymphomas**" observed in the Sankyo experiments probably represented histological changes due to subcellular processing of massive amounts of drug and were not **neoplastic**. Armed with the new findings and committed to going forward, Merck, therefore, did what had to be done: It presented all its data to the FDA and sought approval for further studies on patients with this condition.

The FDA consented, and Merck's clinical trials on lovastatin resumed in 1982. The early results suggested that this compound dramatically reduces LDL levels with few side effects. The company continued its work, moving through the drug-development process. By 1987, the FDA approved Mevacor (alias lovastatin) for use in patients whose cholesterol levels could not be adequately controlled by diet or by using other drugs, such as inhibitors of the intestinal resorption of cholesterol **derivatives** or absorption of the parent compound from dietary sources.

Despite the FDA's approval, Merck had to stipulate in its product label that no clinical outcome benefit could be inferred from those findings—all they could say was that statin safely lowered LDL cholesterol levels in blood. Merck still faced a fundamental question: did statin necessarily protect against cardiovascular disease? To find out, Merck sponsored the Scandinavian Simvastatin Survival Study (the "4S study" for short), which was completed in 1994. In a group of patients diagnosed with "moderate" hypercholesterolemia, 2,223 patients received a placebo, and 2,221 took simvastatin, a second-generation statin from Merck produced by the synthetic modification of lovastatin. The results of this study, a milestone in cardiology and <u>evidence-based medicine</u>[5], were conclusive. The group of patients taking simvastatin not only showed statistically significant decreases in total blood cholesterol and LDL cholesterol of 25 and 35 percent, respectively, but also a 42 percent decrease in death rate. Since then, the association between cholesterol reduction by statins and the improvement of survival in coronary heart disease patients was established.

These stunning results and the successful trials with Mevacor drew other pharmaceutical companies into the statin market, with the approval of pravastatin (Pravachol) in 1991, fluvastatin (Lescol) in 1994, atorvastatin (Lipitor) in 1997, cerivastatin (Baycol/Lipobay) in 1998, and rosuvastatin (Crestor) in 2003. All commercial statins are mevastatin-analogs that have a common structure resembling HMG-CoA.

5. Adding Applications

Akira Endo's decades-old adventure continues. In the mid-1990s, the U.K. Heart Protection Study—sponsored by the U.K. Medical Research Council, the British Heart Foundation, Merck and Hoffman-La Roche—examined 20,000 volunteers who were 40 to 80 years old. These subjects were considered at high risk of cardiovascular disease because of factors such as diabetes, but their physicians did not consider them candidates for statin therapy because their blood LDL-cholesterol levels were within the normal range. Nonetheless, this study put these people on either 40 milligrams per day of simvastatin or a **placebo** for an average of 5.5 years. The results were impressive. In those individuals with diabetes but no obvious arterial disease who were put on simvastatin, the risk of a heart attack or stroke decreased by about 20 percent. Rory Collins, who together with Richard Peto, headed this study, estimates that up to 20 million people worldwide would be eligible for statin therapy. On TheHeart.org, Collins noted that "even if an extra 10 million people took them, we would save 50,000 lives a year" and prevent untold numbers of **debilitating** heart attacks and strokes.

Other work shows the potential for still broader applications of statins. In April 2008, for example, Beatrice A. Golomb, a professor of medicine at the San Diego School of Medicine and director of the University of California, San Diego's statin study, and colleagues reported that **statins** lower blood pressure. Pending their confirmation or otherwise, these findings point to further expansion of the types of patients who stand to gain from being prescribed statins. Stroke prevention, not just of the occlusive but also of the hemorrhagic variety, is an obvious target in that statins may alleviate not just one but both of the main predisposing factors, atherosclerosis, and high blood pressure.[6]

The applications of statins might not stop here, however. Some studies suggest that these drugs can also help prevent **Alzheimer's dementia**, age-related bone loss, and even prostate cancer. Stated plainly, the discovery of statins and the new insights into cardiovascular and other diseases that have and continue to come from their implementation represents one of the most significant accomplishments of the biomedical sciences in the 20th century.

Word Study

1. Alzheimer's dementia ['æltshaimǝz dɪ'menʃǝ] *n.* 阿尔茨海默型痴呆症
2. analogue ['ænǝlɒg] *n.* 类似物
3. angina [æn'dʒaɪnǝ] *n.* 心绞痛
4. antimetabolite [ˌæntɪmɪ'tæbǝlaɪt] *n.* 抗代谢物, 抗代谢药
5. atheroma [ˌæθǝ'rǝʊmǝ] *n.* [医] 粥样斑, 粥样斑块
6. atheromatous [ˌæθe'rǝʊmǝtǝs] *adj.* 动脉粥样化的
7. atherosclerosis [ˌæθǝrǝʊsklɪ'rǝʊsɪs] *n.* [医] 动脉粥样硬化, 动脉硬化
8. autosomal-dominant [ˌɔ:tǝ'sǝʊmǝl 'dɒmɪnǝnt] *adj.* 常染色体显性的
9. biosynthesis [ˌbaɪǝʊ'sɪnθɪsɪs] *n.* 生物合成
10. cardioprotective [kɑ:daɪɒprǝʊ'tektɪv] *adj.* 心脏保护的
11. cardiovascular [ˌkɑ:diǝʊ'væskjǝlǝ(r)] *adj.* 心血管的
12. cholesterol [kǝ'lestǝrɒl] *n.* 胆固醇
13. cholesteryl ester [kɒ'lestǝrǝl 'estǝ(r)] *n.* 胆固醇酯
14. coagulation [kǝʊˌægju'leɪʃn] *n.* 凝固, 凝结
15. coronary ['kɒrǝnri] *adj.* 冠状的
16. debilitating [dɪ'bɪlɪteɪtɪŋ] *adj.* 使衰弱的
17. deficiency [dɪ'fɪʃnsi] *n.* 缺乏, 不足, 缺陷
18. deleterious [ˌdelǝ'tɪǝriǝs] *adj.* 有害的
19. derivative [dɪ'rɪvǝtɪv] *n.* 派生物, 衍生物

20. eligible ['elɪdʒəbl] *adj.* 符合条件的,合格的

21. encapsulate [ɪn'kæpsjuleɪt] *v.* 封进内部

22. engorged [en'gɔːdʒd] *adj.* 塞满的,过饱的

23. enzyme ['enzaɪm] *n.* 酶

24. estrogen ['iːstrədʒən] *n.* 雌激素

25. feedback ['fiːdbæk] *n.* 反馈

26. filter ['fɪltə(r)] *v.* 过滤,渗透

27. fungus ['fʌŋɡəs] *n.* 真菌,霉菌

28. hypercholesterolemia [haɪpə(ː)kəlestərəu'liːmjə] *n.* [医]高胆固醇血症

29. immune system [ɪ'mjuːn 'sɪstəm] *n.* 免疫系统

30. *in vivo* [ɪn 'viːvəu] *adv.*(拉)[生物]在活的有机体内

31. inhibitor [ɪn'hɪbɪtə(r)] *n.* 抑制剂,抑制物

32. interfere [ˌɪntə'fɪə(r)] *v.* 干涉,妨碍

33. lipid ['lɪpɪd] *n.* 脂质

34. lipoprotein ['lɪpəprəutiːn] *n.* 脂蛋白

35. lymphoma [lɪm'fəumə] *n.* 淋巴瘤

36. mechanism ['mekənɪzəm] *n.*(生物体内的)机制

37. methyl ['meθɪl] *n.* 甲基

38. mevalonic acid [mevə'lɒnik 'æsɪd] *n.* 甲羟戊酸

39. myocardial infraction [ˌmaɪəu'kɑːdɪəl ɪn'frækʃn] *n.* 心肌梗死

40. neoplastic [ˌniːəu'plæstɪk] *adj.* 肿瘤的

41. occlusive [ɒ'kluːsɪv] *adj.* 闭塞的

42. off-target ['ɒf 'tɑːɡɪt] *adj.* 脱靶

43. oxidize ['ɒksɪdaɪz] *v.* 氧化

44. pharmacological [ˌfɑːməkə'lɒdʒɪkl] *adj.* 药理学的

45. placebo [plə'siːbəu] *n.* 安慰剂

46. plaque [plæk] *n.*(医)斑(块)

47. precursor [pri'kɜːsə(r)] *n.* 前体

48. receptor [rɪ'septə(r)] *n.* [生化]受体

49. reductase [rɪ'dʌkteɪs] *n.* 还原酶

50. selective [sɪ'lektɪv] *adj.* 选择性的,选择的

51. species ['spiːʃiːz] *n.* 种类,物种

52. statin ['stætɪn] *n.* 他汀(一类降血脂药物的统称)

53. steady-state [s'tediːst'eɪt] *adj.* 恒定的,不变的

54. testosterone [te'stɒstərəun] *n.* 睾酮

55. therapeutically [ˌθerə'pjuːtɪkəli] *adv.* 在治疗上,有疗效地

56. toxicity [tɒk'sɪsəti] *n.* 毒性

57. toxicological [ˌtɒksɪkə'lɒdʒɪkl] *adj.* 毒理学的

Notes

1. 在理解 "By feedback inhibiting the pacemaker enzyme that catalyzes the first committed and rate-limiting step in the pathway, cholesterol downregulates its own synthesis." 这一句时,需要注意两个

词的用法：①"pacemaker"原义为"领跑者、起搏器、标兵"，通读全句可发现，HMG-CoA 还原酶对于胆固醇生物合成的途径非常重要和关键，该词在此句中用于比喻该酶的关键作用；②在"first committed and rate-limiting step"中，"committed"在通用英语中的释义为"尽心尽力的、坚定的"，而在生物合成途径的多步骤反应说明中，该词具有"定向的"之意，即该催化反应对于整个生物合成途径起到基团定向的作用，所以"first committed and rate-limiting step"译为"第一个定向及限速的步骤"。整句可译为：胆固醇正是通过反馈性抑制 HMG-CoA 还原酶，此催化合成途径中第一个定向及限速步骤的关键酶，用于降低自身的合成水平。

2. niche-carving："niche"源自法语，本义为"壁龛"，是一种在外墙上凿出的边界清晰的小神龛，后来被引来形容大市场中的缝隙市场。在经济学中，"niche market"是指"高度专门化的需求市场"。此外，"niche"还可指"山体凹进的地方、悬崖上的石缝"，人们在登山时，常常要借助这些微小的缝隙作为支点，一点点向上攀登。因此，"carve a niche"具有"开辟一席之地"之意。虽然"niche"在生物学中可表示"生态位"（一个生物所占环境的最小单位），但结合上下文，此处显然不能使用这一释义。所以，"niche-carving"译为"开创性的、独特的"。

3. dock：该词作为名词使用时，意为"码头、船埠、船坞、港区"等；作为动词使用则有"（使船）靠码头、进港，（航天器）在太空对接，将电子设备（如电脑、数码相机）相接"等意。在药学专业词汇中，"dock"的意思为药物与其作用靶点（如酶、受体）的可供结合口袋在空间结构上匹配，或通过计算机模拟的方法模拟药物与靶点（如酶、受体）的可供结合口袋的结合状态。在药物分子设计方向一般译为"对接"，如"molecular docking"译为"分子对接"。

4. heterozygous familial hypercholesterolemia：杂合子型家族性高胆固醇血症。家族性高胆固醇血症（familial hypercholesterolemia, FH）是一种常染色体显性遗传病，由低密度脂蛋白在肝脏代谢有关的基因发生致病性突变所致。其主要特征为血清低密度脂蛋白胆固醇水平明显升高，多部位形成皮肤黄色瘤，以及早发动脉粥样硬化性心血管疾病。

5. evidence-based medicine：循证医学，即遵循证据的医学。其核心思想是任何医疗决策的确定都应基于客观的临床科学研究依据。具体工作包括作出系统评价（systematic review）和利用证据进行循证医学的实践。

6. Stroke prevention, not just of the occlusive but also of the hemorrhagic variety, is an obvious target in that statins may alleviate not just one but both of the main predisposing factors, atherosclerosis, and high blood pressure. 该句为复杂长句，应找出其中的主干"Stroke prevention ... is an obvious target in that statins may alleviate ... the main predisposing factors"，即"由于他汀类药物可以减轻卒中的主要易感因素，预防卒中是他汀类药物的明确目标"。梳理主干后，便于找出不同的从句对应修饰的部分，利用括号注释的方式可以简化中文译文的复杂性，从而得到整句的译文：由于他汀类药物可以减轻卒中的两个主要易感因素（动脉粥样硬化和高血压），因此预防卒中（包括预防血栓和出血性卒中）是他汀类药物的明确目标。

Exercises

1. Decide whether each of the following statements is true (T) or false (F) according to the passage.

(1) The published reports from the *Framingham Heart Study* in 1961 revealed that high blood cholesterol level increased the risk of cardiovascular diseases.

(2) Diet is the exclusive source of cholesterol in human body.

(3) HDL is the good form of cholesterol that transports cholesterol from liver to the blood.

(4) Mevastatin docks onto HMG-CoA reductase to block the conversion from mevalonic acid to cholesterol.

(5) Mevastatin showed similar cholesterol-lowering effect in rats over short-term and long-term trails.

(6) High expression of LDL receptors on liver cells help to further decrease circulating level of LDL cholesterol.

2.   Questions for oral discussion

(1) Why was HMG-CoA reductase considered as a potential therapeutic target for the development of drugs used to treat coronary artery disease?

(2) What are the upside and downside of cholesterol?

(3) What are statins' effects on HDL and LDL? And by what mechanism?

(4) In terms of new drug R&D, what insight can you get from the therapeutic expansion of statins?

3.   Choose the best answer to each of the following questions

(1) During the development of atherosclerosis, _____.

   A. excess LDLs only accumulate on the outer layer of the arterial wall

   B. oxidation of LDLs causes changes in the arterial wall that are totally different from those caused by pathogenic infection

   C. immune system is involved to drive the formation of plaques

   D. coagulation is promoted due to the stabilization of the plaques

(2) Akira Endo decided to screen fungal cultures to search for potential inhibitors of HMG-CoA reductase because _____.

   A. some other researchers had adopted the same method

   B. at that time it was well known that fungi were capable of producing antimetabolites targeting HMG-CoA reductase

   C. he just wanted to try his luck to see if there was any fungal species surviving on cholesterol

   D. he theorized that some fungal species could produce inhibitors of HMG-CoA reductase to compete with other fungal species surviving on cholesterol

(3) As to the cholesterol-lowering effects of statins, which of the following statements is true?

   A. Statins lower the levels of both HDLs and LDLs in the blood.

   B. Statins lower the level of LDLs while leaving HDLs unaffected.

   C. Statins increase the level of HDLs through some mechanisms that haven't been fully elucidated.

   D. Statins increase the entry of LDLs from liver cells to the cholesterol pool.

(4) Why was consistent lowering of total cholesterol not observed for mevastatin over longer trials in rats?

   A. Because mevastatin actually didn't work in rats with high cholesterol level.

   B. Because the decrease in LDL was compensated for by the increase in HDL, resulting in unnoticeable change in total blood cholesterol.

   C. Because LDL represents the major fraction of total cholesterol in rats.

   D. Because mevastatin was tested at low doses.

(5) As a result of the diminished production of cholesterol in liver cells by the inhibition of HMG-CoA reductase, _____.

   A. more LDLs enter the cholesterol pool

   B. circulating LDLs are depleted

   C. expression of hepatic LDL receptors is downregulated

   D. total cholesterol level is increased due to the increase in HDL level

(6) Which of the following is not one of the reasons for Merck to choose patients with familial

hypercholesterolemia when resuming its clinical trial of lovastatin?

A. Mevastatin already showed favorable results in similar patients.

B. The disease only affects a small population.

C. People with familial hypercholesterolemia face much higher risk of cardiovascular disease.

D. For those patients, the benefits of lovastatin may outweigh the risks even considering the possibility of causing cancer.

(7) Why did Merck conduct the Scandinavian Simvastatin Survival Study?

A. To prove that statins actually protect against cardiovascular disease.

B. To prove that mevastatin could safely lower LDL cholesterol in blood.

C. To prove that simvastatin works better than mevastatin in lowering cholesterol.

D. To prove that statin therapy is necessary for the general population.

(8) What can be concluded from the U.K. Heart Protection Study in the mid-1990s?

A. Simvastatin significantly reduced the risk of heart attack or stroke even in those individuals without obvious atherosclerosis.

B. Only people with very high risk of cardiovascular disease can benefit from statin therapy.

C. People with normal blood LDL-cholesterol levels are not eligible for stain therapy although they have other risk factors of cardiovascular disease.

D. Stains could also lower blood pressure.

(9) For other statins like pravastatin, atorvastatin, cerivastatin and rosuvastatin that were approved after lovastatin, _____ .

A. they all have similar structure

B. they work on different stages of the pathway of cholesterol biosynthesis

C. they have the same safety profile

D. they are all screened from fungal cultures

(10) According to the passage, which of the following is not a possible indication expansion of statins?

A. Alzheimer's dementia.   B. Stroke.

C. Age-related bone loss.   D. Lymphoma.

4. Fill in the blanks with the words given below in their proper forms.

> placebo,   alleviate,   mortality,   precursor,   downregulate,   isolate
> coagulation,   analogue,   express,   heterozygous,   homozygous

(1) In the controlled clinical trial, patients were randomly assigned to simvastatin 40 mg daily versus _____ .

(2) Mcvalonic acid is the immediate _____ of cholesterol in the biosynthetic pathway known as the mevalonate pathway.

(3) Mevastatin is a close structural _____ of lovastatin and both agents have the same biochemical and pharmacological activities.

(4) The number of functional LDL receptors _____ on the surface of hepatocytes is the primary determinant of plasma LDL-cholesterol levels.

(5) Acute coronary syndrome commonly results from atherosclerotic plaque rupture, followed by platelet and _____ cascade activation, which leads to a thrombus formation in the coronary arteries.

(6) Familial hypercholesterolemia (FH) can be inherited from one parent (_____ FH), or, in rare

instances, from both (_____ FH).

(7) Mevastatin (Compactin) is a hypolipidemic agent that was _____ from the *Penicillium citrinum* by Akira Endo in the 1970s.

(8) Statins may _____ both of the main predisposing factors, atherosclerosis and high blood pressure, of stroke.

(9) Obesity and diabetes are 2 of the 4 metabolic risk factors (in addition to high blood pressure and dyslipidemia) that are estimated to account for 60% of cardiovascular disease _____ worldwide.

(10) Gene expression analysis showed that genes in the cholesterol synthesis pathway were _____ in mice on a high-carbohydrate diet, low-fat diet, and *de novo* cholesterol synthesis was reduced.

5.   Translate the following sentences and paragraphs into Chinese.

(1) Cholesterol biosynthesis is a complex process involving more than 30 enzymes. The pathway was a natural target in the search for drugs to reduce plasma cholesterol concentrations, in the hope that these treatments would reduce the risk of coronary heart disease.

(2) Feedback suppression of cholesterol synthesis in the liver by dietary cholesterol is mediated through changes in the activity of HMG-CoA reductase that catalyzes the conversion of HMG-CoA to mevalonate. Changes in reductase activity are closely related to changes in the overall rate of cholesterol synthesis.

(3) However, early attempts to reduce cholesterol biosynthesis were disastrous. Triparanol, which inhibits a late step in the pathway, was introduced into clinical use in the mid-1960s, but was withdrawn from the market shortly after because of the development of cataracts and various cutaneous adverse effects.

(4) HMG-CoA reductase is the rate-limiting enzyme in the cholesterol biosynthetic pathway. In contrast to desmosterol and other late-stage intermediates, hydroxymethyl glutarate is water soluble and there are alternative metabolic pathways for its breakdown when HMG-CoA reductase is inhibited, so that there is no build-up of potentially toxic precursors. HMG-CoA reductase was, therefore, an attractive target.

(5) In April 1980, after animal safety studies had been performed, Merck began clinical trials of lovastatin in healthy volunteers. Lovastatin was shown to be dramatically effective for lowering LDL cholesterol in healthy volunteers, with no obvious adverse effects.

(6) Lovastatin is a fermentation product. Simvastatin is a semisynthetic derivative of lovastatin, and pravastatin is derived from the natural product compactin by biotransformation, whereas all other HMG-CoA reductase inhibitors are totally synthetic products. All commercial inhibitors of HMG-CoA reductase are mevastatin-analogs that have a common structure resembling HMG-CoA.

(7) The mechanism of the reduction in plasma cholesterol by statins is not simply reduction in cholesterol biosynthesis. Inhibition of HMG-CoA reductase reduces levels of mevalonate, which leads to a reduction in the regulatory sterol pool, which in turn causes upregulation of HMG-CoA reductase, other enzymes of cholesterol biosynthesis, and most importantly the LDL receptor. Although the LDL receptor was not the original target that the discoverers of compactin and lovastatin were aiming at, the work of Brown and Goldstein and others showed that induction of this receptor is crucial to the effectiveness of the statin drug class.

Value-Oriented Reflective Reading

The Creation of Synthetic Crystalline Bovine Insulin

Fifty years ago, a great achievement in life science occurred in China—the complete synthesis of crystalline (结晶的) bovine insulin—which gave Chinese scientists a sense of great elation and pride. In 1958, Shanghai Institute of Biochemistry, Chinese Academy of Sciences and Perking University proposed that China should artificially synthesize insulin and obtained the support of the Chinese government. The project started in 1959, however, at that time, there was a lack of adequate equipment, the raw materials of amino acids and other necessary reagents. Consequently, synthesis of such a large compound represented a formidable (难对付的) task. The strategy adopted was to involve as many capable scientists as possible with eventually several hundreds of participants from eight different institutes participating in the project. People worked day and night preparing amino acids and other reagents, purifying solvents and synthesizing small peptides.

In order to accomplish this task three teams were chosen to work together synergistically (协同地) in Shanghai: Prof. Qiyi Xing of Perking University was to lead his group to Shanghai and combine with Prof. You Wang's group in Shanghai Institute of Organic Chemistry, Chinese Academy of Sciences where they were to be responsible for the synthesis of chain A; Prof. Jingyi Niu of Shanghai Institute of Biochemistry, Chinese Academy of Sciences and his team would complete the synthesis of chain B; and Prof. Chenglu Zhou's team in Shanghai Institute of Biochemistry, Chinese Academy of Sciences would be responsible for the split and recombination of chain A and B.

In August of 1964, Prof. Jingyi Niu successfully synthesized chain B and assembled it with chain A of natural insulin into semi-synthesized bovine insulin. In May of 1965, the combined team of Perking University and Shanghai Institute of Organic Chemistry finished the synthesis of Chain A of insulin. At the same time, Prof. Chenglu Zhou's team greatly increased the yield of the recombination of chain A and B. And finally, the fully synthetic bovine insulin came into production on September 17, 1965. This is the first totally synthetic insulin in crystallized form with full biological activity, immunogenicity and chemical property in the world.

This work was published in *Scientia Sinica* which aroused a great deal of international interest. *Science* magazine reported this achievement in July, 1966. Prof. Henry Norman Rydon, a celebrated statesman in peptide chemistry reviewed in *New Scientist* magazine the reasons why the competitors of the Chinese scientists had failed to obtain insulin with full activity and commented that the achievement of the Chinese scientists was "a truly seminal (影响深远的) piece of work which would stimulate and encourage work directed towards the synthesis of larger, more typical, proteins".

The synthesis of a complete and active insulin in only six years was a fantastic achievement given that it was predicted to take much longer. Why was such a brilliant and awesome achievement first accomplished in China, a developing country where the basis of scientific research was relatively weak, rather than in developed countries such as America and Germany? Besides the timely decision-making and strategic planning of the scientific administrative department in the government, the most important determinants might be the laudable mentality of Chinese scientists at that time, which can be summed up into "insulin spirit", which includes four aspects: (1) selfless dedication. All people involved in the project devoted all themselves into the demands of the project without considering their own interest; (2) honesty. Every intermediate in more than 200 steps of the synthetic procedure had to be rigorously identified, so even a slight problem on these identification procedures might lead to total failure of the whole project; (3) close cooperation. The three teams organized from three different institutes had clear assignment of their responsibilities and worked synergistically for the common aim of the project, so that high efficiency was achieved; (4) the spirit of welcoming challenges. To synthesize a protein consisting of 51 amino acids was a formidable task, so it was the spirit of welcoming a challenge that helped the Chinese scientists gain the respect of the world. Today, the "insulin spirit" is still of great value in constructing our research systems and managing research projects. Most importantly, it has become the source of confidence and strength of every Chinese researcher.

Questions for oral discussion:

1. Why was synthetic crystalline bovine insulin regarded as a great achievement in life science?

2. What were the difficulties and challenges faced by Chinese scientists during project implementation? And how were they conquered?

3. As students of medical and pharmaceutical sciences, what can you learn from the "insulin spirit"?

Text B
Discovery of Insulin, and the Making of a Medical Miracle

Background

Insulin is a hormone that regulates the amount of glucose (sugar) in the blood and is required for the body to function normally. Insulin is produced by β-cells in the **pancreas**, also called the **islets of Langerhans**. These cells continuously release a small amount of insulin into the body, but release surges of the hormone in response to a rise in the blood glucose level.

Certain cells in the body change the food ingested into energy, or blood glucose, that cells can use. Every time a person eats, the blood glucose rises. Raised blood glucose triggers the cells in the islets of Langerhans to release the necessary amount of insulin. Insulin allows the blood glucose to be transported from the blood into the cells. Cells have an outer wall, called a membrane, which controls what enters and exits the cell. Researchers do not yet know exactly how insulin works, but they do know insulin binds to receptors on the cell membrane. The binding of insulin to receptors activates a set of transport molecules so that glucose and proteins can enter the cell. The cells can then use glucose as energy to carry out their functions. Once transported into the cell, the blood glucose level is returned to normal within hours.

Without insulin, the blood glucose builds up in the blood, and the cells are starved of their energy source. Some of the **symptoms** that may occur include **fatigue**, constant infections, **blurred** eye sight, **numbness**, **tingling** in the hands or legs, increased thirst, and slowed healing of **bruises** or cuts. The cells will begin to use fat, the energy source stored for emergencies. When this lasts for too long a time, the body produces **ketones**, chemicals produced by the liver. Ketones can poison and kill cells if they build up in the body over an extended period of time. This can lead to serious illness and coma.

People who do not produce the necessary amount of insulin have diabetes. There are two general types of diabetes. The most severe type, known as Type I or juvenile-onset diabetes, is when the body does not produce any insulin. Type I diabetics usually inject themselves with different types of insulin three to four times daily. Dosage is taken based on the person's blood glucose reading, taken from a glucose meter. Type II diabetics produce some insulin, but it is either not enough or their cells do not respond normally to insulin. The symptoms usually occur in **obese** or middle aged and older people. Type II diabetics do not necessarily need to take insulin, but they may inject insulin once or twice a day.

How Insulin Almost Wasn't Discovered

Before the discovery of insulin, diabetes was a feared disease that most certainly led to death. Patients wasted away, grew weak, and suffered indescribably before their inevitable death. They had **insatiable** thirst and hunger, but trying to satisfy their hunger only made things worse, and they continued to lose weight. Doctors knew that sugar worsened the condition of diabetic patients and that the most effective treatment was to put the patients on very strict diets where sugar intake was kept to a minimum. At best, this treatment could buy patients a few extra years, but it never saved them. In some cases, the **harsh** diets even caused patients to die of starvation.

During the nineteenth century, observations of patients who died of diabetes often showed that the pancreas was damaged. In 1869, a German medical student, Paul Langerhans, found that within the pancreatic tissue that produces digestive juices, there were clusters of cells whose function was unknown. Some of these cells were eventually shown to be insulin-producing beta cells. Later, in honor of the person who discovered them, the cell clusters were named the islets of Langerhans.

In 1889 in Germany, physiologist Oskar Minkowski and physician Joseph von Mering showed that if the pancreas was removed from a dog, the animal got diabetes. But if the duct through which the pancreatic juices flow to the intestine was **ligated**—surgically tied off so the juices couldn't reach the intestine - the dog developed minor digestive problems but no diabetes. So, it seemed that the pancreas must have at least two functions:

- to produce digestive juices;
- to produce a substance that regulates the sugar glucose.

This hypothetical internal secretion was the key. If a substance could actually be **isolated**, the mystery of **diabetes** would be solved. Progress, however, was slow.

In 1920, an unknown Canadian surgeon named Frederick Banting approached Professor John Macleod, the head of the University of Toronto's **physiology** department, with an idea about finding that secret. He theorized that the pancreatic digestive juices could be harmful to the secretion of the pancreas produced by the islets of Langerhans. He therefore wanted to ligate the pancreatic ducts in order to stop the flow of **nourishment** to the pancreas. This would cause the pancreas to **degenerate**, making it shrink and lose its ability to secrete the **digestive** juices. The cells thought to produce an antidiabetic secretion could then be extracted from the pancreas without being harmed. Unfortunately, Macleod, a leading figure in the study of diabetes in Canada, didn't think much of Banting's theories and rebuffed his suggestion. Despite this, Banting managed to convince Macleod that his idea was worth trying. Macleod gave Banting a laboratory with a minimum of equipment and ten dogs. Banting also got an assistant, a medical student by the name of Charles Best. The experiment was set to start in the summer of 1921.

Banting and Best began their experiments by removing the pancreas from a dog. This resulted in the following:

- Its blood sugar rose.

- It became thirsty, drank lots of water, and urinated more often.
- It became weaker and weaker.

The Dog Had Developed Diabetes

Experimenting on another dog, Banting and Best surgically ligated the pancreas, stopping the flow of nourishment, so that the pancreas degenerated. After a while, they removed the pancreas, sliced it up, and froze the pieces in a mixture of water and salts. When the pieces were half-frozen, they were ground up and filtered. The isolated substance was named "isletin".

The **extract** was injected into the diabetic dog. Its blood glucose level dropped, and it seemed healthier and stronger. By giving the diabetic dog a few injections a day, Banting and Best could keep it healthy and free of symptoms. Banting and Best showed their result to Macleod, who was impressed, but he wanted more tests to prove that their pancreatic extract really worked. For the increased testing, Banting and Best realized that they required a larger supply of organs than their dogs could provide, and they started using pancreases from cattle. With this new source, they managed to produce enough extract to keep several diabetic dogs alive. The new results convinced Macleod that they were onto something big. He gave them more funds and moved them to a better laboratory with proper working conditions. He also suggested that they should call their extract "insulin." Now, the work proceeded rapidly. In late 1921, a third person, biochemist Bertram Collip, joined the team. Collip was given the task of trying to purify the insulin so that it would be clean enough for testing on humans. During the intensified testing, the team also realized that the process of shrinking the pancreases had been unnecessary. Using whole fresh pancreases from adult animals worked just as well.

In 1922 the insulin was tested on Leonard Thompson, a 14-year-old diabetes patient who lay dying at the Toronto General Hospital. He was given an insulin injection. At first he suffered a severe **allergic** reaction, and further injections were canceled. The scientists worked hard on improving the extract, and then a second dose of injections was administered to Thompson. The results were spectacular. The scientists went to the other wards with diabetic children, most of them **comatose** and dying from diabetic **ketoacidosis**. They reacted just as positively as Leonard to the insulin extract.

Banting and Macleod were awarded the Nobel Prize in 1923 for the practical extraction of insulin. They were incensed that the other members of their team were not included, and they immediately shared their prize money with Best and Collip. They sold the original **patent** to the University of Toronto for one half-dollar. They were not looking for fame or fortune; they wanted to keep sick children from dying. They did eventually benefit financially, but that was the last thing on their minds.

Very soon after the discovery of insulin, the medical firm Eli Lilly started large-scale production of the extract. As early as 1923, the firm was producing enough insulin to supply the entire North American continent. Although insulin doesn't **cure** diabetes, it's one of the biggest discoveries in medicine. When it came, it was like a miracle. People with severe diabetes and only days left to live were saved. And as long as they kept getting their insulin, they could live an almost normal life.

Working with Human Insulin

In 1982, the Eli Lilly Corporation produced human insulin (Humulin®) that became the first approved genetically engineered pharmaceutical product. This important achievement was the result of a vast network of basic and applied scientific advances that began in the 1950s with the classic structural studies on DNA by Watson and Crick and on insulin by Sanger.[1] Without needing to depend on animals, researchers could produce genetically engineered insulin in unlimited supplies. It also did not contain any of the animal contaminants. Using human insulin also took away any concerns about transferring any potential animal diseases into the insulin. While companies still sell a small amount of insulin produced from animals—mostly **porcine**—from the 1980s onwards, insulin users increasingly moved to a form of human insulin created through recombinant DNA technology.

Insulin is a protein consisting of two separate chains of amino acids, an A above a B chain, that are held together by disulfide bonds. The insulin A chain consists of 21 amino acids, and the B chain has 30. Before becoming an active insulin protein, insulin is first produced as **preproinsulin**. This is one single long protein chain with the A and B chains not yet separated, a section in the middle linking the chains together, and a signal sequence at one end telling the protein when to start secreting outside the cell. After preproinsulin, the chain evolves into **proinsulin**, still a single chain but without the signaling sequence. Then comes the active protein insulin, the protein without the section linking the A and B chains. At each step, the protein needs specific enzymes to produce the next form of insulin.

Lilly has prepared human insulin by two different means—initially, by a chain combination procedure and, since 1986, by transforming human proinsulin into human insulin. In the first method, the two insulin chains are produced separately. Manufacturers need the two mini-genes: one that produces the A chain and one for the B chain. Since the exact DNA sequence of each chain is known, they synthesize each mini-gene's DNA and insert them into **plasmids**. The **recombinant**, newly formed, plasmids are then transformed into bacterial cells. During a fermentation process, the millions of bacteria harboring the recombinant plasmid replicate roughly every 20 minutes through cell division, and each expresses the insulin gene.[2] After multiplying, the cells are taken out of the fermentation tanks and broken open to extract the protein chains. The two chains are then mixed together and joined by disulfide bonds through the reduction-reoxidation reaction. Although the chain combination procedure worked quite well, the proinsulin approach required fewer processing steps and, consequently, superseded the chain method in 1986. The sequence that **codes** for proinsulin is inserted into the non-**pathogenic** *E. coli* bacteria. The bacteria go through the fermentation process where they reproduce and produce proinsulin. Then the connecting sequence between the A and B chains is **spliced** away with an enzyme, and the resulting insulin is purified.

The Future

The future of insulin holds many possibilities. Since insulin was first synthesized, diabetics needed to regularly inject the liquid insulin with a **syringe** directly into their bloodstream. This allows the insulin to enter the blood immediately. For many years it was the only way known to move the intact insulin protein into the body. In the 1990s, researchers began to make inroads in synthesizing various devices and forms of insulin that diabetics can use in an alternate drug delivery system.

Manufacturers are currently producing several relatively new drug delivery devices. An insulin pen looks like a writing pen. A **cartridge** holds the insulin, and the tip is the needle. The user sets a dose, inserts the needle into the skin, and presses a button to inject the insulin. With pens, there is no need to use a vial of insulin. However, pens require inserting separate tips before each injection. Another downside is that the pen does not allow users to mix insulin types, and not all insulin is available.

The insulin pump allows a controlled release in the body. This is a computerized pump, about the size of a beeper, that diabetics can wear on their belt or in their pocket. The pump has a small flexible tube that is inserted just under the surface of the diabetic's skin. The diabetic sets the pump to deliver a steady, measured dose of insulin throughout the day, increasing the amount right before eating. This mimics the body's normal release of insulin. Manufacturers have produced insulin pumps since the 1980s but advances in the late 1990s and early twenty-first century have made them increasingly easier to use and more popular. Researchers are exploring the possibility of **implantable** insulin pumps. Diabetics would control these devices through an external remote control.

Researchers are exploring other drug-delivery options. Ingesting insulin through pills is one possibility. The challenge with edible insulin is that the stomach's high acidic environment destroys the protein before it can move into the blood. Researchers are working on coating insulin with special materials that would protect the drugs from the stomach's acid.

In 2001 promising tests are occurring on inhaled insulin devices, and manufacturers could begin producing the products within the next few years. Since insulin is a relatively large protein, it does not **permeate** into the lungs. Researchers of inhaled insulin are working to create insulin particles that are small enough to reach the deep lung. The particles can then pass into the bloodstream. Researchers are testing several inhalation devices much like that of an asthma inhaler.

Insulin **patches** are another drug delivery system in development. Patches would release insulin continuously into the bloodstream. The challenge is finding a way to have insulin pass through the skin. **Ultrasound** is one method researchers are investigating. These low frequency sound waves could change the skin's **permeability** and allow insulin to pass.

Other research has the potential to discontinue the need for manufacturers to synthesize insulin. Researchers are working on creating the cells that produce insulin in the laboratory. The thought is that physicians can someday replace the non-working pancreatic cells with insulin-producing cells. Another hope for diabetics is gene therapy. Scientists are working on correcting the insulin gene's mutation so that diabetics would be able to produce insulin on their own.

Word Study

1. allergic [ə'lɜːdʒɪk] *adj.* 过敏的
2. blur [blɜː(r)] *v.* 弄脏,使……模糊
3. bruise [bruːz] *n.* 淤青,擦伤; *v.* 碰伤,擦伤,挫伤
4. cartridge ['kɑːtrɪdʒ] *n.* 笔芯
5. code [kəʊd] *n.* 密码; *v.* 把……编码
6. comatose ['kəʊmətəʊs] *adj.* 昏睡状态的,昏迷的
7. cure [kjʊə(r)] *n.* 治疗,治愈,疗法; *v.* 治愈
8. degenerate [dɪ'dʒenəreɪt] *v.* 退化
9. diabetes [ˌdaɪə'biːtiːz] *n.* 糖尿病
10. digestive [daɪ'dʒestɪv] *adj.* 消化的
11. extract ['ekstrækt] *n.* 榨出物,浓缩物,提取物; [ɪk'strækt] *v.* 拔出,榨出,提取
12. fatigue [fə'tiːg] *n.* 疲劳,疲乏
13. harsh [hɑːʃ] *adj.* 粗糙的,严厉的,严酷的,刺耳的
14. implantable [ɪm'plɑːntəbl] *adj.* 可移植的,可植入的
15. insatiable [ɪn'seɪʃəbl] *adj.* 不知足的,贪得无厌的

16. islet ['aɪlət] *n.* 小岛

17. islets of Langerhans 胰岛（又称"朗格尔汉斯岛"）

18. isolate ['aɪsəleɪt] *v.* 分离

19. ketoacidosis ['ketəʊæsɪ'dəʊsɪs] *n.* 酮酸中毒

20. ketone ['kiːtəʊn] *n.* 酮

21. ligate [lɪ'geɪt] *v.* 绑，扎；连接

22. nourishment ['nʌrɪʃmənt] *n.* 营养

23. numbness [nʌmnəs] *n.* 麻木

24. obese [əʊ'biːs] *adj.* 肥胖的

25. pancreas ['pæŋkriəs] *n.* 胰腺

26. patch [pætʃ] *n.* 贴剂

27. patent ['pætnt] *n.* 专利，特许

28. pathogenic ['pæθə'dʒenɪk] *adj.* 致病的

29. permeability [ˌpɜːmiə'bɪləti] *n.* 弥漫，渗透

30. permeate ['pɜːmieɪt] *v.* 弥漫，渗透

31. physiology [ˌfɪzi'ɒlədʒi] *n.* 生理学

32. plasmid ['plæzmɪd] *n.* 质粒

33. porcine ['pɔːsaɪn] *adj.* 猪的

34. preproinsulin [priːprəʊ'ɪnsjʊlɪn] *n.* 前胰岛素原

35. proinsulin [prəʊ'ɪnsjʊlɪn] *n.* 胰岛素原

36. recombinant [rɪ'kɒmbɪnənt] *n.* 重组体，重组子；*adj.*（基因）重组的

37. splice [splaɪs] *v.* 拼接，剪接

38. symptom ['sɪmptəm] *n.* 症状

39. syringe [sɪ'rɪndʒ] *n.* 注射器

40. tingling [tɪŋɡlɪŋ] *n.* 刺痛感

41. ultrasound ['ʌltrəsaʊnd] *n.* 超声

Notes

1. This important achievement was the result of a vast network of basic and applied scientific advances that began in the 1950s with the classic structural studies on DNA by Watson and Crick and on insulin by Sanger. 译为：这一重要成就归功于 20 世纪 50 年代以来在基础和应用科学领域取得的一系列研究成果，其中包括沃森和克里克对 DNA 的结构研究和桑格对胰岛素结构的研究。"that began in the 1950s"为修饰"advances"的定语从句。"classic structural studies on...by...and on...by..."包含两个并列的结构。

2. During a fermentation process, the millions of bacteria harboring the recombinant plasmid replicate roughly every 20 minutes through cell division, and each expresses the insulin gene. 译为：在发酵过程中，数以百万计的携带重组质粒的细菌几乎每 20 分钟就会通过细胞分裂增殖一代，每一个细菌细胞都会表达胰岛素基因。"harboring the recombinant plasmid"为"bacteria"的后置定语。"each expresses..."中的 each 指的是前面提到的"millions of bacteria"。

Supplementary Parts

1. Medical and Pharmaceutical Terminology (3): Common Morphemes in English Terms for Biology and Biochemistry

Morpheme	Meaning	Example
acet	醋酸,乙酸,醋	acetone　丙酮
aden	腺	adenosine　腺苷
allo-	异	allopurinol　别嘌呤醇
andr	雄	androgen　雄性激素
angul	角	triangular　三角(形的)
anthrop	人	anthropometry　人体测量学
arachid	花生	arachidonic acid　花生四烯酸
aspar	天冬	asparagine　天冬酰胺
bio	生物,生命	biology　生物学
chol	胆	cholecalciferol　胆钙化醇
cinchon	金鸡纳	cinchona　金鸡纳树(皮)
clon	克隆	monoclonal　单克隆的,单细胞系的
corn	角	cornification　角(质)化
cyt	细胞	cytochrome　细胞色素
de-	脱,使……失去	denaturation　变性
dem	人	demography　人口学,人口统计学
endo-	内	endopeptidase　内肽酶
estr	雌	estrogen　雌激素
exo-	外	exopeptidase　外肽酶
fem	雌	female　女性的,雌性的
gamet	配子	gametocide　杀配子剂
gen	基因	genome　染色体基因,基因组
gluc	甘,葡萄糖	glucokinase　葡糖激酶
glyc	甘,甜	glycolysis　糖酵解
gon	角	goniometer　测角仪,测角计,测角器
heter	异	heteroduplex　异源双链体,异源双链
hydro	水	hydrolase　水解酶类
iso-	异构	isomerase　异构酶类
kerat	角	keratin　角蛋白
ket	酮	ketogenic amino acid　生酮氨基酸
kin	动	kinase　激酶
lact	乳	lactate　乳酸盐
lino	亚麻	linolenate　亚麻酸
lipo	脂肪	lipoprotein　脂蛋白
mal	苹果	malate　苹果酸
malt	麦芽	maltase　麦芽糖酶
mono	单	monooxygenase　单加氧酶
mort	死	mortality　死亡率
necr	死	necrology　死亡统计学,死亡通知

Morpheme	Meaning	Example
ped	儿童	pediatrics　儿科学
pent	戊	pentose　戊糖
pept	肽	peptidyl site　肽酰位
phosph	磷	phospholipase　磷脂酶
phyll	叶	chlorophyll　叶绿素
phyt	植物	phytosterol　植物固醇
poly	多	polypeptide　多肽
pyridox	吡哆	pyridoxamine　吡哆胺
pyruv	丙酮酸	pyruvate kinase　丙酮酸激酶
rib	核	riboflavin　核黄素（维生素 B_2）
spor	孢子	sporicide　杀孢子剂
tel	末端	telomerase　端粒酶
term	终端	terminator　终止子
thym	胸腺	thymine (T)　胸腺嘧啶
trans	转	transaldolase　转醛醇酶
ur	尿	uracil (U)　尿嘧啶
vit	生命	vital　生命的,生机的
vivi	生命	vivisect　活体解剖
zyg	合子	zygote　合子
zym	酶	zymogen　酶原

(1) Decompose the following words and translate them into Chinese.

1) aminopeptidase　_____

2) amyloid　_____

3) argininemia　_____

4) fructokinase　_____

5) gelatinous　_____

6) glutamine　_____

7) histidinuria　_____

8) mannitol　_____

9) nucleoprotein　_____

10) proteinuria　_____

11) steatosis　_____

12) tyrosinosis　_____

(2) Fill in the blanks with the missing word root, prefix or suffix.

1) _____ometry　人体测量学

2) _____purinol　别嘌呤醇

3) mono_____al　单克隆的,单细胞系的

4) _____ogen　雌激素

5) _____lysis　糖酵解

6) _____merase　异构酶类

7) _____protein　脂蛋白

8) _____iatrics　儿科学

9) chloro_____　叶绿素

10) _____peptide　多肽

11) _____aldolase　转醛醇酶

12) _____gen　酶原

2. English-Chinese Translation Skills: 药学英语语篇特点与翻译

　　药学英语语篇是关于药学以及相关学科的文献,这就决定了药学英语语篇区别于其他类型的语篇,具有不同的语言功能、语言特点和表达方式,以及在传播中构建的作者与读者之间的人际关系。根据系统功能语言学的情景语境理论,药学英语语篇有三个变量,即语场(field)、语旨(tenor)和语式(mode)。简单来说,语场是指语篇话题(subject matter)、内容以及场地(setting)等情境因素;语旨是指交际双方的社会角色;语式是指语言活动所采用的媒介(medium)或渠道(channel)。这三个变量相互影响,构成一个整体。翻译药学英语语篇时,要首先了解语篇作者是在讨论某个具体内容时如何选择语言表达方式,要构建何种读者和作者之间关系。这样才能够准确判断原文的交际意图、正式程度、交际对象和交际重点等,做到翻译得体。如下文所示。

　　例: The Structure of DNA Allows for Its Repair and Replication with Near-Perfect Fidelity

　　The capacity of living cells to preserve their genetic material and to duplicate it for the next generation results from the structural complementarity between the two halves of the DNA molecule. The basic unit of DNA is a linear polymer of four different monomeric subunits, deoxyribonucleotides, arranged in a precise linear sequence. It is this linear sequence that encodes the genetic information. Two of these polymeric strands are twisted with each other to form the DNA double helix, where each monomeric subunit in one strand pairs specifically with the complementary subunit in the opposite strand. In the enzymatic replication or repair of DNA, one of the two strands serves as a template for the assembly of another, structurally complementary DNA strand. Before a cell divides, the two DNA strands separate and each serves as a template for the synthesis of a complementary strand, generating two identical double-helical molecules, one for each daughter cell. If one strand is damaged, continuity of information is assured by the information present on the other strand.

　　翻译前仔细分析该语篇,可以发现该段是关于 DNA 结构的自身修复和复制的内容。从语篇的语场来看,该段文字语言规范,结构严谨,专业性词汇密度高,属于专业性较强的学术文献;从语篇的语旨来看,该段文字作者以客观、科学的方式介绍研究信息或主要观点,属于同行之间的学术交流,本着尊重科学的严谨态度,没有刻意构建轻松愉快的作者 - 读者关系,从语篇的语式来看,该段文字采用书面语的形式,句式规范,逻辑性强,在实际应用的过程中应该还配有其他模态,比如图片、模型、PPT 等。翻译前对语篇进行分析对正确翻译原文、确定翻译风格具有重要意义。

　　参考译文: DNA 的结构允许其以几近完美精准度的方式进行自身修复和复制。

　　活细胞保持其遗传物质和为下一代复制的能力来源于 DNA 分子两条单链之间的结构互补性。DNA 的基本单位是由四种不同脱氧核糖核苷酸单体亚单位精密排列成的线性序列。正是这种线性序列能够编码遗传信息。两条聚合 DNA 单链互相缠绕而形成 DNA 双螺旋结构,在这里一条链上每一个单体亚基都能在另一条链中找到其特定的互补的亚基。在 DNA 的酶复制或修复过程中,两条链中一条充当另一条的装配模板,即结构互补 DNA 链。在细胞分裂前,两条 DNA 链分离,每个 DNA 分子作为模板用以合成另一条互补链,生成两个相同的双螺旋分子,一个子细胞含有一个双螺旋分子。如果一条链被破坏了,遗传信息的连续性可以确保由另一条链得以呈现。

　　从参考译文可以看出,译文真实反映了原文作者传递的信息内容,译文语言规范,结构严谨,专业词汇使用正确。阅读译文可以感受到原文作者与读者的沟通是建立在具有共同学科知识基础上,作者在介绍专业信息的同时希望读者能够理解并做出相应回应,体现出学术交流平等的直接关系。从译文语言媒介来看,语言简洁,句式短小精悍,没有主观性形容词,书面语特征明显,语言风格与原文基本吻合。

　　就语篇体裁而言,药学英语语篇也有多种形式,如医药科普文章、医药广告、药典、药品说明书、医药实验报告、质量标准等,不同的语篇体裁具有不同的语篇特点和语境意义,正确分析并理解不同语篇体裁是做好药学英语翻译的重要前提之一。

（欧田苗　唐　漫　陈　菁　史志祥　龚长华）

Unit Four

Pharmacology

Pharmacology is concerned with all facets of the interaction of chemicals with biological systems. When such interactions are applied to the cure or amelioration of disease, the chemicals are usually called drugs.

Most drugs produce effects by combining with biological receptors. The chemical bonds that form between drug molecule and receptor are usually reversible. The ease with which drug and receptor interact is influenced by the degree of complementarity of their respective three-dimensional structures. For this reason, minor chemical modification of a drug may produce profound changes in its pharmacological activity.

Pharmacology is a hybrid science. It freely draws upon the intellectual resources of all the basic medical sciences and contributes to every aspect of clinical medicine. Today receptor theory serves as a unifying concept for the explanation of the effects of chemicals on biological systems, whether these chemicals be of exogenous (pharmacological) or endogenous (physiological) origin. In general, a drug produces a particular effect by combining chemically with some specific molecular constituent (receptor) of the biological system upon which it acts. The function of the receptor molecule in the biological system is thereby modified to produce a measurable effect.

药理学是全面研究化学物质与生物系统之间相互作用的一门学科。当这些相互作用被用于治疗或减轻疾病症状时,这些化学物质即称为药物。

大多数药物通过与生物受体相结合而产生药效。药物分子与受体之间的化学偶联作用往往是可逆的。药物与受体相互作用易受它们各自的三维结构的互补程度影响。因此,即使是细微的化学修饰也可能引起药物药理学活性的重大改变。

药理学是一门交叉科学,它最大限度地综合了各个基础医学科学的知识资源,并且有助于临床医学的每一方面。当今,受体理论作为一个共识的概念,用于解释化学物质对生物系统的作用,无论这些化学物质是外源性的(药理的)还是内源性的(生理的)来源。总之,药物通过与其作用(影响)的生物系统的某些特定分子成分(受体)的化学结合而产生特定的作用,从而使生物系统中受体分子的功能改变而产生明显的作用。

Text A
The Scope of Pharmacology

In its **entirety**, pharmacology **embraces** the knowledge of the history, source, physical and chemical properties, compounding, biochemical and physiological effects, mechanisms of action, absorption, distribution, metabolism and **excretion**, and therapeutic and other uses of drugs. Since a drug is broadly defined as any chemical agent that affects living processes, the subject of pharmacology is obviously quite extensive.

For the physician and the medical student, however, the scope of pharmacology is less expansive than indicated by the above definitions. The clinician is interested primarily in drugs that are useful in the prevention, diagnosis, and treatment of human disease, or in the prevention of pregnancy. His study of the pharmacology of these drugs can be reasonably limited to those aspects that provide the basis for their rational clinical use. Secondarily, the physician is also concerned with chemical agents that are not used in therapy but are commonly responsible for household and industrial poisoning as well as environmental pollution. His study of these substances is justifiably restricted to the general principles of prevention, recognition, and treatment of such toxicity or pollution. Finally, all physicians share in the responsibility to help resolve the continuing sociological problem of the abuse of drugs.

A brief consideration of its major subject areas will further clarify how the study of pharmacology is best approached from the standpoint of the specific requirements and interests of the medical students and practitioners. At one time, it was essential for the physician to have a broad botanical knowledge, since he had to select the proper plants from which to prepare his own crude medicinal preparations. However, fewer drugs are now obtained from natural sources, and, more importantly, most of these are highly purified or standardized and differ little from synthetic chemicals. Hence, the interests of the clinician in pharmacognosy are correspondingly limited. Nevertheless, scientific curiosity should stimulate the physician to learn something about the sources of drugs, and this knowledge often proves practically useful as well as interesting. He will find the history of drugs of similar value.

The preparing, compounding, and dispensing of medicines at one time lay within the province of the physician, but this work is now delegated almost completely to the pharmacist.[1] However, to write intelligent prescription orders, the physician must have some knowledge of the physical and chemical properties of drugs and their available dosage forms, and he must have a basic familiarity with the practice of pharmacy. When the physician shirks his responsibility in this regard, he invariably fails to translate his knowledge of pharmacology and medicine into prescription orders and medication best suited for the individual patient.

Pharmacokinetics deals with the absorption, distribution, metabolism, and excretion of drugs. These factors, coupled with dosage, determine the concentration of a drug at its sites of action and, hence, the intensity of its effects as a function of time. Many basic principles of biochemistry and enzymology and the physical and chemical principles that govern the active and passive transfer and the distribution of substances across biological membranes are readily applied to the understanding of this important aspect of pharmacology.[2]

The study of the biochemical and physiological effects of drugs and their mechanisms of action is termed as pharmacodynamics. It is an experimental medical science that dates back only to the later half of the nineteenth century. As a border science, pharmacodynamics borrows freely from both the subject matter and the experimental techniques of physiology, biochemistry, microbiology, immunology, genetics, and pathology. It is unique mainly in that attention is focused on the characteristics of drugs. As the name implies, the subject is a dynamic one. The student who attempts merely to memorize the pharmacodynamic properties of drugs is foregoing one of the best opportunities for correlating the entire field of preclinical medicine. For example, the actions and effects of the saluretic agents can be fully understood only in terms of the basic principles of renal physiology and of the pathogenesis of edema. Conversely, no greater insight into normal and abnormal renal physiology can be gained than by the study of the pharmacodynamics of the saluretic agents.

Another **ramification** of pharmacodynamics is the correlation of the actions and effects of drugs with their chemical structures. Such structure-activity relationships are an **integral** link in the analysis of drug action, and **exploitation** of these relationships among established therapeutic agents has often led to the development of better drugs. However, the correlation of biological activity with chemical structure is usually of interest to the physician only when it provides the basis for summarizing other pharmacological information.

The physician is understandably interested mainly in the effects of drugs in man. This emphasis on clinical pharmacology is justified, since the effects of drugs are often characterized by significant **interspecies** variation, and since they may be further modified by disease. In addition, some drug effects, such as those on mood and behavior, can be adequately studied only in man. However, the pharmacological evaluation of drugs in man may be limited for technical, legal, and **ethical** reasons, and the choice of drugs must be based in part on their pharmacological evaluation in animals. Consequently, some knowledge of animal pharmacology and comparative pharmacology is helpful in deciding the extent to which claims for a drug based upon studies in animals can be reasonably **extrapolated** to man.[3]

Pharmacotherapeutics deals with the use of drugs in the prevention and treatment of disease. Many drugs stimulate or depress biochemical or physiological function in man in a sufficiently **reproducible** manner to provide relief of symptoms or, ideally, to alter favorably the course of disease. Conversely, **chemotherapeutic** agents are useful in therapy because they have only minimal effects on man but can destroy or eliminate **parasites**. Whether a drug is useful for therapy is crucially dependent upon its ability to produce its desired effects with only tolerable undesired effects. Thus, from the standpoint of the physician interested in the therapeutic uses of a drug, the **selectivity** of its effects is one of its most important characteristics. Drug therapy is rationally based upon the correlation of the actions and effects of drugs with the physiological, biochemical, microbiological, **immunological**, and **behavioral** aspects of disease. Pharmacodynamics provides one of the best opportunities for this correlation during the study of both the preclinical and the clinical medical sciences.

Toxicology is the aspect of pharmacology that deals with the adverse effects of drugs. It is concerned not only with drugs used in therapy but also with the many other chemicals that may be responsible for household, environmental, or industrial **intoxication**. The adverse effects of the pharmacological agents employed in therapy are properly considered an integral part of their total pharmacology. The toxic effects of other chemicals are such an extensive subject that the physician must usually confine his attention to the general principles applicable to the prevention, recognition, and treatment of drug poisonings of any cause.

Word Study

1. approach [ə'prəʊtʃ] *vt.*（着手）探讨/处理,（开始）对付
2. behavioral [bɪ'heɪvjərəl] *adj.* 关于行为的,关于态度的
3. botanical [bə'tænɪkl] *adj.* 植物的,植物学的; *n.* 植物性药材
4. chemotherapeutic [ˌkeməʊˌθerə'pju:tɪk] *adj.* 化学治疗的; *n.* 化学治疗剂
5. clinician [klɪ'nɪʃn] *n.* 临床医生
6. conversely [kən'vɜ:sli] *adj.* 相反的,逆的,颠倒的
7. delegate ['delɪɡeɪt] *v.* 授权,把……委托给; *n.* 代表
8. diagnosis [ˌdaɪəɡ'nəʊsɪs] *n.* 诊断（法）
9. edema [ɪ'di:mə] *n.* 浮肿,水肿

10. embrace [ɪmˈbreɪs] *vt.* 包含，包括

11. entirety [ɪnˈtaɪərəti] *n.* 全部，整体

12. ethical [ˈeθɪkl] *adj.* 伦理的，道德的，（药品）合乎规格的，凭处方出售的

13. excretion [ɪkˈskriːʃn] *n.* 排泄（物），分泌（物）

14. exploitation [ˌeksplɔɪˈteɪʃn] *n.* 利用，开发，剥削

15. extrapolate [ɪkˈstræpəleɪt] *v.* 推断，推知；extrapolate to 推广到……

16. genetics [dʒəˈnetɪks] *n.* 遗传学

17. immunological [ˌɪmjunəˈlɒdʒɪkl] *adj.* 免疫的，免疫学的

18. integral [ˈɪntɪɡrəl] *adj.* 完整的，整体的，组成的

19. interspecies [ɪntəˈspiːʃiːz]] *n.* 种类之间，种间

20. intoxication [ɪnˌtɒksɪˈkeɪʃn] *n.* 中毒，醉酒

21. invariably [ɪnˈveəriəbli] *adv.* 不变地，永恒地；总是

22. justifiably [dʒʌstɪˈfaɪəbli] *adv.* 正当地，有理地，情有可原地

23. parasite [ˈpærəsaɪt] *n.* 寄生生物

24. pathology [pəˈθɒlədʒi] *n.* 病理学，病理，病状

25. pharmacognosy [ˌfɑːməˈkɒgnəsɪ] *n.* 生药学，药材学

26. pharmacotherapeutics [fɑːməkʌθerəpˈjuːtɪks] *n.* 药物治疗学，药物疗法

27. practitioner [prækˈtɪʃənə(r)] *n.* 从业者（尤指医生、律师等），职业医生，开业者

28. preclinical [priːˈklɪnɪkəl] *adj.* 临床用以前的，临床前的

29. pregnancy [ˈpregnənsi] *n.* 怀孕，怀胎，怀孕期

30. province [ˈprɒvɪns] *n.* 范围，领域，分科

31. ramification [ˌræmɪfɪˈkeɪʃn] *n.* 分枝，细节，分歧

32. renal [ˈriːnl] *adj.* 肾（脏）的

33. reproducible [ˌriːprəˈdjuːsəbl] *adj.* 能再现的，能再复制的，能再生产的，能繁殖的

34. saluretic [səluˈretɪk] *adj.*（促）尿食盐排泄的；*n.*（促）尿食盐排泄剂

35. selectivity [səˌlekˈtɪvəti] *n.* 选择，精选，选择性

36. shirk [ʃɜːk] *v.* 逃避（义务、责任等），推掉

Notes

1. The preparing, compounding, and dispensing of medicines at one time lay within the province of the physician, but this work is now delegated almost completely to the pharmacist. 译为：药物的制备、合成与配制一度属于医生的职责，但这项工作现在几乎完全委托给药剂师。"lay within the province of"：属于……的职责范围之内。

2. Many basic principles of biochemistry and enzymology and the physical and chemical principles that govern the active and passive transfer and the distribution of substances across biological membranes are readily applied to the understanding of this important aspect of pharmacology. 译为：生物化学和酶学方面的许多基本原理以及控制物质在生物膜之间主动转运、被动转运及分布的一些物理和化学原理，可以用来帮助我们理解药理学中这一重要部分。

3. Consequently, some knowledge of animal pharmacology and comparative pharmacology is helpful in deciding the extent to which claims for a drug based upon studies in animals can be reasonably extrapolated to man. 译为：因此，掌握一些动物药理学和比较药理学方面的知识有助于确定针对以动物实验为基础研制的某种药物的想法可在多大程度上合理地外推到人体。

Exercises

1.   Decide whether each of the following statements is true (T) or false (F) according to the passage.

(1) Pharmacodynamics, which is concerned with the study of the biochemical and physiological effects of drugs and their mechanisms of action, is an experimental medical science.

(2) It's unreasonable for a physician to be interested mainly in the effects of drugs on human beings, for the pharmacological evaluation of drugs in them may be limited due to technical, legal, and ethical reasons.

(3) As the effects of drugs are often characterized by significant interspecies variation and may be further modified by disease, clinical pharmacology has never been emphasized.

(4) The physician is not interested in drugs that are useful in the prevention, diagnosis, and treatment of human disease, but in chemical agents that are commonly responsible for household and industrial poisoning as well as environmental pollution.

(5) A drug is said to be useful in therapy if it has the ability to produce its desired effects with only tolerable undesired effects.

(6) Toxicology deals not only with drugs used in therapy but also with many other chemicals that may be responsible for household, environmental, or industrial intoxication.

2.   Questions for oral discussion.

(1) How do you understand pharmacology in a broad sense or less expansive sense?

(2) What are the traditional major subject areas in the study of pharmacology from the viewpoint of the specific requirements and interests of medical students and practitioners?

(3) How is pharmacodynamics defined in this passage?

(4) Why is it understandable that the physician is interested mainly in the effects of drugs on human beings?

3.   Choose the best answer to each of the following questions.

(1) Which of the following most comprehensively summarizes the scope of pharmacology?

    A. The effects of drugs on man.

    B. The correlation of biological activity with chemical structure.

    C. The history, source, physical and chemical properties, compounding, biochemical and physiological effects, mechanisms of action, absorption, distribution, metabolism and excretion.

    D. The prevention, recognition, and treatment of drug poisonings.

(2) Which of the following is what a clinician is primarily interested in according to the text?

    A. Drugs which can be reasonably limited to those aspects that provide the basis for their rational clinical use.

    B. Chemical agents that are not used in therapy but are commonly responsible for household and industrial poisoning as well as environmental pollution.

    C. Drugs which are useful in the prevention, diagnosis and treatment of human disease, or in the prevention of pregnancy.

    D. Drugs which help resolve the continuing abuse of drugs.

(3) Why was the physician not interested in pharmacognosy?

    A. He didn't have to select the proper plants for his prescription.

    B. He had a broad botanical knowledge.

    C. No drug was obtained from natural sources.

D. Natural drugs had little difference with synthetic ones.

(4) Which of the following is helpful for studying pharmacology for medical students and practitioners?

A. To have a broad botanical knowledge.

B. To select a plant and its preparation.

C. To have the ability to purify natural plants.

D. To have curiosity that stimulates them to learn about sources of drugs.

(5) What are the tasks related to medicines almost completely delegated to the pharmacists now?

A. The physical and chemical properties of medicines.

B. The preparing, compounding, and dispensing of medicines.

C. Dosage forms of medicines available.

D. The therapeutic and other uses of medicines.

(6) Drug selectivity depends on _____ .

A. pharmacokinetic properties

B. pharmacodynamic properties

C. medicinal chemical properties

D. all of the above

(7) What time of history does pharmacodynamics date back to?

A. The second half of the seventeenth century.

B. The second half of the eighteenth century.

C. The second half of the nineteenth century.

D. The second half of the twentieth century.

(8) What does the research on pharmacodynamics focus on?

A. Study of clinical effects of drugs.

B. Study of the process of drugs in the body.

C. Study of the effect and the mechanism of drugs on the body.

D. Study of the correlation of the actions and effects of drugs with their chemical structure.

(9) In the preclinical study, which of the following is true when drugs are selected?

A. It has to be based in part on legal reasons.

B. It has to be based in part on ethical reasons.

C. It has to be based in part on the pharmacological evaluation in man.

D. It has to be based in part on the pharmacological evaluation in animals.

(10) Why are chemotherapeutic agents useful in therapy?

A. They stimulate or depress biochemical or physiological function in man in a sufficiently reproducible manner to provide relief of symptoms or, ideally, to alter favorably the course of disease.

B. They can produce desired effects with only tolerable undesired effects.

C. They may have some side effects on man which are tolerable but can destroy or eliminate parasites.

D. The selectivity of their effects is one of their most important characteristics.

4. Fill in each of the following blanks with an appropriate word or expression according to the meaning of the sentence(s).

(1) The clinician is interested primarily in drugs that are useful in the prevention, _____ and treatment of human disease, or in the prevention of pregnancy.

(2) A brief consideration of its major subject areas will further clarify how the study of pharmacology is

best approached from the standpoint of the specific requirements and interests of the medical students and _____.

(3) _____ deals with the absorption, distribution, metabolism , and excretion of drugs.

(4) _____ is an experimental medical science that dates back only to the second half of the nineteenth century.

(5) Pharmacodynamics borrows freely from both the subject matter and the experimental techniques of physiology, biochemistry,_____, immunology, genetics and pathology.

(6) Another _____ of pharmacodynamics is the correlation of the actions and effects of drugs with their chemical structures.

(7) _____ deals with the use of drugs in the prevention and treatment of disease.

(8) Drug therapy is rationally based upon the correlation of the actions and effects of drugs with the physiological, biochemical, microbiological, _____, and behavioral aspects of disease.

(9) It is concerned not only with drugs used in therapy but also with many other chemicals that may be responsible for household, environmental, or industrial _____.

(10) Chemotherapeutic agents are useful in therapy because they have only minimal effects on man but can destroy or eliminate _____.

5. Translate the following sentences and paragraphs into Chinese.

(1) Such structure-activity relationships are an integral link in the analysis of drug action, and exploitation of these relationships among established therapeutic agents has often led to the development of better drugs.

(2) The student who attempts merely to memorize the pharmacodynamic properties of drugs is foregoing one of the best opportunities for correlating the entire field of preclinical medicine.

(3) However, the pharmacological evaluation of drugs in man may be limited for technical, legal, and ethical reasons, and the choice of drugs must be based in part on their pharmacological evaluation in animals.

(4) At one time, it was essential for the physician to have a broad botanical knowledge, since he had to select the proper plants from which to prepare his own crude medicinal preparations.

(5) Since a drug is broadly defined as any chemical agent that affects living processes, the subject of pharmacology is obviously quite extensive.

(6) Pharmacokinetics deals with the absorption, distribution, metabolism, and excretion of drugs. These factors, coupled with dosage, determine the concentration of a drug at its sites of action and, hence, the intensity of its effects as a function of time. Many basic principles of biochemistry and enzymology and the physical and chemical principles that govern the active and passive transfer and the distribution of substances across biological membranes are readily applied to the understanding of this important aspect of pharmacology.

(7) The study of the biochemical and physiological effects of drugs and their mechanisms of action is termed as pharmacodynamics. It is an experimental medical science that dates back only to the later half of the nineteenth century. As a border science, pharmacodynamics borrows freely from both the subject matter and the experimental techniques of physiology, biochemistry, microbiology, immunology, genetics, and pathology. It is unique mainly in that attention is focused on the characteristics of drugs. As the name implies, the subject is a dynamic one. The student who attempts merely to memorize the pharmacodynamic properties of drugs is foregoing one of the best opportunities for correlating the

entire field of preclinical medicine. For example, the actions and effects of the saluretic agents can be fully understood only in terms of the basic principles of renal physiology and of the pathogenesis of edema. Conversely, no greater insight into normal and abnormal renal physiology can be gained than by the study of the pharmacodynamics of the saluretic agents.

Value-Oriented Reflective Reading

From Heaven to Hell: Heroin's Double-Edged Sword

Opium was placed on this earth to alleviate suffering. A soldier, injured in battle, is given a dose of morphine intramuscularly to reduce the pain of his shattered leg. Or a cancer victim sips a "Brompton's cocktail" (containing mostly heroin) throughout the day to reduce the intense and chronic pain produced by tumors throughout her body. Modern medicine has changed the morphine molecule to produce heroin and codeine (可待因), and has produced synthetic drugs, including hydrocodone (氢可酮), oxycodone (羟考酮), meperidine (哌替啶), and methadone (美沙酮), which the brain interprets as morphine. Chemists have even produced drugs such as fentanyl (芬太尼), a narcotic 1,000 times as potent as morphine. Once consumed, these opiate drugs move from the bloodstream into the brain and bind to receptor sites on specific cells. The brain responds by shutting off its response to pain, reducing anxiety and allowing the recipient to relax and feel peace. Pain relievers that work in this manner are called narcotics. A narcotic does not decrease the response at the site of the injury, but rather fools the brain into thinking that the pain is less.

Pain researchers tell us that the reduction in the brain's perception of pain is an important effect of the narcotic drugs like heroin, but that it is in some ways incidental to (附带于) the true value of narcotics in the management of pain. What seems to be just as important is the ability of narcotics to reduce anxiety, produce a sense of well-being, and even euphoria (兴奋). These effects counteract the crisis of the situation that produced the pain; the soldier rests easier and is less panicked about his battle injury, and the cancer ridden patient is less grief stricken with her slow, painful death.

Human suffering is not limited to these situations, however. Suffering is part of every person's life, from the grief of losing loved ones to the loss of physical health, to the pain of social and political injustice. Every one of us has or will endure (忍受) suffering at some point in our lives. How one responds to this suffering is often the key to a successful life. If we have the tools to move through the suffering, we become stronger and better able to endure the next blow that comes our way. If we lack the tools to endure suffering, either by our genetic nature or by our upbringing, we may wind up susceptible to becoming addicted, especially to a drug like heroin.

A factor that plays a role in the rise of heroin is the growing abuse of prescription painkillers such as oxycodone and hydrocodone. People who become dependent on or misuse these drugs may start looking for a stronger, cheaper high. Heroin is both. But it's also more dangerous. The heroin addict's experience in withdrawal (戒断) is exactly the opposite of the experience of a heroin high. He is filled with pain, anxiety, remorse, and grief. In addition, his heroin habit has seriously crippled his ability to tolerate the normal ups and down so of life. This double-edged sword is the crux of heroin addiction. In using narcotics to fight normal human strife (困难), the addict has lost all of the internal skills needed to manage and fight the creeping return of drug withdrawal.

Detox (戒毒) is usually the first phase of treatment for heroin addiction. During heroin detox, the addict will overcome physical dependence on the drug. Dependence is one of the physical side effects of heroin use. It's associated with cravings and withdrawal. He may be provided with medications, such as clonidine, to ease some symptoms of heroin withdrawal. Some people who are severely addicted to heroin are poor candidates for heroin detox. They have a high risk of relapse during the counseling phase of treatment. For them, maintenance medication can lower the risk of relapse. Maintenance medications such as methadone and buprenorphine ease withdrawal symptoms and cravings caused by heroin. They work in a similar way to heroin, binding to cells in the brain called opioid receptors. These medicines are safer and longer-lasting than heroin. Naltrexone (纳曲酮) blocks those receptors so opioids like heroin don't have any effect. This makes using them less enjoyable.

While taking a maintenance medication, they may attend counseling in order to learn to live without heroin. They can find a job, go to school and form healthy relationships with people who don't use heroin. Once they have a stable history of sobriety from heroin, they can taper off of the maintenance medication.

Questions for oral discussion:

1. How do narcotics relieve pain?
2. Why is heroin a double-edged sword?
3. What measures can be taken to prevent drug addiction?

Text B
Adverse Drug Reactions

Adverse drug reactions are unwanted effects caused by normal therapeutic doses. Drugs are great mimics of diseases, and adverse drug reactions present with diverse clinical signs and symptoms. The classification proposed by Rawlins and Thompson divides reactions into type A and type B.

Type A reactions, which constitute the great majority of adverse drug reactions, are usually a consequence of the drug's main pharmacological effect (e.g. bleeding from **warfarin**) or a low therapeutic index (e.g. nausea from **digoxin**), and they are therefore predictable. They are dose-related and usually mild, although they may be serious or even fatal (e.g. **intracranial** bleeding from warfarin). Such reactions are usually due to incorrect dosage (too much or too long), for the individual patient or to disordered pharmacokinetics, usually impaired drug elimination. The term "side-effects" is often applied to minor type A reactions.

Type B (**idiosyncratic**) reactions are not predictable from the drug's main pharmacological action, are not dose-related and are severe, with a considerable mortality. The underlying **pathophysiology** of type B reactions is poorly if at all understood, and often has a genetic or immunological basis. Type B reactions occur infrequently (1 : 1,000–1 : 10,000 treated subjects being typical).

Three further minor categories of adverse drug reactions have been proposed.

1. Type C—continuous reactions due to long-term drug use (e.g. **neuroleptic**-related **tardive dyskinesia** or **analgesic nephropathy**);

2. Type D—delayed reactions (e.g. alkylating agents leading to **carcinogenesis**, or **retinoid**-associated **teratogenesis**);

3. Type E—end-of-use reactions such as **adrenocortical** insufficiency following **withdrawal**

of **corticosteroids**, or withdrawal **syndromes** following discontinuation of treatment with **clonidine**, **benzodiazepines**, **tricyclic antidepressants** or beta-adrenoreceptor **antagonists**.

There are between 30,000 and 40,000 medicinal products available directly or on prescription in the UK. A recent survey suggested that approximately 80% of adults take some kind of medication during any 2-week period. Exposure to drugs in the population is thus substantial, and the incidence of adverse reactions must be viewed in this context.[1] Type A reactions are believed to be responsible for up to 3% of acute hospital **admissions** and 2%–3% of consultations in general practice[2]. In hospital, clinically significant adverse reactions are estimated to complicate 10%–20% of all admissions, prolonging hospital stay and causing suffering and an **appreciable** number of **fatalities**, as well as wasting resources. They are the most frequent and severe in **neonates**, the elderly, women, patients with **hepatic** or renal disease, and individuals with a history of previous adverse drug reactions. Adverse drug reactions often occur early in therapy (during the first 1–10 days). The drugs most commonly **implicated** are digoxin, antimicrobials, **diuretics**, potassium salt **replacements**, analgesics, **sedatives** and major **tranquilizers**, insulin, aspirin, **glucocorticosteroids**, **antihypertensives** and warfarin.

Factors involved in the etiology of adverse drug reactions can be classified as follows:

1. patient factors

Intrinsic:

Age—neonate, **infant** and elderly

Sex—**hormonal** environment

Genetic abnormalities (e.g. enzyme or receptor **polymorphisms**)

Previous adverse drug reactions, **allergy**, **atopy**

Presence of organ dysfunction- disease

Personality and habits—alcoholic, drug **addict**, **nicotine**, **compliance**

Extrinsic:

Environment—sun

Xenobiotics (e.g. drugs, **herbicides**)

Malnutrition

2. Prescriber factors

Incorrect drug or drug combination

Incorrect route of administration

Incorrect dose

Incorrect duration of therapy

3. Drug factors

Drug-drug interactions

Pharmaceutical—**batch** problems, shelf-life, incorrect dispensing

Adverse Drug Reaction Monitoring/Surveillance Pharmacovigilance

The evaluation of drug safety is complex, and there are many methods for monitoring adverse drug reactions. Each of these has its own advantages and shortcomings, and no single system can offer the absolute security that public opinion expects. The ideal method would identify adverse drug reactions with a high degree of sensitivity and specificity and respond rapidly. It would detect rare but severe adverse drug reactions, but would not be overwhelmed by common ones, the incidence of which would quantify together with predisposing factors.[3] Continued surveillance is **mandatory** after a new drug has been marketed, as it is inevitable that the preliminary testing of medicines in humans during drug development, although excluding many ill effects, cannot identify uncommon adverse effects. A variety of early detection methods have been introduced to identify adverse drug reactions as swiftly as possible.

Phase I/II/III Trials

Early (phase I/II) trials are important for assessing the **tolerability** and dose-response relationship of new therapeutic agents. However, these studies are very insensitive at detecting adverse reactions because they are performed on relatively few subjects (perhaps 200–300). This is illustrated by the failure to detect the serious toxicity of several drugs (e.g. **practolol**, **benoxaprofen**, **temafloxacin**, **felbamate**, **dexfenfluramine** and **fenfluramine**, **troglitazone**) before marketing. However, phase III clinical trials can establish the incidence of common adverse reactions and relate this to therapeutic benefit. Analysis of the reasons given for dropping out of phase III trials is particularly valuable in establishing whether common events such as headache, **constipation**, **lethargy** or male sexual dysfunction are truly drug related. The Medical Research Council Mild Hypertension Study unexpectedly identified **impotence** as being more commonly associated with **thiazide** diuretics than with **placebo** or beta-adrenoreceptor antagonist therapy in this way.

The problem of adverse drug reaction recognition is much greater if the reaction resembles **spontaneous** disease in the population, such that physicians are unlikely to attribute the reaction to drug exposure.[4] The numbers of patients that must be exposed to enable such reactions to be detected are probably greater than those quoted by more than one or two orders of **magnitude**.

Word Study

1. addict ['ædɪkt] *n.* 沉溺,成瘾(者)
2. admission [əd'mɪʃn] *n.* 住院,入院
3. adrenocortical [ə,driːnəʊ'kɔːtɪkəl] *adj.* 肾上腺皮质的
4. allergy ['ælədʒi] *n.* 过敏
5. analgesic [,ænəl'dʒiːzɪk] *n.* 止痛剂,镇痛剂
6. antagonist [æn'tægənɪst] *n.* 拮抗剂
7. antidepressant [,æntɪdɪ'presnt] *n.* 抗抑郁药
8. antihypertensive ['ænti:haɪpə'tensɪv] *n.* 抗高血压药
9. appreciable [ə'priːʃəbl] *adj.* 可感知的,很可观的
10. atopy ['ætəpɪ] *n.* 特异反应性,特应性
11. batch [bætʃ] *n.* 一批,批处理,批次
12. benoxaprofen [benɒk'sæprəfn] *n.* 苯洛芬
13. benzodiazepines [,benzɒdai'æzə,pɪnz] *n.* 苯二氮䓬类药物
14. carcinogenesis [kɑːsɪnəʊ'dʒenɪsɪs] *n.* 癌变
15. clonidine ['klɒnɪdiːn] *n.* 可乐定(一种降压药)
16. compliance [kəm'plaɪəns] *n.* 依从性
17. constipation [,kɒnstɪ'peɪʃən] *n.* 便秘
18. consultation [,kɒnsl'teɪʃn] *n.* 咨询,会诊
19. corticosteroids [,kɔːtɪkəʊs'tɪrɔɪd] *n.* 皮质甾类,皮质类固醇类

20. dexfenfluramine [ˌdeksˈfenflʊərəˌmiːn] *n.* 右芬氟拉明

21. digoxin [daɪˈɡɒksɪn] *n.* 地高辛

22. diuretic [ˌdaɪjuˈretɪk] *n.* 利尿剂

23. dyskinesia [ˌdɪskɪˈniːʒə] *n.* 运动障碍

24. extrinsic [eksˈtrɪnsɪk] *adj.* 外在的

25. fatality [fəˈtæləti] *n.* 死亡, 病死

26. felbamate [ˈfelbəˌmeit] *n.* 非氨酯

27. fenfluramine [fenˈflʊərəmiːn] *n.* 芬氟拉明

28. glucocorticosteroids [ɡˈluːkəʊkɔːtɪkɒstɪrɔɪdz] *n.* 皮质类固醇类, 糖皮质激素类

29. hepatic [hɪˈpætɪk] *adj.* 肝的

30. herbicide [ˈhɜːbɪsaɪd] *n.* 除草剂

31. hormonal [hɔːˈməʊnl] *adj.* 激素的

32. idiosyncratic [ˌɪdiəsɪŋˈkrætɪk] *adj.* 特质的, 特殊的, 异质的

33. implicate [ˈɪmplɪkeɪt] *vt.* 牵涉, 意味着, 暗示

34. impotence [ˈɪmpətəns] *n.* 阳痿

35. infant [ˈɪnfənt] *n.* 婴儿, 幼儿

36. intracranial [ˌɪntrəˈkreɪniəl] *adj.* 头盖内的, 颅内的

37. intrinsic [ɪnˈtrɪnsɪk] *adj.* 内在的

38. lethargy [ˈleθədʒi] *n.* 嗜睡, 倦怠

39. magnitude [ˈmæɡnɪtjuːd] *n.* 大小, 量级

40. malnutrition [ˌmælnjuˈtrɪʃn] *n.* 营养不良

41. mandatory [ˈmændətəri] *adj.* 命令的, 强制性的, 法定的

42. monitor [ˈmɒnɪtə(r)] *v.* 监控, 监测, 监视

43. neonate [ˈniːəʊneɪt] *n.* 新生儿

44. nephropathy [nəˈfrɒpəθɪ] *n.* 肾病

45. neuroleptic [njʊərəˈleptɪk] *n.* 精神抑制药, 安定药

46. nicotine [ˈnɪkətiːn] *n.* 尼古丁

47. pathophysiology [ˈpæθəʊfɪzɪˈɒlədʒɪ] *n.* 病理生理, 病理生理学

48. pharmacovigilance [fɑːməkʌˈvɪdʒɪləns] *n.* 药物警戒

49. placebo [pləˈsiːbəʊ] *n.* 安慰剂

50. polymorphism [ˌpɒlɪˈmɔːfɪzəm] *n.* 多态性, 多形性

51. practolol [ˈpræktəlɒl] *n.* 普拉洛尔

52. replacement [rɪˈpleɪsmənt] *n.* 补充

53. retinoid [ˈretɪnɔɪd] *n.* 类视黄醇

54. sedative [ˈsedətɪv] *n.* 镇静剂

55. spontaneous [spɒnˈteɪniəs] *adj.* 自发的, 本能, 自然产生的

56. surveillance [sɜːˈveɪləns] *n.* 监视, 监督

57. syndrome [ˈsɪndrəʊm] *n.* 症候群, 综合征

58. tardive [ˈtɑːdɪv] *adj.* 迟缓的, 迟发的

59. temafloxacin [ˌteməˈflɒksəsin] *n.* 替马沙星

60. teratogenesis [ˌterətəˈdʒenɪsɪs] *n.* 畸形生长, [胚]畸形发生

61. thiazide [ˈθaɪəzaɪd] *n.* [药]噻嗪化物, 噻嗪类(利尿药)

62. tolerability [tɒlərə'biliti] *n.* 容忍度

63. tranquillizer ['træŋkwəlaɪzə(r)] *n.* 安定剂,镇定剂

64. tricyclic [traɪ'saɪklɪk] *adj.* 三环的

65. troglitazone [trəuglɪ'teɪzəun] *n.* 曲格列酮

66. warfarin ['wɔ:fərɪn] *n.* 华法林,双香豆素(抗凝剂)

67. withdrawal [wɪð'drɔ:əl] *n.* 撤退,退回,取消

68. xenobiotics [zenəbaɪ'ɒtɪks] *n.* 外源性物质

Notes

1. Exposure to drugs in the population is thus substantial, and the incidence of adverse reactions must be viewed in this context. 译为:可见人群中暴露药物是多见的,因此在这种情况下必须注意不良反应的发生。"exposure to..." 意思是"暴露于……","in this context" 意思是"在这种情况下"。

2. consultations in general practice,译为:会诊,全科医疗。

3. It would detect rare but severe adverse drug reactions, but would not be overwhelmed by common ones, the incidence of which would quantify together with predisposing factors. 译为:它(这种方法)能够检测罕见且严重的药物不良反应,而不是只是顾及一般的不良反应,并且可以对这些罕见且严重的反应的发生率及易感因素进行量化。"the incidence of which..." 为非限制性定语从句。

4. The problem of adverse drug reaction recognition is much greater if the reaction resembles spontaneous disease in the population, such that physicians are unlikely to attribute the reaction to drug exposure. 译为:如果药物不良反应与人群的自发性疾病相似,以至于医生不大可能将其归因于药物暴露,那么对不良反应的认识问题就更加重要。在这句话中,"such that" 相当于 "to such an extent that"(到……程度,以至于……)。

Supplementary Parts

1. Medical and Pharmaceutical Terminology (4): Common Morphemes in Terms of English for Pharmacology

Morpheme	Meaning	Example
adreno	肾上腺	adrenoceptor 肾上腺受体 adrenergic (药物或其作用)类似肾上腺素的
alg	痛	analgesia 镇痛
alges/i	对痛的感受性	hyperalgesia 痛觉过敏
anti	抗	anti-anemic drug 抗贫血药 antitussive 止咳药
carcino	癌	carcinogenicity 致癌性;致癌力
chem/o	化学,药	chemotherapy 化学疗法
chrono	时间	chronopharmacology 时辰药理学
contra	对抗	contraceptive 避孕药
dynam	动力	pharmacodynamic 药(物)效(应)动力学,药效学
erg/o	工作,能力	adrenergic 肾上腺素能的
esthesi/o	感受	anesthesia 麻醉
hist/o	组织	histology 组织学
hypn/o	睡眠	hypnotic 催眠药
idi/o	自己,个人	idiosyncracy 特异反应性,特异性

Morpheme	Meaning	Example
-ia	症	insomnia 失眠症
		hypoglycemia 低血糖（症）
immuno	免疫	immunopharmacology 免疫药理学
mut	突变	mutagenicity 致突变性
narc/o	麻木	narcosis 麻醉，昏迷状态
neuro	神经	neuropharmacology 神经药理学
pharmac/o	药	pharmacognosy 生药学
-phylaxis	保卫，保护	anaphylactic 过敏性的
pyr/o	热，发热	pyrogenic 致热的
rhythm	规律，节律	antiarrhythmic drug 抗心律失常药
somn/i	睡眠	insomnia 失眠
sopor/i	沉睡	soporific 催眠的
spasm/o	痉挛	spasmodic 痉挛的
terato	畸形	teratogenicity 致畸性
-therapy	治疗	thermotherapy 热疗法
ton/o	紧张	atony 张力缺乏，弛缓
tox/o	毒	toxin 毒素
toxic/o	毒	toxicology 毒理学
tuss/i	咳嗽	antitussive 镇咳药

Word-matching.

1) histology		A. 抗贫血药
2) antiarrhythmic drug		B. 致突变性
3) anesthesia		C. 肾上腺素能的
4) anaphylactic		D. 特异反应性
5) spasmodic		E. 痉挛的
6) idiosyncracy		F. 抗心律失常药
7) antianemic drug		G. 麻醉
8) mutagenicity		H. 异染色体
9) teratogenicity		I. 利胆剂
10) adrenergic		J. 组织学
11) allosome		K. 过敏性的
12) cholagogue		L. 致畸性

2. English-Chinese Translation Skills: 药学英语翻译中的直译与意译

直译（literal translation）和意译（free translation）是英汉翻译两种不同的方法。所谓"直译"，就是在不失原文语言形式和语篇风格，比较完整地按照原文意义翻译，直译不是"逐字翻译"也不是"词典翻译"，直译的重点在于译文的"准确"，但也要求译文通顺。所谓"意译"就是为了完整表达原文内容，抛弃原文语言形式，按照译入语的习惯重新造句，意译不是乱译或者漏译、错译，意译的重点在于"通顺"，但也不失意义正确。药学英语语篇属于科技文献，注重客观事实，在翻译时主要采用直译法。举例如下。

例1：Type B (idiosyncratic) reactions are not predictable from the drug's main pharmacological action, are not dose-related and are severe, with a considerable mortality.

参考译文：B 型不良反应（特异性反应）无法从药物的主要药理作用预测到，与药物剂量无关，且较严重，死亡率高。

药学英语原文结构复杂，加上英汉语言结构上的差异，翻译时要适当调整译文语言结构，使得译文通畅，这种译法还属于直译。举例如下。

例 2：Several of the traditional diseases that were major causes of death before the antibiotic era, e.g. tuberculosis and diphtheria, are now re-emerging in resistant form, adding to the problems posed by infections in which antibiotic resistance has long been a problem, and those like West Nile virus and severe acute respiratory syndrome (SARS) that have been recognized in recent years. Not only has the development of resistance to established antibiotics become a challenge, so too has the ability of microorganisms to take advantage of changing practices and procedures in medicine and surgery.

参考译文：在抗生素时代之前一些曾经是主要死因的传统疾病，如肺结核和白喉，现在又以抗性形式出现，这加剧了由长期存在的抗生素耐药性带来的感染问题，以及那些类似于西尼罗河病毒和严重急性呼吸综合征（SARS）等近年来人们才有所认识的疾病带来的问题。这不仅对已有抗生素耐药性的发展是一种挑战，而且对微生物在药物和手术方面利用不断改变的实践和操作能力也是一种挑战。

说明：例句原文由两个小句组成，专业词汇多，句子结构复杂。第一小句的主句是 Several of the traditional diseases are now re-emerging in resistant form. 主语 diseases 后面有 that 引导的定语从句，主句后面有非谓语动词 adding to... 作状语，而且在这个状语中又包含有两个定语从句。第二小句又是一个特殊英语句型 Not only..., so too...。译文很好地将原文复杂结构进行拆分，用短小句子将原文的意思一层层表述出来，既忠实原文，又符合汉语表达习惯。

另外，药学英语语篇中含有很多化学、医学、药学名称，这些词的处理肯定是直接翻译。一般来讲，医药名词的翻译具有单一性，基本属于词典翻译。举例如下。

例 3：Identification:

A: *Infrared Absorption* <197K>

B: *Ultraviolet Absorption* <197U>

Solution: 5 μg per ml.

Medium: 0.1*N* hydrochloric acid in methanol (1 in 100).

C: it responds to *Thin-layer Chromatographic Identification Test* <201>, a test solution in methanol containing about 1 mg per ml and a solvent system consisting of a mixture of methylene chloride and methanol (4 : 1) being used.

参考译文：

鉴别：

A. 红外吸收（附录 197K ）

B. 紫外吸收（附录 197U ）

溶液：5 μg/ml

介质：0.1 mol/L 盐酸的甲醇溶液（1 → 10 ）

C. 薄层色谱法（附录 201），每 1 ml 中约含供试品 1 mg 的甲醇溶液作为供试品溶液，二氯甲烷 - 甲醇（4：1）为展开剂。

这种"词典翻译"法也不是完全照词典释义，也是要根据原文内容，对术语在词典中的释义进行选择，这类翻译大多出现在药典、药品说明书、医药实验报告中。

（李晨睿　张予阳　史志祥　龚长华）

Medicinal Chemistry

Medicinal chemistry is a discipline mainly concerned to new drug research.

Before the twentieth century, medicines consisted mainly of herbs and potions, and it was not until the mid-nineteenth century that the first serious efforts were made to isolate and purify the active principles of those remedies (i.e. the pure chemicals responsible for the medicinal properties). The success of these efforts led to the birth of many of the pharmaceutical companies we know today. Since then, many naturally occurring drugs have been obtained and their structures determined (e.g. morphine from opium, cocaine from coca leaves, quinine from the bark of the cinchona tree).

These natural products sparked off a major synthetic effort where chemists made literally thousands of analogues in an attempt to improve on what nature had provided. Much of this work was carried out on a trial and error basis, but the results obtained revealed several general principles behind drug design.

In recent years, medicinal chemistry has undergone a revolutionary change. Rapid advances in the biological sciences have resulted in a much better understanding of how the body functions at the cellular and the molecular level. As a result, most research projects in the pharmaceutical industry or university sector now begin by identifying a suitable target in the body and designing a drug to interact with that target. An understanding of the structure and function of the target, as well as the mechanism by which it interacts with potential drugs, is crucial to this approach.

药物化学是一门以新药研究为主的学科。

20 世纪以前,药物主要是草药和汤药。直到 19 世纪中期,人们才重视并努力尝试从这些药物中分离和纯化有效成分(即产生药效的单体化合物)。这些尝试的成功催生了今天所熟知的许多制药公司。从那时起,许多天然来源的药物不断被发现,它们的化学结构也进一步被确定(例如,从鸦片中获得吗啡,从古柯叶中获得可卡因,从金鸡纳树的树皮中获得奎宁)。

这些天然产物的获得激发了合成化学家们进行大规模合成的尝试和努力,他们合成了成千上万的类似物以改善这些天然产物的性质。虽然这些工作绝大多数都基于反复实验摸索,但获得的结果揭示了药物设计的一些基本原理。

近年来,药物化学发生了革命性的变化。生物科学的快速发展使得人们更深入地了解机体如何在细胞和分子水平上发挥功能。因此,制药行业或大学的大多数研究项目现在都是从确定体内合适的靶点开始,然后设计一种可与该靶点相互作用的药物。明确靶点的结构和功能,以及其与潜在药物相互作用的机制,对药物研发至关重要。

Generally speaking, the stages for bringing a drug to the market can be identified drug discovery, design and development. Many of these stages run concurrently and are dependent on each other. For example, preclinical trials are usually carried out in parallel with the development of a manufacturing process. Even so, this project is a very time-consuming and expensive process which can take 15 years or more, involve the synthesis of over 10,000 compounds, and cost in the region of $800 million.

一般来说,一个药物推向市场大致可分为药物的发现、设计和开发等阶段。各阶段中的许多工作能同时运行并相互依赖。例如,(药物开发阶段的)临床前试验通常与生产工艺开发并行进行。即便如此,研发一个新药仍然是一个非常耗时且昂贵的过程,通常需要合成 1 万多种化合物,花费大约 8 亿美元,耗时 15 年或更久。

Text A
Lead Compounds

When any medicinal chemistry project can get underway, a lead compound is required. A lead compound will have some properties considered therapeutically useful. The property sought will depend on the tests used to detect the lead compound, which in turn depends on the drug development. The level of biological activity may not be particularly high, but that does not matter. The lead compound is not intended to be used as a clinical agent. It is the starting point from which a clinically useful compound can be developed. Similarly, it also does not matter whether the lead compound is toxic or has undesirable side effects. Again, drug design aims to improve the desirable effects of the lead compound and to remove the undesirable effects.

The suggested properties for a lead compound are that it should have a molecular weight of 100–350 amu and a Clog$P$ (Clog$P$ is a measure of how **hydrophobic** a compound is) value of 1–3. In general, there is an average increase in molecular weight of 80 amu and an increase of 1 in Clog$P$ when going from a lead compound to the final drug. Studies also show that a lead compound generally has fewer aromatic rings and hydrogen bond acceptors compared with the final drug. Such considerations can be taken into account when deciding which lead compound to use for a research project if several such structures are available.

Another approach in making this decision is to calculate the binding or **ligand** "**efficiency**" of each potential lead compound. This can be done by dividing the free energy of binding for each molecule by the number of non-hydrogen atoms present in the structure.[1] The better the ligand efficiency, the lower the molecular weight of the final optimized structure is likely to be. Moreover, if you have a choice of lead compounds, the most suitable one is not necessarily the most **potent**.

In order to search for lead compounds, a suitable test is required. This could be a test that reveals a physiological effect in a tissue preparation, organ or test animal. Alternatively, it could be a cellular effect, resulting from the interaction of a lead compound with a particular target, such as a receptor or an enzyme; or a molecular effect, such as the binding of a compound with a receptor. In the latter situation, the molecular target is considered important to a particular disease state, and in such cases, the lead compound may not have the desired physiological activity at all. For example, there have been several examples where the natural **agonist** for a receptor was used as the lead compound in order to design a receptor **antagonist**. Here, the crucial property of the lead compound was that it should be recognized and bound to the binding site of the target receptor. The lead compound was then modified to bind as an antagonist rather than as an agonist. For example, the chemical messenger histamine was used as the lead compound in developing the anti-ulcer agent cimetidine. Histamine is an agonist that activates histamine receptors in the stomach wall to increase the release of gastric acid. Cimetidine acts as an antagonist at these receptors, thus reducing the levels of gastric acid released and allowing the body to heal the ulcer.

Lead compounds can be obtained from a variety of different sources such as the flora and fauna of the natural world, or synthetic compounds made in the laboratory. There is also the potential of designing lead compounds using computer modeling or NMR spectroscopic studies.

The natural world is particularly rich in potential lead compounds. For example, plants, trees, snakes, lizards, frogs, fungi, corals and fish have all yielded potent lead compounds which have either resulted in clinically useful drugs or have the potential to do so. There is a good reason why nature should be so rich in potential lead compounds. Years of evolution have resulted in the "selection" of biologically potent natural compounds that have proved useful to the natural host for a variety of reasons. For example, a fungus that produces a toxin can kill off its microbiological competitors and take advantage of available nutrients.

Large numbers of novel structures are synthesized in research laboratories across the world for a diverse range of synthetic projects. This is a potential source of lead compounds, and pharmaceutical companies will often enter into arguments with research teams in order to test their compounds. Many of these structures may have been synthesized in research topics unrelated to medicinal chemistry, but are still potential lead compounds. The history of medicinal chemistry has many examples of lead compounds that were discovered from synthetic projects that had no medicinal objective in mind.[2] For example, Prontosil was manufactured as a dye, but was the lead compound for the development of the sulfonamides.

Strategies in the Search for New Lead Compounds

A retrospective analysis of the ways leading to discovery of new drugs suggests that there are five types of successful strategies leading to new lead compounds.

The first strategy consists of systematic screening of sets of compounds arbitrarily chosen for their diversity, by selected biological assays. This approach was useful in the past for the discovery of new antibiotics such as streptomycin and for the identification of Compactin as 3-hydroxy-3-methyl glutaryl coenzyme A (HMG-CoA)[3] reductase inhibitor. Presently, as high throughput screening (HTS), it is applied in a very general manner to synthetic as well as to natural compounds. Experience gathered has confirmed that high throughput screening allows for the rapid identification of numerous hits, and the literature is full of success stories obtained with that approach. Among them, one could mention the discovery of insulin mimetics, presence of opioid receptor-like (ORLI) receptor[4] agonists, protein tyrosine phosphatase-lB inhibitors, selective neuropeptide Y5 receptor antagonists, selective cyclooxygenase-2 (COX-2) inhibitors, and corticotropin releasing factor (CRF) receptor modulators. Yet the HTS strategy for drug discovery has several limitations. It suffers from inadequate diversity, has low hit rates, and often leads to compounds with poor bioavailability or toxicity profiles.

The second strategy is based on the modification and improvement of existing active molecules. The objective is to start with known active principles and, by various chemical transformations, prepare new molecules (sometimes referred to as "me-too compounds") for which an increase in potency, a better specific activity profile, improved safety, and a formulation that is easier to handle by physicians and nurses or more acceptable to the patient are claimed. A typical illustration of this approach is found in the series of lovastatin analogues (lovastatin, simvastatin, pravastatin, fluvastatin, atorvastatin, rosuvastatin, etc.).

In the pharmaceutical industry, motivations for this kind of research are often driven by competitive and economic factors. Indeed, if the sales of a given medicine are high and if a company is in a monopolistic situation protected by patents and trademarks, other companies will want to produce similar medicines, if possible with some therapeutic improvements. They will, therefore, use the already commercialized drug as a lead compound and search for ways to modify its structure and some of its physical and chemical properties while retaining or improving its therapeutic properties.

The third approach resides in the **retroactive** exploitation of various pieces of biological information that sometimes results from new discoveries made in biology and medicine and sometimes is just the fruits of more or less serendipitous observations. Examples are the chance discoveries of the **vasodilating** activity of **nitroglycerol**, the antibiotic activity of Penicillium notatum, and the clinical observation of the activity of **sildenafil** on erectile dysfunction. Research programs based on the exploitation of clinical observations of side effects are of great interest in the discovery of new tracks as they are based on information about activities observed directly in man and not in animals.[5] They can also detect new therapeutic activities even when no pharmacological models in animals exist.

The fourth route to new active compounds is a rational design based on the knowledge of the molecular cause of the pathological dysfunction. The approaches that we have described above owe a great deal to chance (screening, fortuitous discoveries). A more scientific approach is based on the knowledge of the incriminated molecular target: enzyme, receptor, ion channel, signaling protein, transport protein, or DNA. Therefore, this approach depends heavily on the progresses made in fundamental research, particularly in the identification and structural elucidation of a new receptor or enzyme subclass involved in a specific disease. Moreover, progress in molecular and structural biology technologies allowed the identification and experimental characterization of several hundred molecular targets and facilitated the design of drugs at a more rational level. Examples of this approach are the design of **captopril** as a hypotensive drug or of cimetidine as a treatment for peptic ulcers.

Finally, the fifth strategy is based on the structural knowledge of the target combined with biophysical technologies of ligand-protein interaction or computational methods. This strategy combines the increasing knowledge that we have on various targets and the new technologies that we can apply to assist the discovery of small molecules interacting both physically and functionally with the target protein. Knowledge of the three-dimensional structures of protein targets has the potential to greatly accelerate drug discovery, but technical challenges and time constraints have traditionally limited its use to lead **optimization**. The application of biophysical technologies is now being extended beyond structure determination into new approaches for lead discovery. For example, structure-activity relationships by nuclear magnetic resonance (NMR) have been widely used to detect ligand binding and to give some indication of the location of the binding site. X-ray crystallography has the advantage of defining ligand-binding sites with greater certainty. High-throughput approaches make this method applicable to screening to identify molecular fragments that bind protein targets and to defining precisely their binding sites. X-ray crystallography can then be used as a rapid technique to guide the elaboration of the fragments into larger molecular weight compounds that might be useful leads for drug discovery. In addition, large panels of biophysical methods, such as protein crystallization, ligand-protein co-crystallization and soaking, ligand-protein H^3 and N^{15}-NMR, surface plasmon resonance, differential scanning fluorimetry and mass **spectrometry**, are currently used. The integration of these techniques with computational chemistry technologies, such as virtual screening, computational drug repurposing and scaffold hopping, support the rational design and optimization of hits.

In summary, the discovery of new lead compounds can be **schematically** classified into five approaches. These consist of the systematic screening, of improvement of already existing drugs, of retroactive exploitation of biological information, of attempts toward rational design, and of the combination of the target protein structural information with biophysical technologies or computational methods. It would be imprudent to compare hastily the merit of each of these approaches. Indeed, "poor" research can end with a universally recognized medicine, and conversely, a brilliant rational demonstration can remain sterile. It is therefore of highest importance, given the random nature of discovery and the virtual impossibility of planned invention of new active principles, that decision-makers in the pharmaceutical industry employ all five strategies described, and that they realize that these strategies are not mutually exclusive. On the other hand, once a lead compound is discovered and characterized, it would be inappropriate not to study its molecular mechanism of action. Every possible effort should be made in this direction. In conclusion, all strategies resulting in identification of lead compounds are good and advisable, provided that the research they induce afterwards is done in a rational manner.

Word Study

1. agonist ['æɡənɪst] *n.* 激动剂
2. antagonist [æn'tæɡənɪst] *n.* 拮抗剂
3. bioavailability [ˌbaɪəʊəˌveɪləˈbɪlɪtɪ] *n.* 生物利用度
4. captopril ['kæptəprɪl] *n.* 卡托普利
5. cimetidine [saɪˈmetɪdiːn] *n.* 西咪替丁（一种抗消化性溃疡药）
6. compactin ['kəmpæktɪn] *n.* 美伐他汀 (mevastatin) 的商品名
7. coral ['kɒrəl] *n.* 珊瑚
8. cyclooxygenase [saɪkˈluːksɪdʒəneɪs] *n.* 环氧合酶
9. efficiency [ɪˈfɪʃnsɪ] *n.* 效率
10. fauna ['fɔːnə] *n.* 动物区系
11. flora ['flɔːrə] *n.* 植物区系
12. high throughput screening (HTS) [haɪ 'θruːpʊt 'skriːnɪŋ] *n.* 高通量筛选
13. hydrophobic [haɪdrəˈfəʊbɪk] *adj.* 疏水的
14. ligand ['laɪɡənd] *n.* 配体，配基
15. lizard ['lɪzəd] *n.* 蜥蜴
16. nitroglycerol [naɪtrəʊɡˈlɪsrɒl] *n.* 硝酸甘油
17. optimization [ˌɒptɪmaɪˈzeɪʃən] *n.* 优化，最佳化
18. potent ['pəʊtnt] *adj.* （药品或化学品）药效强的，强效的
19. prontosil ['prɒntəsl] *n.* 百浪多息（一种磺胺类药的商品名）
20. retroactive [ˌretrəʊˈæktɪv] *adj.* 追溯的，有追溯力的
21. schematically [skiːˈmætɪklɪ] *adv.* 用示意图地，大略地
22. sildenafil ['sɪldnəfɪl] *n.* 西地那非
23. spectrometry [spekˈtrɒmɪtrɪ] *n.* 光谱测定法，频谱测定法
24. tyrosine ['taɪrəsiːn] *n.* 酪氨酸
25. ulcer ['ʌlsə] *n.* 溃疡
26. vasodilating [væsəʊdaɪˈleɪtɪŋ] *adj.* ［生理］血管舒张的，引起血管舒张的

Notes

1. This can be done by dividing the free energy of binding for each molecule by the number of non-hydrogen atoms present in the structure. 译为：这可以用每个分子的结合自由能除以该分子结构中非氢原子的数量计算得到。句中 "this" 指的是上句提到的 ligand "efficiency"，即配体效率，用以评价分子中的每个非氢原子对结合能或活性的贡献。"divide A by B" 意思是 "用 A 除以 B"。

2. The history of medicinal chemistry has many examples of lead compounds that were discovered from synthetic projects that had no medicinal objective in mind. 译为：药物化学史上有多例先导化合物是从非药物研发为目的的合成项目中发现的。注意该句中第一个定语从句中含有另外一个定语从句，翻译时要正确处理定语从句的表述。

3. 3-hydroxy-3-methyl glutaryl coenzyme A (HMG-CoA)，译为：3- 羟基 -3- 甲基戊二酰单酰辅酶 A，英文简称 HMG-CoA。

4. opioid receptor-like (ORLI) receptor，译为：阿片受体样受体。

5. Research programs based on the exploitation of clinical observations of side effects are of great interest in the discovery of new tracks as they are based on information about activities observed directly in man and not in animals. 译为：基于对药物副作用临床观察的研究项目对于发现新药具有重要意义，因为它们是建立在直接在人类而非动物身上观察到生物活性信息基础上的。句中 "new tracks" 引申为新药，"be of interest in" 译为 "对……有意义"。

Exercises

1. Decide whether the following statements are true (T) or false (F) according to the passage.

(1) The level of biological activity of a lead compound must be particularly high.

(2) It is suggested that a lead compound should have a molecular weight of 100–350 amu and a Clog$P$ value of 1–3.

(3) If you have a choice of lead compounds, the most suitable one is exactly the most potent one.

(4) The natural agonist for a receptor can not be used as the lead compound in order to design a receptor antagonist.

(5) Structures that have been synthesized in research topics unrelated to medicinal chemistry are also potential lead compounds.

(6) Rational approach for lead discovery depends heavily on the progresses made in fundamental research, such as the identification of a new receptor involved in a specific disease.

2. Questions for oral discussion.

(1) What considerations should be taken into account when deciding which lead compound to use for a research project?

(2) What drugs are obtained by structural modification and optimization based on existing active molecules?

(3) What can serve as source(s) of a potential compound?

(4) Why does the author say "It would be imprudent to compare hastily the merit of each of these approaches"?

3. Choose the best answer to each of the following questions.

(1) Clog$P$ is a measure of how _____ a compound is.

A. hydrophobic   B. hydrophobicity

C. hydrophilic   D. hydrophilicity

(2) Generally speaking, a lead compound has _____ hydrogen bond acceptors compared with the final drug.

A. more   B. fewer

C. equal   D. less

(3) The plural form of "fungus" is _____.

A. fungus   B. funguses

C. fungi   D. fungis

(4) Which of the following is the advantage of HTS approach for discovering lead compound?

A. High hit rate.   B. Inadequate diversity.

C. Rapid identification of numerous hits.   D. Leading to compounds with poor bioavailability.

(5) According to the passage, which of the following drug was discovered by rational drug design?

A. Antibiotic streptomysin.

B. HMG-CoA reductase inhibitor compactin.

C. Anti-impotence drug sildenafil.

D. Histamine H2 receptor antagonist cimetidine.

(6) The molecules that were prepared by structural modification of an existing drug are referred to as a _____.

A. lead compound   B. drug candidate

C. me-too compound   D. commercialized drug

(7) Which of the following techniques has the advantage of defining ligand-binding sites with greater certainty?

A. Nuclear magnetic resonance.   B. X-ray crystallography.

C. High throughput screening.   D. Mass spectrometry.

(8) Which of the following words can optimally replace "commercialized" in the sentence "they will therefore use the already commercialized drug as a lead compound "?

A. marketed   B. approved

C. clinical   D. profitable

4. **Fill in each of the following blanks with an appropriate word or expression according to the meaning of the sentences.**

(1) Drug design aims to _____ the desirable effects of the lead compound and to _____ the undesirable effects.

(2) Ligand efficiency of a compound is calculated by dividing the free energy of binding for the molecule by the number of _____ present in the structure.

(3) Cimetidine acts as an _____ at histamine receptors, thus reducing the levels of gastric acid released and allowing the body to heal the ulcer.

(4) Prontosil was the lead compound for the development of the _____.

(5) Research programs based on the exploitation of clinical observations of side effects are _____ in the discovery of new lead compound.

(6) All strategies _____ identification of lead compounds are *a priori* equally good and advisable.

(7) In the pharmaceutical industry, motivations for "me-too" compound research are often driven by _____ factors.

(8) The better the ligand efficiency, _____ the molecular weight of the final optimized structure is likely to be.

5. Translate the following sentences into Chinese.

(1) The therapeutically useful property of a lead compound sought will depend on the tests used to detect the lead compound, which in turn depends on the drug's target.

(2) Such factors, viz., the molecular weight, a ClogP value, and the numbers of aromatic rings and hydrogen bond acceptors, can be taken into account when deciding which lead compound to use for a research project if several such structures are available.

(3) The crucial property of the lead compound was that it should be recognized and bound to the binding site of the target receptor.

(4) In the history of medicinal chemistry, there are many examples of lead compounds that were discovered from synthetic projects that had no medicinal objective in mind.

(5) Experience gathered has confirmed that high throughput screening allows for the rapid identification of numerous hits, and the literature is full of success stories obtained with that approach.

(6) The third approach resides in the retroactive exploitation of various pieces of biological information that sometimes results from new discoveries made in biology and medicine and sometimes is just the fruits of more or less serendipitous observations.

(7) The progress in molecular and structural biology technologies allowed the identification and experimental characterization of several hundred molecular targets and facilitated the design of drugs at a more rational level.

Value-Oriented Reflective Reading

The Green Wormwood Makes a Powerful Eastern Medicine—A Gift from Traditional Chinese Medicine to the World

On October 4, 1971, in a lab of the Institute of Chinese Materia Medica, China Academy of Chinese Medical Sciences, researchers held their breaths as they waited for the final results of an experiment on the antimalarial properties of a sample of ether-based neutral extract of artemisinin. Finally, the results came out: The sample inhibited plasmodium parasites at a rate of 100 percent! The lab erupted with excitement and the head of the research team, Tu Youyou, broke into a gratified smile.

On May 23, 1967, a national meeting on collaboration on malaria control research was held in Beijing. It marked the beginning of then 39-year-old Tu Youyou's work to develop a traditional Chinese medicine (TCM) for malaria that would span half a century. The five decades witnessed hundreds of experiments with a mixture of failures, successes and hopes in the tortuous search for artemisinin. Every breakthrough and discovery along the way was the product of the wisdom and hard work of numerous researchers. In November 1978, a meeting on the assessment of the research outcome in artemisinin-based malaria treatment finally declared the birth of artemisinin. After years of experiments and improvements, in 1986, artemisinin was certified as a new drug by the Ministry of Health. In 1999, it joined the list of the World Health Organization. The powerful Eastern medicine finally made its way to the world, freeing hundreds of millions of people from the pain of the disease.

On December 10, 2015, at the Stockholm Concert Hall in the capital of Sweden, Tu Youyou received the diploma, medal and cash award of the Nobel Prize in Physiology or Medicine from Swedish King Carl XVI Gustaf. The concert hall reverberated with the sound of a warm standing ovation. By then, it had been 44 years since the experiment on the antimalarial properties of an artemisinin sample achieved success. The malaria expert who had worked on the front line of research for decades finally won China's first Nobel Prize in science for domestically-conducted scientific research with her outstanding contribution to malaria treatment.

Together with her team, the pharmacologist derived artemisinin from sweet wormwood, which she found cited in a fourth-century TCM text as an ingredient to cure fever, developing a crucial drug that has significantly reduced mortality rates among malaria patients in recent decades.

"The discovery of artemisinin has led to development of a new drug that has saved the lives of millions of people, halving the mortality rate of malaria during the past 15 years," said Professor Hans Forssberg, a member of the Nobel committee for physiology or medicine, when presenting Tu's scientific contributions.

According to the WHO, more than 240 million people in sub-Saharan Africa have benefited from artemisinin, and more than 1.5 million lives are estimated to have been saved since 2000 thanks to the drug. Apart from its contribution to the global fight against malaria, TCM played a vital role in the deadly outbreak of severe acute respiratory syndrome across China in 2003.

Questions for oral discussion:

1. How many years have passed since Tu Youyou's work on an anti-malaria drug and artemisinin was approved by the WHO?

2. On what basis did Tu's team develop the new drug for curing malaria?

3. What can we learn from the article?

Text B
General Principles of Antiviral Agents

Antiviral drugs are useful in tackling viral diseases where there is a lack of an effective vaccine or where infection has already taken place. The life cycle of a virus means that for most of its time in the body, it is within a host cell and is effectively disguised both from the immune system and from circulating drugs.[1] As it also uses the host cells that for most of its time in multiply, the number of potential drug targets that are unique to the virus is more limited than those for invading microorganisms. Thus, the search for effective antiviral drugs has proved more challenging than that for antibacterial drugs. Indeed, the first antiviral agents appeared relatively late on in the 1960s and only three clinically useful antiviral drugs were in use during the early 1980s. Early antiviral drugs included **idoxuridine** and **vidarabine** for **herpes** infections, and **amantadine** for **influenza** A.

Since then, progress has accelerated for two principal reasons: i) the need to tackle the AIDS pandemic and ii) the increased understanding of viral infectious mechanisms resulting from viral genomic research.

In the early 1980s, diseases such as **pneumonia** and **fungal infection** were only associated with patients whose immune response had been weakened. The problem soon reached epidemic proportions and it was discovered that a virus (the human **immunodeficiency** virus—HIV) was responsible. It was found that this virus infected T-cells which are crucial to the immune response—and was therefore directly attacking the immune system. With a weakened immune system, infected patients were proved susceptible to a whole range of opportunistic secondary diseases resulting in the term acquired immune deficiency syndrome (AIDS). This discovery led to a major research effort into understanding the disease and counteracting it—an effort which kick-started more general research into antiviral chemotherapy. Fortunately, the tools needed to carry out effective research appeared on the scene at about the same time with the advent of viral genomics.[2] The full genome of any virus can now be determined quickly and compared with those of other viruses, allowing the identification of how the genetic sequence is split into genes. This, in turn, helps to identify viral proteins as potential drug targets. Standard genetic engineering methods permit the production of pure copies of the target protein by inserting the viral gene into a bacterial cell thus providing sufficient quantities of the protein to be isolated, and studied.

HIV has been studied extensively over the last 20 years and a vast research effort has resulted in a variety of antiviral drugs which have proved successful in slowing down the disease, but not eradicating it. At present, most clinically useful antiviral drugs act against two targets: the viral **reverse transcriptase** and **protease**.

Reverse Transcriptase Inhibitor

Reverse transcriptase is an important enzyme in the process of HIV replication. Under normal circumstances, there is no such enzyme in human cells. In the course of animal research, it has found an inhibitor of the enzyme, which makes it possible to study anti HIV drugs targeting reverse transcriptase. Reverse transcriptase inhibitors are mainly divided into **nucleosides** and non-nucleosides.

The Nucleoside Reverse Transcriptase

As the enzyme reverse transcriptase is unique to HIV, it serves as an ideal drug target. Nevertheless, the enzyme is still a DNA **polymerase** and care has to be taken that inhibitors do not have a significant inhibitory effect on cellular DNA polymerases. Various nucleoside-like structures have proved useful as antiviral agents. The vast majority of these are not active themselves, but are phosphorylated by three cellular enzymes to form an active **nucleotide triphosphate**. Cellular enzymes are required to catalyse all three phosphorylations because HIV does not produce a viral kinase.[3]

Zidovudine was the first drug to be approved for use in the treatment of AIDS but was developed originally as an anticancer agent. It is an analogue of **deoxythymidine** where the sugar 3'-hydroxyl group has been replaced by an **azido** group. On conversion to the triphosphate, it inhibits reverse transcriptase. Furthermore, the triphosphate is attached to the growing DNA chain. Since the sugar unit has an **azide** substituent at the 3' position of the sugar ring, the nucleic acid chain cannot be extended any further.

Other approved drugs of this class include didanosin, lamivudine, emtricitabine, stavudine, zalcitabin, abacavir, etc.

Non-nucleoside Reverse Transcriptase Inhibitors (NNRTIs)

The NNRTIs are generally hydrophobic molecules that bind to an **allosteric** binding site which is hydrophobic in nature.[4] Since the allosteric binding site is separate from the substrate binding site, the NNRTIs are non-competitive, reversible inhibitors. They include first-generation NNRTIs, such as **nevirapine**, and **delavirdine**, as well as second-generation drugs, such as efavirenz, etravirine[5], rilpivirine[6].

X-ray crystallographic studies on inhibitor-enzyme complexes show that the allosteric binding site is adjacent to the substrate binding site. Binding of a NNRTI to the allosteric site results in an induced fit which locks the neighbouring substrate-binding site into an inactive conformation. Unfortunately, rapid resistance emerges as a result of mutations in the NNRTI binding site—the most common being the replacement of Lys-103 with **asparagine**. This mutation is called K103N and is defined as a pan-class resistance mutation. The resistance problem can be countered by combining an NNRTI with an NRTI from the start of treatment. The two types of drugs can be used together as the binding sites are distinct.

As a classic inhibitor of first generation NNRTI, nevirapine was developed from a lead compound discovered through a random screening programme and has a rigid butterfly-like conformation that makes it chiral. One "wing" interacts through hydrophobic and van der Waals interactions with aromatic residues in the binding site, while the other wing interacts with aliphatic residues. The other NNRTI inhibitors bind to the same pocket and appear to function as π electron donors to aromatic side chain residues.

Second-generation NNRTIs were developed specifically to find agents that were active against resistant variants, as well as wild-type viruses. This development has been helped by X-ray crystallographic studies which show how these structures bind to the binding site.

In the second-generation NNRTIs, efavirenz is a **benzoxazinone** structure which has activity against many mutated variants but has less activity against the mutated variant K103N. Nevertheless, activity drops less than for nevirapine and a study of X-ray structures of each complex revealed that the cyclopropyl group of efavirenz has fewer interactions with Tyr-181 and Tyr-188 than does nevirapine. Consequently, mutations of these amino acids have a lesser effect on efavirenz than they do on nevirapine. Efavirenz is also a smaller structure and can shift its binding position when K103N mutation occurs, allowing it to form hydrogen bonds to the main peptide chain of the binding site.

Protease Inhibitors

The HIV protease enzyme is an example of an enzyme family called the aspartyl proteases—enzymes which catalyse the cleavage of peptide bonds and which contain an **aspartic** acid in the active site that is crucial to the catalytic mechanism. The enzyme is relatively small and can be obtained by synthesis. Alternatively, it can be cloned and expressed in fast-growing cells then purified in large quantities. The enzyme is crystallized with or without an inhibitor bound to the active site, making it an ideal target for structure-based drug design.

In the mid 1990s, the use of X-ray crystallography and molecular modeling led to the structure-based design of a series of inhibitors which act on the viral enzyme HIV protease. Like the reverse transcriptase inhibitors, protease inhibitors (PIs) have a short-term benefit when they are used alone, but resistance soon develops. Consequently, combination therapy is now the accepted method of treating HIV infections. When protease and reverse transcriptase inhibitors are used together, the antiviral activity is enhanced and viral resistance is slower to develop.

Unlike the reverse transcriptase inhibitors, the protease inhibitors are not prodrugs and do not need to be activated. Therefore, it is possible to use *in vitro* assays involving virally infected cells in order to test their antiviral activity. The protease enzyme can also be isolated, allowing enzyme assays to be carried out. In general, the latter are used to measure IC_{50} levels as a measure of how effectively novel drugs inhibit the protease enzyme. The IC_{50} is the concentration of drug required to inhibit the enzyme by 50%. Thus, the lower the IC_{50} value, the more potent the inhibitor. However, a good PI does not necessarily mean a good antiviral drug. In order to be effective, the drug has to cross the cell membrane of infected cells, and so *in vitro* whole-cell assays are often used alongside enzyme studies to check cell absorption. EC_{50} values are a measure of antiviral activity and represent the concentration of compounds required to inhibit 50% of the cytopathic effect of the virus in isolated lymphocytes. Another complication is the requirement for anti-HIV drugs to have a good oral bioavailability (i.e. to be orally active). This is a particular problem with the PIs. Most PIs are designed from peptide lead compounds. Peptides are well known to have poor **pharmacokinetic** properties (i.e. poor absorption, **metabolic susceptibility**, rapid **excretion**, limited access to the central nervous system, and high plasma protein binding).[7] This is mainly due to high molecular weight, poor water solubility, and susceptible peptide linkages. Potent PIs were discovered relatively quickly, but that these had a high peptide character. Subsequent work was then needed to reduce the peptide character of these compounds in order to retain high activity, whilst gaining acceptable levels of oral bioavailability and half-life.

Up to now, there are three types of HIV protease inhibitors: the original peptide inhibitors, peptide-like inhibitors and non peptide inhibitors. Most of the drugs used in clinic are peptide-like inhibitors, which are the largest class of HIV protease inhibitors.

Saquinavir was the first PI to reach the market. It is still used clinically but suffers from poor oral bioavailability and susceptibility to drug resistance. Various efforts have been made to design simpler analogues of saquinavir which have lower molecular weight, less peptide character, and, consequently, better oral bioavailability. These efforts led to plenty of approved PIs including **ritonavir, lopinavir, indinavir, nelfinavir, amprenavir,** tipranavir[8], etc.

Clinically useful PIs are generally less well absorbed from the gastrointestinal tract than reverse transcriptase inhibitors, and are also susceptible to first pass metabolic reactions involving the cytochrome P450 isozyme (CYP3A4). This metabolism can result in drug-drug interactions with many of the other drugs given to AIDS patients to combat opportunistic diseases (e.g. rifabutin[9], **ketoconazole, rifampin,** and **astemizole**).

An alternative approach to inhibiting the protease enzyme would be to prevent its formation in the first place. Studies are in progress to design protein-protein binding inhibitors that will prevent the association of the two protein subunits that make it up. Another interesting approach is to design prodrugs of toxic compounds that are only activated by HIV protease. The prodrugs would contain a moiety that acts as a substrate for HIV-protease, such that the toxin is only released in HIV-infected cells. The toxin would then attack cellular targets and eliminate those cells.

Inhibitors of Other Targets

Beyond reverse transcriptase and protease inhibitors, other agents under study for the treatment of HIV include **integrase** inhibitors, and cell entry inhibitors.

Blocking entry of a virus into a host cell is particularly desirable, because it is so early in the life cycle. Enfuvirtide[10] was approved in March 2003 as the first member of a new class of fusion inhibitors.

The first integrase inhibitor to reach the market in 2007 was raltegravir. The keto-enol system in its chemical structure is important for activity as it acts as a chelating group for two magnesium ion cofactors in the enzyme's active site.[11]

Word Study

1. allosteric [ˌæləˈsterɪk] *adj.* 变构的
2. amantadine [əˈmæntəˌdiːn] *n.* 金刚烷胺
3. amprenavir [æmpriˈneɪvɜː] *n.* 安泼那韦
4. asparagine [əˈspærəˌdʒiːn] *n.* 天冬酰胺
5. aspartic [əˈspɑːtik] acid *n.* 天冬氨酸
6. astemizole [ˈæstəmɪəʊl] *n.* 阿司咪唑
7. azide [ˈeɪzaɪd] *n.* 叠氮化物
8. azido [ˈæzɪdəʊ] *n.* 叠氮基
9. benzoxazinone [ˈbenzɒksɑːzɪnwʌn] *n.* 苯并噁嗪酮
10. delavirdine [deleɪvɜːˈdaɪn] *n.* 地拉韦定
11. deoxythymidine [diːɒksɪθɪˈmaɪdaɪn] *n.* 脱氧胸苷
12. efavirenz [ɪfeɪˈvaɪərenz] *n.* 依非韦伦
13. excretion [ɪkˈskriːʃn] *n.* 排泄，排泄物；分泌，分泌物
14. fungal infection [ˈfʌŋɡl ɪnˈfekʃn] *n.* 真菌感染
15. genomics [dʒiˈnɒmɪks] *n.* 基因组学
16. herpes [ˈhɜːpiːz] *n.* 疱疹
17. idoxuridine [ˌaɪdɒksjʊˈrɪdiːn] *n.* 碘苷；[药]疱疹净
18. immunodeficiency [ɪˌmjuːnəʊdɪˈfɪʃnsi] *n.* 免疫缺陷
19. indinavir [ɪndɪˈneɪvə] *n.* 茚地那韦
20. influenza [ˌɪnfluˈenzə] *n.* 流行性感冒
21. integrase [ˈɪntɪɡreɪs] *n.* [生化]整合酶
22. ketoconazole [ˌkɪtəʊˈkəʊnəˌzəʊl] *n.* 酮康唑
23. lopinavir [ləpɪˈneɪvə] *n.* 洛匹那韦
24. metabolic [ˌmetəˈbɒlɪk] *adj.* 代谢的
25. nelfinavir [nelfɪˈneɪvə] *n.* 奈非那韦
26. nevirapine [nevɪˈræpaɪn] *n.* 奈韦拉平
27. nucleoside [ˈnjuːklɪəˌsaɪd] *n.* [生化]核苷
28. nucleotide triphosphate [ˈnjuːklɪəˌtaɪd traɪˈfɒsfeɪt] *n.* 核苷三磷酸，三磷酸核苷
29. pharmacokinetic [fɑːməkəʊkaɪˈnetɪk] *adj.* 药代动力学的
30. pneumonia [njuːˈməʊniə] *n.* 肺炎
31. polymerase [ˈpɒlɪməreɪs] *n.* 聚合酶
32. protease [ˈprəʊtieɪz] *n.* 蛋白酶
33. reverse transcriptase [rɪˈvɜːs trænˈskrɪpteɪz] *n.* 逆转录酶
34. rifampin [raɪˈfæmpɪn] *n.* 利福平
35. ritonavir [riːtəʊˈneɪvaɪər] *n.* 利托那韦
36. susceptibility [səˌseptəˈbɪləti] *n.* 易受影响（或伤害等）的特性
37. vidarabine [vaɪˈdærəbaɪn] *n.* 阿糖腺苷
38. zidovudine [zaɪˈdɒvjuˌdiːn] *n.* 齐多夫定

Notes

1. The life cycle of a virus means that for most of its time in the body, it is within a host cell and is effectively disguised both from the immune system and from circulating drugs. 译为：病毒的生命周期使其在体内的大部分时间都处在宿主细胞内，可以有效地躲过免疫系统和流通药物的攻击。句中动词 "means" 意思是 "to have sth. as a result"，即 "产生……的结果"，这里翻译为 "使……"。

2. Fortunately, the tools needed to carry out effective research appeared on the scene at about the same time with the advent of viral genomics. 译为：幸运的是，开展有效抗病毒研究所需的技术几乎与病毒基因组学分析同时兴起。"appeared on the scene"，意思是 "到场，出现"；"with the advent of..."，意思是 "随着……的出现"。

3. The vast majority of these are not active themselves, but are phosphorylated by three cellular enzymes to form an active nucleotide triphosphate. Cellular enzymes are required to catalyse all three phosphorylations because HIV does not produce a viral kinase. 译为：这些（药物）绝大多数本身没有活性，但可被三种细胞酶磷酸化，形成活性的三磷酸核苷。细胞酶需要催化所有这三个磷酸化过程，因为 HIV 不产生病毒激酶。"kinase"，激酶，通常指催化底物进行磷酸化的酶。多数核苷类抗病毒药物都需要利用宿主细胞内的激酶进行三磷酸化后，才具有抗病毒作用，为前药（prodrug）。

4. The NNRTIs are generally hydrophobic molecules that bind to an allosteric binding site which is hydrophobic in nature. 译为：NNRTIs 通常是疏水分子，可以与（逆转录酶的）疏水性变构位点结合。"allosteric binding site"，变构位点，即 substrate binding site（酶底物的结合位点）之外的配体结合位点。substrate binding site 也称作 "orthosteric site（正构位点）"。

5. etravirine n. 依曲韦林，是一种非核苷逆转录酶抑制剂（NNRTIs），具有抗 HIV 的作用。

6. rilpivirine n. 利匹韦林，是一种有效和特异性的二芳基嘧啶（DAPY）非核苷逆转录酶抑制剂（NNRTIs），被用于治疗 HIV-1 感染。

7. Peptides are well known to have poor pharmacokinetic properties (i.e. poor absorption, metabolic susceptibility, rapid excretion, limited access to the central nervous system, and high plasma protein binding). 译为：众所周知，多肽具有较差的药代动力学性质（例如，不易吸收、易被代谢、消除快、难以进入中枢神经系统、血浆蛋白结合率高）。

8. tipranavir, n. 替拉那韦，是非肽 HIV 蛋白酶抑制剂（NPPI），具有抗病毒作用。

9. rifabutin n. 利福布汀，为一个含有螺哌嗪基的利福霉素衍生物，具广谱抗菌活性。其作用机制与利福平一样，可与微生物的 DNA 依赖性 RNA 多聚酶 β 亚基形成稳定的结合，抑制该酶活性，从而抑制细菌 RNA 的合成。在国外已被批准用于预防和治疗 HIV 感染者鸟分枝杆菌复合群（Mycobacterium avium complex, MAC）的广泛播散性感染，也用于多重耐药结核病的治疗。

10. enfuvirtide n. 恩夫韦肽，是一种抗 HIV-1 融合的抑制肽，用于成人及 6 岁以上儿童的抗艾滋病药品。

11. The keto-enol system in its chemical structure is important for activity as it acts as a chelating group for two magnesium ion cofactors in the enzyme's active site. 译为：其（raltegravir，雷特格韦）化学结构中的酮 - 烯醇片段能够与酶活性位点的两个镁离子辅基螯合，因此对其活性至关重要。

Supplementary Parts

1. Medical and Pharmaceutical Terminology (5): Common Morphemes of Colors in Medical and Pharmaceutical English Terms

Morpheme	Meaning	Example
erythro-	红	erythrocyte 红细胞
rubro-		rubriblast 原红细胞
xantho-	黄	xanthoma 黄色瘤
cyano-	蓝	cyanosis 发绀；苍白病，黄萎病
chloro-	绿	chlorophyll 叶绿素
vio-	紫	viomycin 紫霉素
albo-	白	albumin 清蛋白，白蛋白
leuko-		leukocyte 白细胞
leuco-		leucocidin 杀白细胞素
melano-	黑	melanoma （恶性）黑素瘤，（良性）胎记瘤
nigro-		nigrometer 黑度计
polio-	灰,白灰	poliomyelitis 脊髓灰质炎（小儿麻痹症）
glauco-	绿灰	glaucoma 青光眼，绿内障
chrom-	色	chromosome 染色体

Word-matching.

1) chlorophyll	A. 红细胞
2) cyanosis	B. 染色体
3) xanthoma	C. 叶绿素
4) chromosome	D. 黑度计
5) nigrometer	E. 杀白细胞素
6) rubriblast	F. 紫霉素
7) leucocidin	G. 清蛋白,白蛋白
8) leukocyte	H. 青光眼,绿内障
9) viomycin	I. 白细胞
10) erythrocyte	J. 黄色瘤
11) albumin	K. 发绀；苍白病,黄萎病
12) glaucoma	L. 原红细胞

2. English-Chinese Translation Skills: 药学英语翻译技巧 (1)：词性转换

词性转换法是翻译中常用手段,这是由英汉两种语言表达差异造成的。词性转换几乎可以在所有词性间进行,例如把原文的名词译为汉语的动词,把原文的副词译为汉语的形容词,或把原文的形容词译为汉语的名词等,举例如下。

例 1：A second major area was the <u>synthesis</u> of simplified fragments of complex drug molecules.

参考译文：第二个主要的发展阶段是<u>合成</u>复杂药物分子的简单片段。

例 2：The institute claimed that phosphate also stabilized penicillin <u>beyond</u> its buffer effect.

参考译文：该研究所声称磷酸盐也能稳定青霉素,其效果<u>超过</u>了它的缓冲作用。

说明：本句原文中的介词 beyond 在译文中用了动词"超过"来表达。若不将 beyond 转译,句子难以有效译出。在英语中的介词或介词短语在许多情况下可以译成汉语中的动词。

例 3：The objective is to start with known active principles and, by various chemical transformations, prepare new molecules (sometimes referred to as "me-too compounds") for which an increase in potency, a better specific activity profile, improved safety, and a formulation that is <u>easier</u> to handle by physicians and nurses or more <u>acceptable</u> to the patient are claimed.

参考译文：目的就是利用已知的活性物质，通过一系列的化学转化，制备药效更强、作用更专一、安全性更高的新的化合物分子（有时也称为"me-too 化合物"），并且形成<u>更容易</u>被医师和护士应用、被患者<u>接受</u>的新剂型。

说明：在上面例句中，easier 和 acceptable 在原文中都是形容词做表语，构成"形容词 +to+ 动词"结构，而汉语中没有这样结构，翻译时就需要结构转换，用符合汉语的语言结构表达原义，译文将 easier 转换成了副词修饰"（被医师和护士）应用"，将 acceptable 转换成了动词"接受"，使得译文更加顺畅。

英汉翻译中词性转换也包括英语表达结构中常见的非谓语动词形式，汉语中没有这种词性，在英译汉时需要根据这些非谓语动词的意义和语法功能进行词性转换，译成准确、通顺的汉语，如下。

例 4：By <u>preserving</u> energy metabolism in cell <u>exposed</u> to hypoxia or ischaemia, trimetazidine prevents a decrease in intracellular ATP level, thereby <u>ensuring</u> the proper functioning of ionic pumps and transmembrane sodium-potassium flow while <u>maintaining</u> cellular homeostasis.

参考译文：曲美他嗪通过保护细胞在缺氧或缺血情况下的能量代谢，阻止细胞内 ATP 水平的下降，从而保证了离子泵的正常功能和透膜钠 - 钾流的正常运转，同时维持细胞内环境的稳定。

说明：在上面例句中，原句有四个非谓语动词形式：preserving, exposed, ensuring 和 maintaining，起着不同语法功能。在翻译时，为了译文通顺就必须根据意义表达需要将这些非谓语动词形式翻译成对应的动词形式，以符合汉语的习惯传递信息。

（亢小辉　赵　岩　翟兴英　史志祥　龚长华）

Unit Six

Pharmaceutics

Unit Six
数字内容

Pharmaceutics is the discipline of pharmacy that deals with the process of turning a new chemical entity or old drugs into a medication to be safely and effectively administered by patients. Pharmaceutics aims to deliver drugs to the target sites and maintain appropriate drug concentrations over time. Branches of pharmaceutics mainly include pharmaceutical formulation, pharmaceutical manufacturing, physical pharmacy, biopharmaceutics and pharmacokinetics. Pharmaceutical formulation involves the design, development, and evaluation of dosage forms and drug delivery systems. Biopharmaceutics and pharmacokinetics study the absorption, distribution, metabolism, and excretion of drugs and metabolites in humans, animals, and tissue cultures.

药剂学是药学的分支学科,主要研究将新型化学药物或已知药物以适当的剂型安全有效地应用于患者。药剂学旨在实现靶部位的定点释药,并在一段时间内维持适当药物浓度。其分支学科主要包括药物制剂、药品生产、物理药学、生物药剂学和药物代谢动力学等。药物制剂包括药物剂型和药物传递系统的设计、开发和评估。生物药剂学和药物代谢动力学研究药物在人体、动物以及组织培养中的吸收、分布、代谢和消除过程。

Text A
Design of Dosage Forms

Drugs are rarely administered as pure chemical substances alone and are almost always given as formulated preparations or medicines. These can range from relatively simple solutions to complex drug delivery systems through the use of appropriate additives or **excipients** in the formulations. The excipients provide varied and specialized pharmaceutical functions. It is the formulation additives that, among other things, solubilize, suspend, thicken, preserve, emulsify, modify dissolution, increase the **compactability** and improve the flavour of drug substances to form various medicines or dosage forms.

1. Principles of Dosage Form Design

The principal objective of dosage form design is to achieve a predictable therapeutic response to a drug included in a formulation which can be manufactured on a large scale with reproducible product quality. To ensure product quality, numerous features are required: chemical and physical stability, with suitable preservation against microbial contamination if appropriate, uniformity of the dose of the drug, acceptability to users, including both prescriber and patient, and suitable packaging and labeling. Ideally, dosage forms should also be independent of patient-to-patient variation, although in practice this feature remains difficult to achieve. However, recent developments are beginning to accommodate this requirement. These include drug delivery systems that rely on the specific metabolic activity of individual patients and implants that respond, for example, to externally applied sound or magnetic fields to trigger a drug delivery function.

Consideration should be given to differences in the bioavailability of drugs (the rate and extent to which they are absorbed) and their biological fate in patients between apparently similar formulations and possible causative reasons. In recent years, increasing attention has therefore been directed towards elimination of variation in bioavailability characteristics, particularly for medicinal products containing an equivalent dose of a drug substance, as it is recognized that formulation factors can influence their therapeutic performance. To optimize the bioavailability of drug substances, it is often necessary to carefully select the most appropriate chemical form of the drug. For example, such selection should address solubility requirements, drug particle size and drug physical form and should consider appropriate additives and manufacturing aids coupled with selection of the most appropriate administration route(s) and dosage form(s). Additionally, suitable manufacturing processes, labelling and packaging are required.

There are numerous dosage forms into which a drug substance can be incorporated for the convenient and efficacious treatment of a disease. Dosage forms can be designed for administration by a variety of delivery routes to maximize therapeutic response. Preparations can be taken orally or injected, as well as being applied to the skin or inhaled. However, it is necessary to relate the drug substance to the clinical indication being treated before the correct combination of drug and dosage form can be made, as each disease or illness often requires a specific type of drug therapy. In addition, factors governing the choice of administration route and the specific requirements of that route which affect drug absorption need to be taken into account when dosage forms are being designed.

Many drugs are formulated into several dosage forms of various strengths, each having selected pharmaceutical characteristics which are suitable for a specific application. One such drug is the **glucocorticoid prednisolone** used in the suppression of inflammatory and **allergic** disorders. Through the use of different chemical forms and formulation additives, a range of effective anti-inflammatory preparations are available, including tablets, <u>gastro-resistant coated tablets</u>[1], injections, eye drops and **enemas**. The extremely low aqueous solubility of the base prednisolone and its acetate salt makes these forms useful in tablet and slowly absorbed intramuscular suspension injection forms, whilst the soluble sodium phosphate salt enables preparation of a soluble tablet form and solutions for eye and ear drops, enemas and intravenous injections. The analgesic paracetamol is also available in a range of dosage forms and strengths to meet the specific needs of the user, including tablets, dispersible tablets, **paediatric** soluble tablets, paediatric oral solution, sugar-free oral solution, oral suspension, double strength oral suspension and suppositories.

In addition, whilst many new drugs based on low molecular weight organic compounds continue to be discovered and transformed into medicinal products, the development of drugs from biotechnology is increasing and the importance of these therapeutic agents is growing. Such active compounds are macromolecular and of relatively high molecular weight, and include materials such as peptides, proteins and viral components. These drug substances present different and complex challenges in their formulation and processing into medicines because of their alternative biological, chemical and structural properties. Nevertheless, the underlying principles of dosage form design remain applicable.

At present, these therapeutic agents are principally formulated into **parenteral** and respiratory dosage forms, although other routes of administration are being considered and researched. Delivery of these biotechnologically based drug substances via these routes of administration imposes additional **constraints**

on the selection of appropriate formulation excipients.

Another growing area of clinically important medicines is that of polymer therapeutics. These agents include designed macromolecular drugs, polymer-drug and polymer-protein conjugates as nanomedicines, generally in injection form. These agents can also provide drug-targeting features (e.g. treating specific cancers) as well as modified pharmacokinetic profiles (e.g. changed drug metabolism and elimination kinetics).

It is therefore apparent that before a drug substance can be successfully formulated into a dosage form, many factors must be considered. These can be broadly grouped into three categories:

(1) Biopharmaceutical considerations, including factors affecting the absorption of the drug substance from different administration routes;

(2) Drug factors, such as the physical and chemical properties of the drug molecules;

(3) Therapeutic considerations, including consideration of the clinical indication to be treated and patient factors.

High-quality and efficacious medicines will be formulated and prepared only when all these factors are considered and related to each other. This is the underlying principle of dosage form design.

2. Biopharmaceutical Aspects of Dosage Form Design

Biopharmaceutics can be regarded as the study of the relationship between the physical, chemical and biological sciences applied to drugs, dosage forms and drug action. Clearly, understanding the principles of this subject is important in dosage form design, particularly with regard to drug absorption, as well as drug distribution, metabolism and excretion. In general, a drug substance must be in solution before it can be absorbed via absorbing membranes and epithelia of the skin, gastrointestinal tract and lungs into body fluids. Drugs are absorbed in two general ways: by passive diffusion and by carrier-mediated transport mechanisms. In passive diffusion, which is thought to control the absorption of many drugs, the process is driven by the concentration gradient existing across the cellular barrier, with drug molecules passing from regions of high concentration to regions of low concentration. Lipid solubility and the degree of ionization of the drug at the absorbing site influence the rate of diffusion. Recent research into carrier-mediated transport mechanisms has provided much information and knowledge, providing guidance in some cases for the design of new drug molecules. Several specialized transport mechanisms are postulated, including active and facilitated transport. Once absorbed, the drug can exert a therapeutic effect either locally or at a site of action remote from the site of administration. In the latter case the drug has to be transported in body fluids.

When the dosage form is designed to deliver drugs via the buccal, respiratory, rectal, intramuscular or subcutaneous routes, the drug passes directly into the circulating blood from absorbing tissues, whilst the intravenous route provides the most direct route of all.[2] When a drug is delivered by the oral route, onset of drug action will be delayed because of the required transit time in the gastrointestinal tract before absorption, the absorption process and factors associated with hepatoenteric blood circulation. The physical form of the oral dosage form will also influence the absorption rate and onset of action, with solutions acting faster than suspensions, which in turn generally act faster than capsules and tablets. Dosage forms can thus be listed in order of the time of onset of the therapeutic effect. However, all drugs irrespective of their delivery route remain foreign to the human body, and distribution, metabolism and elimination processes commence immediately following drug absorption until the drug is eliminated from the body via the **urine, faeces, saliva**, skin or lungs in unchanged or metabolized form.

3. Drug Factors in Dosage Form Design

Each type of dosage form requires careful study of the physical and chemical properties of drug substances to achieve a stable, efficacious product. These properties, such as dissolution, crystal size and **polymorphic** form, solid-state stability and drug–additive interaction, can have profound effects on the physiological availability and physical and chemical stability of the drug. Through combination of such information and knowledge with that from pharmacological and biochemical studies, the most suitable drug form and additives can be selected for the formulation of chosen dosage forms.

Variations in physicochemical properties, occurring, for example, between batches of the same material or resulting from alternative treatment procedures, can modify the formulation requirements, as well as processing and dosage form performance. For instance, the fine milling of poorly water-soluble drug substances can modify their wetting and dissolution characteristics, important properties during granulation and product performance respectively.[3] Careful evaluation of these properties is therefore important in dosage form design and processing, as well as for product performance.

4. Therapeutic Considerations in Dosage Form Design

The nature of the clinical indication, disease or illness for which the drug is intended is an important factor when one is selecting the range of dosage forms to be prepared. Factors such as the need for systemic or local therapy, duration of action required, and whether the drug will be used in emergency situations need to be considered. In the vast majority of cases, a single drug substance is prepared in a number of dosage forms to satisfy both the particular preferences of the patient or physician and the specific needs of a certain clinical situation. For example, many **asthmatic** patients use **inhalation aerosols**, from which the drug is rapidly available to the **constricted** airways following deep inhalation for rapid emergency relief, and oral products for chronic therapy.

Interest has grown in the design of drug-containing formulations which deliver drugs to specific 'targets' in the body (e.g. the use of **liposomes** and nanoparticles), as well as providing drugs over longer periods at controlled rates. Alternative technologies for preparing particles with the required properties-crystal engineering-provide new opportunities. Supercritical fluid processing using carbon dioxide as a solvent or antisolvent is one such method,[4] allowing fine-tuning of crystal properties and particle design and fabrication. Undoubtedly, these new technologies and others, as well as **sophisticated** formulations, will be required to deal with the advent of gene therapy and the need to deliver such labile macromolecules to specific targets and cells in the body. Interest is also likely to be directed to individual patient requirements such as age, weight and physiological and metabolic factors, features which can influence drug absorption and bioavailability, and the increasing application of diagnostic agents will play a key role in this area.

5. Summary

The formulation of drugs into dosage forms requires the interpretation and application of a wide range of information and knowledge from several study areas. Whilst the physical and chemical properties of drugs and additives need to be understood, the factors influencing drug absorption and the requirements of the disease to be treated also have to be taken into account when potential delivery routes are being identified. The formulation and associated preparation of dosage forms demand the highest standards, with careful examination, analysis and evaluation of wide-ranging information by pharmaceutical scientists to achieve the objective of creating high-quality, safe and efficacious dosage forms.

Word Study

1. aerosol ['eərəsɒl] *n.* 气雾剂
2. allergic [ə'lɜːdʒɪk] *adj.* 过敏的
3. asthmatic [æs'mætɪk] *adj.* 哮喘的
4. biopharmaceutical [baɪɒfɑːməs'juːtɪkl] *adj.* 生物药剂学的
5. buccal ['bʌkəl] *adj.* 颊的,口(腔)的
6. commence [kə'mens] *v.* 开始,着手
7. compactability [kəmpæktə'bɪlɪtɪ] *n.* 可压性,紧实性
8. conjugate ['kɒndʒəgeɪt] *n.* 偶联物,轭合物
9. constraint [kən'streɪnt] *n.* 约束,强制
10. constricted [kən'strɪktɪd] *adj.* 狭窄的,收缩的
11. enema ['enəmə] *n.* 灌肠剂
12. epithelia [ˌepə'θiːlɪə] *n.* (*pl.*) 上皮细胞(单数 epithelium)
13. excipient [ɪk'sɪpɪənt] *n.* 辅料,赋形剂
14. faeces ['fiːsiːz] *n.* 粪便,排泄物
15. glucocorticoid [gluːkəʊ'kɔːtɪkɔɪd] *n.* 糖(肾上腺)皮质激素
16. hepatoenteric [hɪpɑː'təʊnterɪk] *adj.* 肝小肠的
17. inhalation [ˌɪnhə'leɪʃn] *n.* 吸入,吸入药剂
18. kinetics [kɪ'netɪks] *n.* 动力学
19. liposomes [lɪ'pʊsəʊmz] *n.* 脂质体
20. metabolism [mə'tæbəlɪzəm] *n.* 新陈代谢
21. milling ['mɪlɪŋ] *n.* 磨,制粉
22. onset ['ɒnset] *n.* 开始
23. paediatric [ˌpiːdi'ætrɪk] *adj.* 儿科的,儿科医学的(＝pediatric＜美＞)
24. parenteral [pə'rentərəl] *adj.* 肠胃外的,不经肠道的,非肠胃的,注射用药物的
25. polymer ['pɒlɪmə(r)] *n.* 聚合体
26. polymorphic [ˌpɒli'mɔːfɪk] *adj.* 多形性的
27. postulate ['pɒstjuleɪt] *vt.* 要求,假定
28. prednisolone [pred'nɪsələʊn] *n.* 泼尼松龙,氢化泼尼松
29. rectal ['rektəl] *adj.* 直肠的
30. saliva [sə'laɪvə] *n.* 唾液
31. sophisticated [sə'fɪstɪkeɪtɪd] *adj.* 精密的,复杂的
32. subcutaneous [ˌsʌbkju'teɪnɪəs] *adj.* 皮下的
33. transit ['trænzɪt] *n.* 运输,经过
34. urine ['jʊərɪn] *n.* 尿,小便

Notes

1. gastro-resistant coated tablets：肠溶片,即 enteric-coated tablets。句中 "gastro-resistant" 的意思是防止在胃部环境中溶解或崩解。在药剂中,通过在片剂外面包裹一层肠溶衣,有利于防止药物在胃

酸中降解,或者避免药物对胃的不利影响。

2. When the dosage form is designed to deliver drugs via the buccal, respiratory, rectal, intramuscular or subcutaneous routes, the drug passes directly into the circulating blood from absorbing tissues, whilst the intravenous route provides the most direct route of all. 译为:当剂型设计为经口腔、呼吸道、直肠、肌肉或皮下途径给药时,药物从吸收组织直接进入血液循环,而静脉注射则是上述所有给药方式中最为直接的一种途径。不同的药物剂型针对不同的疾病产生不同的药物吸收,静脉注射直接将药物注射入血液,不存在吸收的过程,是最为直接的给药途径。

3. The fine milling of poorly water-soluble drug substances can modify their wetting and dissolution characteristics, important properties during granulation and product performance respectively. 译为:对水溶性差的药物进行精细研磨,可以改变它们的润湿性和溶出性,这两个性质分别对于制粒过程和产品性能至关重要。这里的"important properties"为"wetting and dissolution characteristics"的同位语,指代前面所述两种特性,其中药物的润湿性是制粒过程中的重要参数,而溶出性又将影响药物的体内溶出行为,继而影响其吸收和生物利用度。

4. Supercritical fluid processing using carbon dioxide as a solvent or antisolvent is one such method. 译为:使用二氧化碳作为溶剂或反溶剂的超临界流体处理就是这样一种技术。超临界流体是一种物质状态,当物质在超过临界温度及临界压力时,气体与液体的性质趋近于类似,最后会达成一个均匀相的流体现象。超临界流体类似气体具有可压缩性,可以像气体一样发生泻流,而且又兼具有类似液体的流动性。超临界流体适合作为工业和实验室过程中的溶剂,而且可以取代许多有机溶剂。二氧化碳和水是最常用的超临界流体。

Exercises

1. Decide whether each of the following statements is true (T) or false (F) according to the passage.

(1) The excipients have been used as many specialized pharmaceutical functions.

(2) Dosage forms should not be independent of patient-to-patient variation.

(3) The most suitable dosage of the drug is often carefully selected in order to obtain the optimize the bioavailability.

(4) The physical form of the oral dosage form will influence the absorption rate and onset of action.

(5) Diagnostic agents are considered to be not suitable for using in the absorption of the drug.

(6) The formulation of drugs into dosage forms requires the interpretation and application of a wide range of information and knowledge from several study areas.

2. Questions for oral discussion.

(1) What is the principal objective of dosage form design?

(2) Why does inhalation therapy work quickly for asthmatic patients compared with oral pathway?

(3) How do you understand biopharmaceutics?

(4) Why can the same drug be prepared into different dosage forms?

3. Choose the best answer to each of the following questions.

(1) The effects of excipients include _____.

   A. solubilizing

   B. modifying dissolution

   C. improving the flavour of drug substances

   D. all of the above

(2) Which of the following belongs to the drug factors in dosage form design?

A. Carrier.   B. Drug loading.

C. Solubility.   D. Inhalation.

(3) The effect of fine milling of poorly water-soluble drug substances is to _____.

A. reduce particle size   B. change wetting property

C. modify dissolution characteristics   D. all of the above

(4) Which of the following is the fastest-release dosage form?

A. Suspension.   B. Capsule.

C. Solution.   D. Tablet.

(5) Which of the following is considered to be the most important aspect when designing the dosage form?

A. Delivery routes.   B. Drug absorption.

C. Compatibility.   D. Bioavailability.

(6) Which of the following routes of administration will involve the absorption of drugs?

A. i.v. injection.

B. i.v. infusion.

C. Subcutaneous injection, transdermal and oral.

D. None of the above.

(7) What factors must be considered before a drug substance can be successfully formulated into a dosage form?

A. Biopharmaceutical considerations, including factors affecting the absorption of the drug substance from different administration routes.

B. Drug factors, such as the physical and chemical properties of the drug substance.

C. Therapeutic considerations, including consideration of the clinical indication to be treated and patient factors.

D. All of the above.

(8) Which of the following statements is false?

A. The analgesic paracetamol has many dosage forms.

B. Drugs are absorbed in two general ways: by passive diffusion and by carrier-mediated transport mechanisms.

C. Inhalation aerosols are the main dosage form for asthmatic patients.

D. For some drugs, the manufacturing processes, labelling and packaging are not required.

(9) According to the route of administration, the dosage form can be divided into _____.

A. subcutaneous and parenteral

B. pulmonary drug delivery system and target drug delivery system

C. parenteral and non-parenteral

D. gastro-resistant coated tablets and injections

(10) Which of the following statements is true?

A. Biopharmaceutics can be regarded as the study of the dosage form and characteristics of drug.

B. Disease or illness for which the drug is intended is an important factor when selecting the range of dosage forms to be prepared.

C. The factors influencing drug absorption and the requirements of the disease to be treated don't need to be taken into account.

D. The drug passes directly into the circulating blood from absorbing tissues when dosage form is designed for i.v. injection.

4. **Please choose an appropriate form of a word from the list below to complete the following sentences based on their meanings.**

> administration, target, damage, formulate, taste, foundation, swallow, dosage, stability, optimization

(1) The study of pharmaceutics provides the scientific _____ for the design and appropriate use of dosage forms and drug delivery systems.

(2) A _____ form is the form that we take our drug in-in other words, a tablet, a syrup, an ointment, or an injection.

(3) Pharmaceutics is a science that applies both drug chemistry and drug biology to the problem of delivering drugs to their _____ tissues.

(4) During the preformulation process, key chemical and physical properties of the drug are studied in order to rationally design a delivery system and predict the fate of the drug *in vivo* after _____ .

(5) Dosage forms should be _____ such that the dose is contained in a unit that can be counted or measured by the patient with reasonable accuracy.

(6) Many drugs are bitter or salty, so we add sweeteners and flavors to mask their _____ .

(7) Parenteral drugs (injections) and drugs for application to mucous membranes must be comfortable enough to prevent tissue _____ or loss of drug from the site.

(8) _____ is defined as the extent to which a product retains the same properties and characteristics that it possessed at the time of its preparation or manufacture.

(9) Drugs that will be used for children or elderly patients should be available in liquid dosage forms that can be easily _____ .

(10) The design of a drug delivery system to control the dissolution or diffusion of a drug allows _____ of how fast, how much and how long the drug moves to the drug target.

5. **Translate the following sentences and paragraphs into Chinese.**

(1) It is the formulation additives that, among other things, solubilize, suspend, thicken, preserve, emulsify, modify dissolution, increase the compactability and improve the flavour of drug substances to form various medicines or dosage forms.

(2) The principal objective of dosage form design is to achieve a predictable therapeutic response to a drug included in a formulation which can be manufactured on a large scale with reproducible product quality.

(3) Ideally, dosage forms should also be independent of patient-to-patient variation, although in practice this feature remains difficult to achieve.

(4) Many drugs are formulated into several dosage forms of various strengths, each having selected pharmaceutical characteristics which are suitable for a specific application.

(5) At present, these therapeutic agents are principally formulated into parenteral and respiratory dosage forms, although other routes of administration are being considered and researched.

(6) Apart from the intravenous route of administration, where a drug is introduced directly into the blood circulation, all other routes of administration involve the absorption of drug from the site of administration into the blood circulation. Drugs must be absorbed in a sufficient quantity and at a sufficient rate to achieve a certain plasma concentration which, in turn, will produce an appropriate concentration of drug at its site(s) of action to elicit the desired therapeutic response.

(7) According to the definition of bioavailability, an administered dose of a particular drug in an oral dosage form will be 100% bioavailable only if: ⅰ) the drug is completely released from the dosage form into solution in the gastrointestinal fluids; ⅱ) the released drug must be completely stable in the gastrointestinal fluids and all of the drug must pass through the gastrointestinal barrier into the mesenteric circulation without being metabolized; ⅲ) all of the absorbed drug must enter the systemic circulation without being metabolized on passing through the liver.

Value-Oriented Reflective Reading

The Story of Inhaled Insulin

"Wait, you can inhale insulin? Isn't that something you have to inject?"

Good question! And the answer is that until the early part of the 21st century, shots were the only way to administer insulin. But an inhalable version of this life-sustaining drug has been in the works for decades, and finally came to market successfully in 2015.

The road to inhalable insulin

For over 85 years after the 1921 discovery of lifesaving liquid insulin, scientists were struggling to find a viable way to get insulin into the bodies of people with diabetes without needles.

Naturally, the idea of an insulin inhaler, similar to an asthma inhaler, was an appealing prospect. But it wasn't until new technologies appeared on the scene in the late 1990s that researchers could really begin to experiment with turning insulin into a concentrated powder with particles sized for inhalation into the lungs.

Exubera, developed by San Francisco-based Nektar Therapeutics, became the first inhaled insulin product to be marketed in 2006 by pharma giant Pfizer. Although you would expect unbridled enthusiasm for an inhalable form of insulin, unfortunately, Exubera was a flop and pulled from market just a year after its introduction in 2007.

Why Exubera failed

In a way, Exubera lived up to its name. Pfizer was positively "exuberant" about the financial gains expected from this new no-needle method for delivering insulin. They were so sure it would be the next 'blockbuster drug' that they plowed ahead, bringing the product to market in complete denial of indications that the inhaler may not appeal to patients.

In fact, we know from reporting in the *Wall Street Journal* (华尔街日报) that Pfizer sought basically zero input from patients on the design of the device, and the few doctors who expressed reservations about the difficulty of use were summarily ignored.

The problem was, the inhaler was large and clunky—a bit larger than a full-size flashlight, making it embarrassing to use in public, to say the least. Not to mention the inconvenience of carrying it around, especially for men who don't typically carry purses. Also, the foil powder packets (measured in 3 or 9 milligrams) were easily mixed up and confusing to patients and doctors to equate to familiar dosing levels.

In the end, Exubera was a $2.8 billion flop—one of the pharmaceutical industry's costliest failures ever. And it seems quite clear that the "unlivable" design of the inhaler was the core problem.

How Afrezza is different

Although commercialization of Exubera was ultimately unsuccessful, innovation with regard to inhaled insulin continued. The newest inhaled insulin, Afrezza, is quite another story. It is made by California-based MannKind Corp. After several attempts to get this through the Food and Drug Administration (FDA), Afrezza finally came to market in early 2015. This followed years of soliciting patient input and whittling the device down to the size of a little whistle dubbed 'Dreamboat'.

Afrezza appears to have key advantages over Exubera. Its delivery system is small, sleek, and dosed in units and provides a simple dosing conversion chart, whereas Exubera's delivery system was large, awkward, and dosed in milligrams. The modifications implemented with Afrezza allow for a more discreet administration process and a dosing regimen that is easier for both prescribers and patients to comprehend.

Summary

As new adverse effects and concerns emerged, and competition from therapeutic alternatives is at an all-time high, Afrezza will continue to face an uphill battle for success.

Whatever, Exubera was unable to succeed, Afrezza still has a chance to positively affect patient care, but time is of the utmost importance. The biggest lesson we learn from the failure of Exubera is: involve patients (the people who will have to live with the drug or device) from the very beginning of product conceptualization, and focus on their real-life concerns throughout.

Questions for discussion:

1. What makes Afrezza different from Exubera?
2. What will be the priority concern when you design a drug or a medical device?
3. Based on the passage, what do you learn from Exubera besides its commercial failure?

Text B
Formulation and Advanced Drug Delivery Systems

"Drugs" taken by a patient exert a biological function by interacting with specific receptors at the site of action. The drug is intended to be delivered to the target site at a certain rate and concentration, which minimizes the side effects and maximizes the therapeutic effect. Human body presents great barriers against drug delivery and targeting which render an otherwise potent drug ineffective *in vivo*. Dosage forms thus serve many purposes including facilitating drug administration and improving drug delivery. Traditional and classical dosage forms mainly include injections, oral formulations (solutions, suspension, tablets, and capsules), topical creams and ointments. Unfortunately, most traditional dosage forms are unable to facilitate adequate drug absorption, gain access to the target site, prevent nonspecific drug distribution and premature metabolism and excretion, or match drug input with the dose requirement. Therefore, alternative routes of drug administration and advanced drug delivery systems are proposed to meet these delivery challenges and improve drug therapy.

Advanced drug delivery systems are defined as a formulation or device that delivers drugs to a specific site in the body at a certain rate. Advanced drug delivery systems usually represent a more sophisticated system that incorporates advanced technologies such as controlled, **pulsatile**, targeted, or bioresponsive drug delivery. This chapter aims to introduce the currently available delivery systems and advanced drug delivery systems under development.

1. Controlled Drug Delivery

Controlled drug delivery is defined as the delivery of drug or active pharmaceutical ingredient (API) in the body at a predetermined rate. A controlled drug delivery system is therefore one that provides **temporal** or **spatial** control or both over drug delivery in the body.

(1) Implant

An implant is a single unit drug delivery system designed for delivering drug at predetermined rate over an extended period of time. For example, drugs can be mixed with either nondegradable or biodegradable polymers. The resulting polymeric matrix can be surgically implanted to achieve controlled drug release *in vivo*. Implants help eliminate the need for continuous intravenous infusion or repeated injections for maintaining therapeutic drug concentrations, which greatly improves patient compliance by reducing or eliminating the patient-involved dosing.[1]

(2) Osmotic Pump

An **osmotic** pump is usually composed of a core tablet surrounded by a semipermeable membrane containing a laser-created hole. The core tablet contains two layers, one with drug and the other with the electrolyte. When the tablet is swallowed, the semipermeable membrane permits the entry of fluid from the stomach and intestines to the tablet, which dissolves/suspends the drug. As pressure increases due to the inward diffusion of water molecules, drug is pumped out of the tablet through the hole. Thus, drug delivery is controlled by the osmotic gradient between the contents of the core tablet and fluids in the gastrointestinal (GI) tract.

2. Advanced Drug Delivery Systems

Representative examples of drug delivery systems designed for different routes of administration are described below.

(1) Buccal Drug Delivery Systems

The buccal and **sublingual** mucosa in the oral cavity provide an excellent alternative for the delivery of drugs. The buccal mucosa offers several advantages for controlled drug delivery: (i) the mucosa is well supplied with both vascular and **lymphatic drainage**; (ii) "first-pass" intestinal/hepatic metabolism and presystemic degradation in the GI tract are avoided; (iii) the area is well suited for a retentive device and is usually acceptable to the patient; and (iv) with the right DDS design, the permeability and the local environment of the mucosa can be controlled and manipulated to accommodate drug permeation.

The most commonly used dosage form through this route is a small tablet, which is designed to dissolve rapidly and be absorbed readily into the systemic circulation. Other dosage forms include gels, adhesive patches for systemic or local mucosal delivery.

(2) Pulmonary Drug Delivery Systems

The respiratory tract including the nasal mucosa, **pharynx**, large and small airway structures (trachea, **bronchi, bronchioles, alveoli**), provides a large mucosal surface for drug absorption, which presents a more convenient way of administration compared with parenteral route.[2] Aerosols are widely used to deliver drugs in the respiratory tract. The deposition of the particles in the respiratory tract is driven by the inhalation regime, the particle size, shape, density, charge, and **hygroscopicity**.

Inhaled medications have been used for years for the treatment of lung diseases, and are widely accepted as the optimal route of administration of first-line therapy for **asthma** and chronic obstructive pulmonary diseases. Aerosols have already been developed to deliver peptide and protein drugs, e.g. gonadotrophin-releasing factor, vasopressin, and insulin. Peptides and proteins easily undergo hydrolysis and degradation in the GI tract due to the presence of various enzymes and stomach acid. Thus, peptide and protein delivery via pulmonary route offers an alternative to parenteral administration, which is considered a better way to deliver proteins and peptides than sticking people with needles.

(3) Transdermal Drug Delivery Systems

The skin has been used for centuries as the site for the topical administration of drugs, but only recently has it been used as a pathway for systemic drug delivery. The skin mainly functions as a barrier to prevent water loss and the entry of external agents. However, some drugs with proper physicochemical properties are proven to penetrate the skin in sufficient amounts to produce a systemic effect. The transdermal route is of particular interest for drugs that have a systemic short elimination half-life or undergo extensive first-pass metabolism, therefore, requiring frequent dosing.[3]

Regarding the fabrication transdermal patches, drugs are often mixed with a polymer matrix or encapsulated within a membrane. An adhesive layer is then impregnated with the drug-containing complex. Placing the patch on the skin allows the drug to diffuse through the skin and into the body. The most widely used so far are **nitroglycerine**-containing patches for **angina,** a transdermal product containing clonidine for **hypertension** as well as the product containing **scopolamine** for motion sickness. A transdermal device containing 17-β-**estradiol** for **postmenopausal** women protects that drug from degradation in the digestive tract.

Current systems can deliver only drugs of proper molecular size and solubility. But with **iontophoresis,** a drug is literally propelled across the skin by a positive electric charge. The use of this system should expand the number of drugs that can be administered transdermally.

3.　Targeted Drug Delivery

Drugs administered by routine parenteral routes are distributed throughout the body and reach nontarget organs/tissues thus leading to extensive adverse effects and low therapeutic efficacy. Most drugs undergo metabolism in the liver and excretion by kidney. As a result, only a small fraction of the administered drug dosage will reach the target (diseased) organ or tissues. The concept of targeted drug delivery was introduced by German chemist Paul Ehrlich more than a century ago. However, making drugs with high therapeutic selectivity or targetability has remained a great challenge for pharmaceutical scientists. The goal of targeted drug delivery is to deliver drugs specifically to diseased organs, tissues and cells while not exposing healthy organs or tissues. Additionally, targeted drug delivery should ensure minimal drug loss during the transit to the target site, protect the drug from metabolism and **premature** clearance, retain the drug at the target site for desired period of time, facilitate the drug transport into target cells and deliver drug to the appropriate intracellular organism.

(1) Carrier-linked Prodrug Strategy

This strategy aims to develop prodrugs by conjugating drug molecules to monoclonal antibodies (mAbs) or ligands for specific recognition and interaction with antigens or receptors expressed on target cell surface. The delivery systems consist of three components: drug, carrier, and the targeting moiety. Carrier-linked prodrugs are obtained by conjugating the drug molecules to low- to high-molecular weight molecules such as sugars, growth factors, antibodies, peptides, natural and synthetic polymers that can transport the drugs to the target site and subsequently release drugs there.

(2) Central Nervous System (CNS) Drug Delivery

Drug delivery to brain remains a great challenge due to the presence of a blood-brain barrier (BBB) regulating the entry of molecules to the brain. <u>The BBB makes the brain inaccessible to CNS-targeted drugs in the systemic circulation, more so for biotherapeutics such as peptides, proteins, and nucleic acids.</u>[4] Transport mechanisms that could be utilized to develop CNS-targeted drug delivery systems include: passive diffusion, active transport, and receptor-mediated transport. The physicochemical properties of the drug molecules are critical to the brain drug delivery. Usually, increasing the hydrophobicity of a drug molecule is likely to increase its transport across the BBB. For low-molecular weight drugs in the range of 400–600 Da, highly lipid soluble molecules such as barbiturate drugs can rapidly cross the BBB into the brain. However, the presence of p-glycoprotein **efflux** pumps will present a major barrier for the passive diffusion of small molecules across the BBB, if those small molecule drugs were substrates for p-**glycoprotein**. Examples include vinblastine, vincristine, and cyclosporine. In addition, drugs that are highly charged or bind strongly to plasma proteins may show low transport efficiency across the BBB.

Over the years, different strategies have been developed to overcome the BBB and achieve brain targeted drug delivery. Polymeric implants, for example, Gliadel® (Guilford Pharmaceuticals, Baltimore, MD), have been developed as an adjunct to surgery for prolonging patient survival with brain tumor. Besides the invasive strategies for local drug delivery to CNS, extensive efforts have been contributed to developing systemic approaches for CNS drug delivery. One strategy to improve poor drug uptake in the brain is to administer compounds as prodrugs that can be shuttled by transporters specifically expressed at the blood-brain barrier. Using this approach, researchers have succeeded in designing drug-carrier conjugates that can specifically interact with glucose transporters (GluT1), amino acid transporters (LAT1) and **choline** transporters, thereby targeting the drugs to the brain.

Word Study

1. alveoli [ˌælˈviəlaɪ] *n.* 肺泡
2. angina [ænˈdʒnə] *n.* 心绞痛
3. asthma [ˈæsmə] *n.* 哮喘
4. bronchi [ˈbrɒŋkaɪ] *n.* 支气管,（尤指肺两侧的）支气管
5. bronchiole [ˈbrɒŋkɪˌəʊl] *n.* 细支气管
6. choline [ˈkəʊliːn] *n.* 胆碱
7. efflux [ˈeflʌks] *n.* 流出，外排
8. estradiol [ˌestrəˈdaɪəʊl] *n.* 雌二醇
9. glycoprotein [ˌglaɪkəʊˈprəʊˌtiːn] *n.* 糖蛋白
10. hygroscopicity [haɪɡrəskɒˈpɪsɪtɪ] *n.* 吸湿性
11. hypertension [ˌhaɪpəˈtenʃn] *n.* 高血压
12. iontophoresis [aɪɒntəfəˈriːsɪs] *n.* 离子导入
13. lymphatic drainage [lɪmˈfætɪk ˈdreɪnɪdʒ] 淋巴引流
14. nitroglycerine [ˌnaɪtrəʊˈɡlɪsəriːn] *n.* 硝酸甘油
15. osmotic [ɒzˈmɒtɪk] *adj.* 渗透的

16. pharynx ['færɪŋks] *n.* 咽

17. postmenopausal [ˌpəʊstmenə'pɔːzəl] *adj.* 绝经后的

18. premature [ˌpriːmə'tʃʊr] *adj.* 过早的，提前的

19. pulsatile ['pʌlsətil] *adj.* 脉冲的，跳动的

20. scopolamine [skəʊ'pɒləmiːn] *n.* 东莨菪碱

21. spatial ['speɪʃl] *adj.* 空间的

22. sublingual [sʌb'lɪŋgwəl] *adj.* 舌下的

23. temporal ['tempərəl] *adj.* 时间的

Notes

1. Implants help eliminate the need for continuous intravenous infusion or repeated injections for maintaining therapeutic drug concentrations, which greatly improves patient compliance by reducing or eliminating the patient-involved dosing. 译为：植入剂有助于减少患者对连续静脉输注或反复注射给药以维持治疗血药浓度的需求，这可通过降低或减少患者参与的给药剂量大大提高患者依从性。

2. The respiratory tract including the nasal mucosa, pharynx, large and small airway structures (trachea, bronchi, bronchioles, alveoli), provides a large mucosal surface for drug absorption, which presents a more convenient way of administration compared with parenteral route. 译为：呼吸道由鼻黏膜、咽、大小气道（气管、支气管、细支气管、肺泡）等结构组成，为药物的吸收提供了较大的黏膜表面，比肠外途径给药更方便。

3. The transdermal route is of particular interest for drugs that have a systemic short elimination half-life or undergo extensive first-pass metabolism, therefore, requiring frequent dosing. 译为：透皮给药途径对于全身消除半衰期短或易于受首过代谢影响的药物特别有意义，因此需要频繁给药。

4. The BBB makes the brain inaccessible to CNS-targeted drugs in the systemic circulation, more so for biotherapeutics such as peptides, proteins, and nucleic acids. 译为：血脑屏障使大脑无法在体循环中接触靶向中枢神经药物，对于生物治疗类药物如多肽、蛋白和核酸的屏障作用更为突出。BBB 意为"血脑屏障"，是 blood-brain barrier 的缩写。"more so" 后面引导的为省略句式，补充完整为 "The BBB makes the brain more inaccessible to biotherapeutics such as peptides, proteins, and nucleic acids"。

Supplementary Parts

1. Medical and Pharmaceutical Terminology (6): Common Morphemes in English Terms for Pharmaceutics

Morpheme	Meaning	Example
aero	气体	aerosol 气溶胶,气雾剂,烟雾剂
amphi	二、两栖	amphiphilic agent 两亲剂
anti	抗	antioxidant 抗氧化剂
de	去、脱	defoamer 消泡剂
lip	脂肪	lipophilic 亲脂性的
lyo	液体	lyophilic 亲液性的
lyt	溶解	carcinolytic 溶癌的
morph	形态、形状	amorphous 无定形的,无组织的

续表

Morpheme	Meaning	Example
oleo	油	oleophilic 亲油性的
philic	亲	amphiphilic agent 两亲剂
phobic	害怕、疏远	hydrophobic 狂犬病的,恐水病的,患恐水病的,疏水的
solv	溶解	dissolve 溶解
therm	热	thermostat 恒温器

(1) Write down different prefixes or suffixes according to the Chinese meanings, and then give one sample word using the same prefix or suffix.

Meaning	Prefix or suffix	Sample word	Meaning
剂,者	ant	coagulant	凝血剂
反对,相反,抗			
霉菌素			
灌肠剂			

(2) Fill in the blanks with the missing word root, prefix or suffix.

1) pro_____   普鲁卡因

2) fungi_____   杀真菌剂

3) _____foamer   去泡剂

4) vermi_____   驱蠕虫药

5) _____in   胰岛素

6) _____philic   亲脂性的

7) _____philic   亲液性的

8) carcino_____   溶癌的

9) _____philic   亲油性的

10) tuberculo_____   结核菌抑制药

11) dis_____   溶解

12) hydro_____   狂犬病的

2. English-Chinese Translation Skills: 药学英语翻译技巧 (2): 句子成分转换

英汉两种语言的句子结构基本相同,有主语、谓语、宾语和定语、状语、补语等,但是不同的句子成分表达方式不完全相同,因此在翻译过程中,常常需要转换句子成分,才能使译文通顺、易懂。句子成分转换法是把英语句子某一成分(如主语)译成汉语句子另一成分(如宾语)等。在多数情况下,词性转换会导致句子成分的转换,句子成分转换法的目的是使译文通顺,更加符合汉语习惯,如下。

例 1：The concentration of drug in blood plasma depends on <u>numerous factors</u>. <u>These</u> include the relative amount of an administered dose that enters the systemic circulation, the rate at which this occurs, the rate and extent of distribution of the drug between the systemic circulation and other tissues and fluids and the rate of elimination of the drug from the body.

参考译文：很多因素决定着血浆中的药物浓度，包括所用药物进入体循环的相对的量，进入的速度，体循环、其他组织及体液之间分布的速度和广度，以及药物从体内排出的速度。

说明：例句原文有两个小句说明决定血浆药物浓度的因素，为了保持语篇结构平衡，numerous factors 作第一小句的宾语，第二句主语用 these，衔接上一小句。在翻译成汉语时，numerous factors 变成了主语，原句第二句主语 these 则省略了，这样的句子成分转换符合汉语言表达习惯。

例 2：Finally, all of the absorbed drug must pass into the systemic circulation <u>without being metabolized on passing through the liver</u>.

参考译文：最后，所有的药物都必须能够进入体循环而不在通过肝脏时被代谢掉。

说明：原例句有两个介词短语 without being metabolized 和 on passing through the liver，语法功能都是状语，在译成汉语时，第二个介词短语保持时间状语功能："在通过肝脏时"，而第一个介词短语则转换成了动词结构"不……被代谢掉"，符合汉语表达习惯。

例 3：Prolonged presence close to the site of the action, improved drug bioavailability, and easier administration of large drug doses <u>belong to</u> the benefits of pellets.

参考译文：微丸有助于延长药物在目标作用部位的作用时间、提高药物的生物利用度，且易于大剂量药物的服用。

说明：原句是一个倒装句结构，谓语动词是 belong to，在翻译成汉语时，为了符合汉语表达习惯，原句的宾语成分 the benefit of pellets 变成了主语，而且省略了谓语成分 belong to，将宾语成分中的名词 benefits 译成了动词"有助于"，避免了类似"微丸的好处包括……"这样生硬的译法。原句主语成分有三个名词词组：prolonged presence close to the site of the action、improved drug bioavailability 和 easier administration of large drug doses，其中，非谓语动词 prolonged 和 improved 作定语，翻译成汉语时都转换成了动词。

句子成分转换是英汉翻译过程中的一个技巧，属于直译策略。药学英语翻译首先还是要对原文句子结构，包括不同语法成分的功能准确理解，不要被句子表层结构限制，拘泥于句子的结构形式，而应把重点放在传达原文逻辑意义上，灵活使用句子成分转换法。

（张维芬　庄　婕　符　垚　史志祥　龚长华）

Unit Seven

Pharmaceutical Analysis

Unit Seven
数字内容

Drug analysis has evolved from a special technique of the 20th century into an ever-maturing science. By utilizing the methodologies and techniques in physics, chemistry, biology and microbiology, pharmaceutical analysis focuses on qualitative and quantitative analysis of drugs, quality control and development of new drugs. This science relates to a wide range of studies, including quality control, clinical pharmacy, analysis of traditional Chinese medicine and natural drugs, drug metabolic analysis, forensic toxicological analysis, doping control and formulation analysis, etc. Pharmaceutical analysis assumes the most important task in drug quality control, which involves physical and chemical inspection of finished drugs, quality control in drug production, quality observation in storage, rapid analysis of preparations formulated in hospitals, establishment of quality standards in the R & D of novel drugs as well as the analysis of drugs *in vivo*. With the vigorous development of pharmaceutical science, the science of pharmaceutical analysis is facing increasing challenges from various related sciences. Instead of being only limited to static quality control of drugs, it has developed into a comprehensive and dynamic analytical study on drug manufacturing, *in-vivo* dynamics and metabolism.

药物分析从 20 世纪初的一种专门技术,逐步发展成为一门日臻成熟的科学。它运用物理学、化学、生物学和微生物学等方法和技术,研究药物的定性和定量分析、药物的质量控制和新药开发。该学科涉及的研究范围包括药品质量控制、临床药学、中药与天然药物分析、药物代谢分析、法医毒物分析、兴奋剂检测和药物制剂分析等。药物分析在药品的质量控制中担任着最主要的任务,包括药物成品的理化检验、药物生物过程中的质量控制、药物贮存过程中的质量控制、医院调配制剂的快速分析、新药研究开发中的质量标准制订以及体内药物分析等。随着药学科学的迅猛发展,各相关学科对药物分析科不断提出新的要求。它已不再仅仅局限于对药物进行静态的质量控制,而是发展到对制药过程、生物体内和代谢过程进行评价和动态分析研究。

Text A
What Do Analytical Chemists Do?

Analytical chemistry is concerned with the chemical characterization of matter and the answers to two important questions: what is it (**qualitative**) and how much is it (**quantitative**). Chemicals make up everything we use or consume, and knowledge of the chemical composition of many substances is important in our daily lives. Analytical chemistry plays an important role in nearly all aspects of chemistry, for example, agricultural, clinical, environmental, **forensic**, manufacturing, **metallurgical**, and pharmaceutical chemistry. The nitrogen content of a fertilizer determines its value. Food must be analyzed for contaminants (e.g. pesticide residues) and for essential nutrients (e.g. vitamin content). The air in cities must be analyzed for carbon monoxide. Blood glucose must be monitored in diabetics (and, in fact, most diseases are diagnosed by chemical analysis). The presence of trace elements from gun powder on a murder defendant's hand will prove a gun was fired. The quality of manufactured products often depends on proper chemical proportions, and measurement of the constituents is a necessary part of quality control. The carbon content of steel will determine its quality. The purity of drugs will determine their efficacy. Here, we will describe the tools and techniques for performing these different types of analysis.

What is Analytical Science?

The above description of analytical chemistry provides an overview of the discipline of analytical chemistry. There have been various attempts to define the discipline more specifically. The late Charles N. Reilley said: "Analytical chemistry is what analytical chemists do." The discipline has expanded beyond the bounds of just chemistry, and many have advocated using the name *analytical science* to describe the field. This term is used in a National Science Foundation report from workshops on "Curricular Developments in the Analytical Sciences." Even this term falls short of recognition of the role of instrumentation development and application. One suggestion is that we use the term analytical science and technology.

The Federation of European Chemical Societies held a contest to define analytical chemistry, and the following suggestion by K. Cammann was selected.

Analytical chemistry provides the methods and tools needed for insight into our material world for answering four basic questions about a material sample:

- What?
- Where?
- How much?
- What arrangement, structure or form?

These questions cover qualitative, spatial, quantitative, and speciation aspects of analytical science. The Division of Analytical Chemistry of the American Chemical Society provides a comprehensive definition of analytical chemistry, which may be found on their website. It is reproduced in most part here:

Analytical chemistry seeks ever improved means of measuring the chemical composition of natural and artificial materials. The techniques of this science are used to identify the substances which may be present in a material and to determine the exact amounts of the identified substance.

Analytical chemists work to improve the reliability of existing techniques to meet the demands for better chemical measurements which arise constantly in our society. They adopt proven methodologies to new kinds of materials or to answer new questions about their composition and their reactivity mechanisms.[1] They carry out research to discover completely new principles of measurement and are at the forefront of the utilization of major discoveries, such as lasers and microchip devices for practical purposes. Their efforts serve the needs of many fields:

- In medicine, analytical chemistry is the basis for clinical laboratory tests which help physicians diagnose disease and chart progress in recovery.

- In industry, analytical chemistry provides the means of testing raw materials and for assuring the quality of finished products whose chemical composition is critical. Many household products, fuels, paints, pharmaceuticals, etc. are analyzed by the procedures developed by analytical chemists before being sold to the consumer.

- Environmental quality is often evaluated by testing for suspected contaminants using the techniques of analytical chemistry.

- The nutritional value of food is determined by chemical analysis for major components such as protein and **carbohydrates** and trace components such as vitamins and minerals. Indeed, even the calories in a food are often calculated from its chemical analysis. Analytical chemists also make important contributions to fields as diverse as forensics, **archaeology**, and space science.[2]

Qualitative and Quantitative Analyses: What does Each Tell Us?

The discipline of analytical chemistry consists of qualitative analysis and quantitative analysis. The former deals with the identification of elements, ions, or compounds present in a sample (we may be interested in whether only a given substance is present), while the latter deals with the determination of how much of one or more constituents is present. The sample may be solid, liquid, gas, or a mixture. The presence of gunpowder residue on a hand generally requires only qualitative knowledge, not of how much is there, but the price of coal will be determined by the percentage of sulfur **impurity** present.

Qualitative tests may be performed by selective chemical reactions or with the use of instrumentation. The formation of a white precipitate when adding a solution of silver nitrate to a dissolved sample indicates the presence of chloride. Certain chemical reactions will produce colors to indicate the presence of classes of organic compounds, for example, ketones. Infrared spectra will give "fingerprints" of organic compounds or their functional groups.

A clear distinction should be made between the terms selective and specific:

- A selective reaction or test is one that can occur with other substances but exhibits a degree of preference for the substance of interest.[3]

- A specific reaction or test is one that occurs only with the substance of interest.

Unfortunately, few reactions are specific but many exhibit selectivity. Selectivity may be achieved by a number of strategies. Some examples are:

- Sample preparation (e.g., **extractions, precipitation**).

- Instrumentation (selective detectors).

- Target **analyte** derivatization (e.g., derivatize specific functional groups with detecting reagents).

- **Chromatography**, which provides powerful separation.

For quantitative analysis, a history of the sample composition will often be known (it is known that blood contains glucose), or else the analyst will have performed a qualitative test prior to performing the more difficult quantitative analysis. Modern chemical measurement systems often exhibit sufficient selectivity that a quantitative measurement can also serve as a qualitative measurement. However, simple qualitative tests are usually more rapid than quantitative procedures. Qualitative analysis is composed of two fields: inorganic and organic. The former is usually covered in introductory chemistry courses, whereas the latter is best left until after the student has had a course in organic chemistry.[4]

In comparing qualitative versus quantitative analysis, consider, for example, the sequence of analytical procedures followed in testing for banned substances at the Olympic Games. The list of prohibited substances includes about 500 different active constituents: stimulants, steroids, beta-blockers, diuretics, narcotics, analgesics, local anesthetics, and sedatives. Some are detectable only as their **metabolites**. Many athletes must be tested rapidly, and it is not practical to perform a detailed quantitative analysis on each. There are three phases in the analysis: the fast-screening phase, the identification phase, and possible quantification phase. In the fast-screening phase, urine samples are rapidly tested for the presence of classes of compounds that will differentiate them from "normal" samples, using various techniques including **immunoassays**, gas chromatography, and liquid chromatography. About 5% of the samples may indicate the presence of unknown compounds that may or may not be prohibited but need to be identified. Samples showing a suspicious profile during the screening undergo a new preparation cycle (possible **hydrolysis**, extraction, derivatization), depending on the nature of the compounds that have been detected. The compounds are then identified using the highly selective combination of **gas chromatography/mass spectrometry (GC/MS)** or liquid chromatography/mass spectrometry (LC/MS). In this technique, complex mixtures are separated by gas chromatography or high performance liquid chromatography (HPLC), and they are then detected by mass spectrometry, which provides molecular structural data on the compounds. The MS data, combined with the time of **elution** from the gas chromatography or HPLC, provide a high probability of the presence of a given detected compound. GC/MS or LC/MS is expensive and time-consuming, and so it is used only when necessary. Following the identification phase, some compounds must be precisely quantified since they may normally be present at low levels, for example, from food, pharmaceutical preparations, or endogenous steroids, and elevated levels must be confirmed. This is done by using quantitative techniques such as **spectrophotometry** or gas chromatography or HPLC.

Word Study

1. analyte ['ænə,laɪt] *n.* 分析物，待测物
2. archaeology [,ɑ:ki'ɒlədʒi] *n.* 考古学
3. carbohydrate [kɑ:bəʊ'haɪdreɪt] *n.* 碳水化合物，糖类
4. chromatography [krəʊmə'tɒgrəfɪ] *n.* 色谱法，色谱，层析，层析法
5. elution [ɪ'lu:ʃən] *n.* 洗脱
6. extraction [ɪk'strækʃn] *n.* 萃取
7. forensic [fə'rɛnsɪk] *adj.* 法医的
8. gas chromatography/mass spectrometry (GC/MS) *n.* 气 - 质联用
9. hydrolysis [haɪ'drɒlɪsɪs] *n.* 水解（作用）
10. immunoassay[,ɪmjʊnəʊ'æseɪ] *n.* 免疫分析
11. impurity [ɪm'pjʊərɪtɪ] *n.* 杂质，不纯
12. late [leɪt] *adj.* 已故的
13. metabolite [me'tæbə,laɪt] *n.* 代谢产物
14. metallurgical [,metə'lɜ:dʒɪkl] *adj.* 冶金的，冶金学的
15. precipitation [prɪ,sɪpɪ'teɪʃən] *n.* 沉淀
16. qualitative ['kwɒlɪtətɪv] *adj.* 定性的
17. quantitative ['kwɒntɪtətɪv] *adj.* 定量的
18. spectrometry [spek'trɒmɪtri] *n.* 光谱分析法
19. spectrophotometry [spɛktrəʊfəʊ'tɒmɪtri] *n.* 分光光度测定法

Notes

1. They adopt proven methodologies to new kinds of materials or to answer new questions about their composition and their reactivity mechanisms. 译为：他们采用经过验证的方法来研究新型材料，或回

答关于其组成及反应机制的新问题。句中 "adopt...to..." 意思是 "使用……来……"。

2. Analytical chemists also make important contributions to fields as diverse as forensics, archaeology, and space science. 译为：分析化学家在法医学、考古学和太空科学等多个领域也作出了重要贡献。句中，"as diverse as..." 强调 "范围很广，覆盖……"。

3. A selective reaction or test is one that can occur with other substances but exhibits a degree of preference for the substance of interest. 译为：选择性反应或检测是指可以和其他物质发生反应但对感兴趣物质显示一定程度的偏好的反应。句中，"one" 指的是 "a reaction or test"。

4. The former is usually covered in introductory chemistry courses, whereas the latter is best left until after the student has had a course in organic chemistry. 译为：前者通常包含在化学导论课程中，而后者最好留到学生上完有机化学课程之后。注意句中的 "The former..., whereas the latter..." 是指 "前者……，而后者……"。

Exercises

1. Decide whether each of the following statements is true (T) or false (F) according to the text.

(1) Analytical chemistry is mainly concerned with two important questions: what is it (qualitative) and how much is it (quantitative).

(2) Measurement of chemical constituents from manufactured products is unnecessary for quality control.

(3) Analytical chemistry seeks ever improved means of measuring the chemical composition of natural and artificial materials.

(4) Infrared spectra will give "fingerprints" of inorganic compounds or their functional groups.

(5) Modern chemical measurement systems often exhibit sufficient selectivity that a quantitative measurement can also serve as a qualitative measurement.

(6) Gas chromatography/mass spectrometry (GC/MS) is a highly selective technique.

2. Questions for oral discussion.

(1) What does analytical chemistry focus on?

(2) What is analytical science?

(3) What is the difference between "selective" and "specific"?

(4) What are the three phases in testing for banned substances at the Olympic Games?

3. Choose the best answer to each of the following questions.

(1) Blood _____ must be monitored in diabetics (and, in fact, most diseases are diagnosed by chemical analysis).

    A. protein   B. pH

    C. glucose   D. hemoglobin

(2) In medicine, analytical chemistry is the basis for _____ laboratory tests which help physicians diagnose disease and chart progress in recovery.

    A. clinical   B. polymer

    C. agricultural   D. fuel

(3) In industry, analytical chemistry provides the means of testing raw materials and for assuring the quality of finished products whose chemical _____ is critical.

    A. composition   B. compound

    C. concentration   D. class

(4) The formation of a white precipitate when adding a solution of silver nitrate to a dissolved sample

indicates the presence of _____ .

    A. nitrate   B. sulfide

    C. chloride   D. sulfate

(5) _____ spectra will give "fingerprints" of organic compounds or their functional groups.

    A. Infrared   B. Ultraviolet

    C. Visible   D. Mass

(6) Chromatography provides powerful _____ .

    A. instrumentation   B. precipitation

    C. extraction   D. separation

(7) The list of prohibited substances at the Olympic Games includes about 500 different active constituents, such as _____ .

    A. stimulants   B. steroids

    C. beta-blockers   D. all of the above

(8) Doping compounds are identified using the highly selective combination of gas _____ -mass spectrometry (GC-MS).

    A. phase   B. concentration

    C. flow   D. chromatography

(9) _____ spectrometry provides molecular structural data on the compounds.

    A. Infrared   B. Mass

    C. Visible   D. Ultraviolet

(10) What does chromato- or chromo- mean?

    A. blood   B. color

    C. electricity   D. light

(11) What does the word root photo- mean?

    A. spectrum   B. light

    C. absorption   D. emission

(12) What does the suffix '-graphy' mean in the word chromatography?

    A. a process or form of writing or drawing   B. an instrument

    C. a photo   D. an object

4. Choose an appropriate word from the list below and write it down in the blanks before its corresponding definition.

> qualitative, quantitative, mass spectrometry, infrared spectroscopy, ultraviolet spectroscopy, chromatography, pharmaceutical, contaminant, structure, nutrition

(1) _____ analysis aims to identify elements, ions and compounds present in a sample.

(2) _____ data are collected through measuring things, and analyzed through numerical comparisons and statistical inferences.

(3) Nuclear magnetic resonance spectroscopy (NMR) is a powerful technique for the characterization of the exact _____ of organic compounds.

(4) _____ is the spectroscopy that deals with the infrared region of the electromagnetic spectrum, that is light with a longer wavelength and lower frequency than visible light.

(5) _____ refers to a quantitative technique used to measure how much a chemical substance absorbs

particular ultraviolet light.

(6) _____ is the collective term for a set of laboratory techniques for the separation of mixtures.

(7) _____ is an analytical technique that sorts ions based on their mass (or "weight").

(8) _____ is the science that interprets the substances in food in relation to maintenance, growth, reproduction, health and disease of an organism.

(9) The _____ industry develops, produces, and markets drugs for use as medications.

(10) In environmental chemistry, _____ is in some cases virtually equivalent to pollution.

5. Translate the following sentences and paragraphs into Chinese.

(1) Qualitative analysis is to identify the elements, ions and compounds contained in a sample while quantitative analysis is to determine the exact quantity.

(2) Analytical chemistry has expanded beyond the bounds of just chemistry, and many have advocated using the name analytical science to describe the field. Even this term falls short of recognition of the role of instrumentation development and application.

(3) Analytical chemists work to improve the reliability of existing techniques to meet the demands for better chemical measurements which arise constantly in our society.

(4) Many household products, fuels, paints, pharmaceuticals, etc. are analyzed by the procedures developed by analytical chemists before being sold to the consumer.

(5) For quantitative analysis, a history of the sample composition will often be known (it is known that blood contains glucose), or else the analyst will have performed a qualitative test prior to performing the more difficult quantitative analysis.

(6) Qualitative tests may be performed by selective chemical reactions or with the use of instrumentation. For example, the formation of a white precipitate when adding a solution of silver nitrate to a dissolved sample indicates the presence of chloride. Infrared spectra will give "fingerprints" of organic compounds or their functional groups.

(7) The first phase in the testing of banned substances is called fast-screening phase, in which qualitative analysis such as GC or LC is adopted to test suspicious samples. In the second phase, GC-MS or LC-MS is employed for further testing of those suspicious samples. Finally, spectrophotometry or GC or HPLC is applied for accurate quantification.

Value-Oriented Reflective Reading

The Nobel Prize in Chemistry 2014

The Royal Swedish Academy of Sciences has awarded the Nobel Prize in Chemistry for 2014 to Eric Betzig, Stefan W. Hell and William E. Moerner "for the development of super-resolved fluorescence microscopy".

Eric Betzig, U.S. citizen. Born 1960 in Ann Arbor, MI, USA. Ph.D. 1988 from Cornell University, Ithaca, NY, USA. Group Leader at Janelia Research Campus, Howard Hughes Medical Institute, Ashburn, VA, USA.

Stefan W. Hell, German citizen. Born 1962 in Arad, Romania. Ph.D. 1990 from the University of Heidelberg, Germany. Director at the Max Planck Institute for Biophysical Chemistry, Göttingen, and Division head at the German Cancer Research Center, Heidelberg, Germany.

William E. Moerner, U.S. citizen. Born 1953 in Pleasanton, CA, USA. Ph.D. 1982 from Cornell University, Ithaca, NY, USA. Harry S. Mosher Professor in Chemistry and Professor, by courtesy, of Applied Physics at Stanford University, Stanford, CA, USA.

For a long time optical microscopy was held back by a presumed limitation: that it would never obtain a better resolution than half the wavelength of light. Helped by fluorescent molecules the Nobel Laureates (获奖者) in Chemistry 2014 ingeniously circumvented this limitation. Their ground-breaking work has brought optical microscopy into the nanodimension. In what has become known as nanoscopy, scientists visualize the pathways of individual molecules inside living cells. They can see how molecules create synapses (突触) between nerve cells in the brain; they can track proteins involved in Parkinson's, Alzheimer's and Huntington's diseases as they aggregate; they follow individual proteins in fertilized eggs as these divide into embryos.

It was all but obvious that scientists should ever be able to study living cells in the tiniest molecular detail. In 1873, the microscopist Ernst Abbe stipulated a physical limit for the maximum resolution of traditional optical microscopy: it could never become better than 0.2 micrometre.

Eric Betzig, Stefan W. Hell and William E. Moerner are awarded the Nobel Prize in Chemistry 2014 for having bypassed this limit. Due to their achievements the optical microscope can now peer into the nanoworld.

Two separate principles are rewarded. One enables the method stimulated emission depletion (STED) microscopy, developed by Stefan Hell in 2000. Two laser beams are utilized; one stimulates fluorescent molecules to glow, another cancels out all fluorescence except for that in a nanometre-sized volume. Scanning over the sample, Eric Betzig and William Moerner, working separately, laid the foundation for the second method, single-molecule microscopy. The method relies upon the possibility to turn the fluorescence of individual molecules on and off. Scientists image the same area multiple times, letting just a few interspersed molecules glow each time. Superimposing these images yields a dense super-image resolved at the nanolevel. In 2006 Eric Betzig utilized this method for the first time.

Today, nanoscopy is used world-wide and new knowledge of greatest benefit to mankind is produced on a daily basis.

Questions for discussion:

1. What are the limitations of traditional optical microscopy? How were the limitations bypassed by the three Nobel Laureates in Chemistry 2014?

2. How does super-resolved fluorescence microscopy benefit the development of medicine ?

3. As a student, how can we be innovative in scientific and technological research?

Text B
Applications of Supercritical Fluid Chromatography Technique in Current Bioanalysis and Pharmaceutical Analysis

In the 21st century, instrumental advances have finally enabled **supercritical fluid chromatography** (SFC) to be used in various analytical fields including bioanalysis and pharmaceutical analysis. Supercritical fluid is employed as primary mobile phase in SFC. Such mobile phase exhibits several unique merits of strong solubility, high diffusion coefficient and low **viscosity** which make SFC a promising method with higher column efficiency and faster separation speed. The commonly used supercritical fluid in SFC is CO_2. CO_2 is an ideal green fluid with low cost, non-toxicity, low critical temperature and pressure, **compatibility** with detectors such as MS. As neat CO_2 is a nonpolar solvent, it is only suitable for separating nonpolar compounds. Therefore, organic modifiers as well as additives are introduced into mobile phase to alter the polarity, so that the SFC method can be **versatile** for nonpolar, polar and ionizable compounds with wide polarity compatibility. SFC can operate either in a normal-phase mode or a reversed-phase mode with the utilization of various types of stationary phases.

In bioanalysis and pharmaceutical analysis, one of the key trends of late years is minimizing the use of hazardous solvents and maximizing the efficiency of the separation process. Although the standardized analytical methods nowadays for the separation of pharmaceutical and biological compounds are still HPLC or GC, scientists have paid more attention to alternative methods, particularly SFC. SFC is not only a green method without hazardous solvents consumption, but also a high-throughput method where samples run from three- to five-times faster than in HPLC. On the other hand, supercritical CO_2 with low viscosity enables high flow rate with minor pressure lifting, which significantly increases the column plate and generates sharper **symmetrical** peaks. Meanwhile, as CO_2 is easily eliminated during **desolvation**, SFC can couple with MS in a straightforward manner to identify the structural formation and improve sensitivity. Consequently, it has replaced HPLC as a favored option in several cases for bioanalysis and pharmaceutical analysis.

The purpose of this article is to share some of the latest achievements of SFC in analyzing compounds of biological and pharmaceutical interest. A brief description of the opportunities and challenges SFC encounters is also discussed.

Historical retrospect of SFC

SFC has evolved since its inception by Klesper in 1962. Although SFC has a long history, it has gone through 'the rise and fall' during its evolution. In the 1960s and 1970s, the development of SFC slowed down because the SFC apparatus had technical difficulties in stabilizing and regulating pressure. During that period, the researchers paid tremendous efforts to develop HPLC because HPLC showed great potential to analyze thermally instable, nonvolatile as well as polar compounds, which GC could not separate. In the 1980s, research activities on SFC gradually increased. The activeness on SFC technology and instrumentation promoted the commercialization of SFC instruments. In 1981, Novontny and Lee's group put forward the idea of a GC-like open **tubular** capillary column SFC system. The system was configured with a delivery pump, an injective valve with a split mechanism, a GC-like oven, an open tubular column, a fixed restrictor and a detector. However, the GC-like SFC system suffered from several intrinsic technical difficulties due to the limitation of the constant restrictor and free induction decay detector, then it gradually withdrew analytical use in the 1990s. In 1982, Gere and Board of Hewlett-Packard converted a HPLC system into an SFC system by adding a backpressure regulator. After that, packed-column SFC became a mainstream player in the analytical field. Further developments of SFC instruments ensured SFC technique complied with modern-day expectations in terms of robustness, resolution and sensitivity. Especially after 2010, state-of-the-art SFC systems not only enhanced reliability, productivity and throughput, but also improved the resolution and identification by tandem MS.

Advances in instrumental development and stationary phase have made SFC one of the most skillful and preferred separation techniques in the analytical field. Nowadays, modern SFC has been considered as a predominant method for bioanalytical and pharmaceutical applications.

Applications of SFC in bioanalysis

In bioanalysis, the application of SFC methodology has extended to the separation and identification of both **endogenous** and **exogenous** molecules including their metabolites. Endogenous compounds in biological samples involve amino acids, proteins, sugars, fatty acids, steroids and lipids, while exogenous compounds are mainly focused on pharmaceutical molecules and their metabolites which will be discussed in the section 'SFC in pharmaceutical analysis'.

Neat supercritical CO_2 is a nonpolar solvent that can be considered as a preferred alternative for the analysis of nonpolar molecules such as lipids. **Lipidomic** analysis is still a challenging task in the biological field. Lisa developed a high-throughput SFC-MS method for lipidomic analysis in tumor tissue, plasma and erythrocytes of kidney cancer patients. This system was compared with direct infusion-MS (DI-MS) and ultrahigh-performance liquid chromatography-MS (UHPLC-MS) in terms of comprehensiveness, sample throughput and validation results. SFC-MS exhibited promising results that 23 lipid classes containing 610 lipid species were identified within 10 min of analysis time. In another study, Bamba summarized the applications of SFC-MS for metabolic profiling of lipids. Even though lipids have numerous analogs with similar structures, SFC-MS proved to be a high-resolution and high-throughput tool for diverse lipids, including carotenoids, **triacylglycerols**, phospholipids, and fat-soluble vitamins.

Moreover, with the addition of modifier **cosolvent**, SFC can also separate polar molecules and even **hydrophilic** metabolites. Wolrab compared SFC-ESI-MS and SFC-APCI-MS for the analysis of polar and ionic compounds represented by amino acids and their metabolites in human serum samples. The respective advantages of the two techniques were observed: SFC-APCI-MS was better suited for amino acids with polar side chains, whereas SFC-ESI-MS was superior for amino acids featuring hydrophobic residues. Zhang reported a SFC-MS method for the separation and analysis of membrane proteins and hydrophobic peptides. A SFC cyanobonded silica column was used to separate the large membrane proteins and a total of 16 out of 26 core proteins could be separated in 15 min. Storbeck utilized UHPLC-MS method to profile steroids in biological samples. They also discussed the limitations and strengths of more frequently used GC-MS and LC-MS. Bamba's group successfully developed a SFC-ESI-MS/MS method for the rapid comprehensive profiling of 25 bile acids and conjugates in biological samples. 25 bile acids were simultaneously identified within 13 min, which was much faster than GC and LC techniques. This method was successfully applied for the study on bile acids metabolism in rat serum.

Applications of SFC in pharmaceutical analysis

With the expansion of SFC technology, its application in pharmaceutical analysis has become a new domain. Pharmaceutical analysis related to SFC methodology focuses on **chiral** separations, natural products isolation, pharmaceutical metabolism and fingerprint study.

Most constituents that play an important role in pharmaceutical and biological fields are chiral molecules. A pair of **enantiomers** may exhibit an entirely different activity or toxicity in biological interactions. In many cases, one enantiomer is effectively active and therapeutic while the other one could be totally inactive or even toxic to humans.

Pharmaceutical analysis of **stereoisomers** represents a tough challenge as they have the same molecular mass. As a consequence, identification of chiral molecules by chromatography methods is required for pharmaceutical analysis. In recent years, the attention of chiral separations has moved from HPLC/UHPLC to SFC/UHSFC. Along with the commercially availability of chiral stationary phases (CSPs), SFC in combination with CSPs has proven to be a suitable alternative to LC in stereoisomer separation, enabling better resolution (higher theoretical plates), high throughput and better enantioselectivity. Toribio's group focused on the enantiomeric separation of omeprazole, a widely used antiulcer drug. The method was carried out on a polysaccharide-based chiral column (Chiralpak AD). When ethanol was added into the mobile phase as the modifier, greatest production rates with purity higher than 99.9% were obtained for S-(–)-omeprazole and R-(+)-omeprazole.[1] Hoke compared packed-column SFC–MS/MS with LC–MS/MS for bioanalytical determination of (R)- and (S)-enantiomers of ketoprofen in human plasma. The samples were prepared with automated 96-well solid-phase extraction.[2] Although the linearity, sensitivity, accuracy and precision were comparable between the two methods, the developed SFC-MS/MS method had a dramatically shorter separation time of 2.3 min per sample, while the other needed 6.5 min. SFC technique has also been applied in the enantioseparation of traditional Chinese medicine. One example is dihydromyricetin, which is a natural **dihydroflavonoid** compound with anti-oxidation, anti-inflammation, hepatoprotective effect and anti-hypertensive activity. Lin investigated the effects of CSPs, cosolvents and flow rates on the separation of dihydromyricetin enantiomers, and the enantioresolution of 5.11was achieved by using a high percentage of modifier in the mobile phase (CO_2/methanol 60 : 40, V/V).[3]

Another portion of pharmaceutical analysis with SFC is found in achiral separations, referring to natural products, vitamins, doping agents, basic drugs and metabolites. In addition to the advantages mentioned above, SFC is also helpful for achiral high-throughput analysis. The investigation of natural products is of vital importance for the study of traditional Chinese medicine. Varieties of natural products have been examined by SFC and a lot of work has been published in this field. In the literature, SFC has been reported for the analysis of natural products including anthraquinones, triterpenoids, artemisinin and coumarins.[4] Vitamins are a class of required nutrients for humans. According to their solubility, vitamins are categorized as fat-soluble vitamins and water-soluble vitamins. It is difficult to implement **simultaneous determination** of fat-soluble and water-soluble vitamins due to the huge structural difference between the two groups. Taguchi developed a SFC method to unify a wide polarity range in a single run, and 17 vitamins varied from fat-soluble to water-soluble were separated in 4 min. More recently, the screening of doping agents have been successfully achieved with SFC technique. Novakova developed a fast and sensitive SFC-MS method for high-throughput screening of 100 doping agents in urine samples. The analysis time was only 7 min and the limits of detection (LODs) for this method were lower than the minimum required performance levels. Besides, SFC is also suitable for the analysis of achiral drugs and metabolites.

Future perspective

Due to the distinct properties of SFC, it has not only been considered as a green approach, but also a high throughput, high-performance, sensitive, versatile method for bioanalytical and pharmaceutical analytical fields. At modern times, the specific areas for SFC technique focus on multidimensional applications and **hyphenation** with advanced detectors, especially MS.

Multidimensional SFC techniques (including 2D SFC system and higher dimensional systems) have been regarded as emerging approaches to distinguish complex sample mixtures in biological and pharmaceutical fields. The resolution and peak capacity can be dramatically enhanced by combining two or more **orthogonal** columns with different separation mechanisms. Several combination modes (e.g., reversed-phase liquid chromatography and SFC, normal-phase liquid chromatography and SFC, GC and SFC) can be constructed by designing heart-cutting or comprehensive modulators. Among these modes, the merits of SFC (e.g., MS compatibility) can be manifest when it is used in the second dimension of 2D system.

Another important trend in SFC is its hyphenation with MS. MS has become the gold rule for the identification and quantification of target compounds in biological and pharmaceutical fields. Compared with conventional detection methods such as UV, diode array detector (DAD) and free induction decay, MS exhibits better sensitivity, high specificity as well as providing detailed information relating to the molecular structure and weight. The above-mentioned techniques can implement several challenges in biological and pharmaceutical separation fields such as:

- Reliable quantification with good sensitivity.
- Increasing peak capacity with high-throughput analysis.
- Identification of **homologous** molecules with similar structures (e.g., drugs and their metabolites, endogenous compounds in biological **matrix**).

Conclusion

In conclusion, SFC has carried out a large panel of work in the field of bioanalysis and pharmaceutical analysis. There is no doubt that SFC exhibits several unique merits in terms of throughput, separation efficiency, separation selectivity, peak capacity, sensitivity and versatility. In the next couple of years, SFC has the potential to replace LC and GC as the reference method. However, evolution is a continual process and future studies involving **kinetic** performance, method validation, matrix effect, system configuration and instrument development are **mandatory** in order to fulfill more applications in bioanalysis and pharmaceutical analysis.

Word Study

1. chiral ['kaɪərəl] *adj.* 手性的
2. compatibility [kəm,pætə'bɪləti] *n.* 兼容性，相容性
3. cosolvent [kəu'sɒlvənt] *n.* 助溶剂
4. desolvation [di:zɒl'veɪʃən] *n.* 去溶剂化
5. dihydroflavonoid [daɪhaɪdrə'flævənɔɪd] *n.* 二氢类黄酮
6. enantiomer [ɪ'næntɪəumə] *n.* 对映体（异构物），对映（异构）体
7. endogenous [en'dɒdʒənəs] *adj.* 内源性的
8. exogenous [ek'sɒdʒənəs] *adj.* 外源性的
9. homologous [hə'mɒləgəs] *adj.* 同源的
10. hydrophilic [,haɪdrə'fɪlɪk] *adj.* 亲水（性）的
11. hyphenation [,haɪfə'neɪʃn] *n.* 用连字符号连接，联用
12. kinetic [kɪ'netɪk] *adj.* 动力学的
13. lipidomic [lɪpɪ'dɒmɪk] *adj.* 脂类组学的
14. mandatory ['mændətəri] *adj.* 义务的，强制性的，强制的
15. matrix ['meɪtrɪks] *n.* 基质

16. orthogonal [ɔː'θɒɡənəl] *adj.* 正交的

17. simultaneous determination [ˌsɪml'teɪnɪəs dɪˌtɜː'mɪ'neɪʃən] *n.* 同时测定

18. stereoisomer [ˌsterɪəʊ'aɪsəmə] *n.* 立体异构体

19. supercritical fluid chromatography 超临界流体色谱

20. symmetrical [sɪ'metrɪkl] *adj.* 对称的

21. triacylglycerol [trɪəsɪlɡliː's'rɒl] *n.* 甘油三酯，三酰甘油

22. tubular ['tjuːbjələ(r)] *adj.* 管子构成的，有管状部分的，管状的

23. versatile ['vɜːsətaɪl] *adj.* 通用的，多功能的，多用途的

24. viscosity [vɪ'skɒsəti] *n.* （液体的）黏性，黏度

Notes

1. When ethanol was added into the mobile phase as the modifier, greatest production rates with purity higher than 99.9% were obtained for *S*-(–)-omeprazole and *R*-(+)-omeprazole. 译为：当在流动相中加入改性剂乙醇，*S*-(–)- 奥美拉唑和 *R*-(+)- 奥美拉唑的纯度可高于 99.9%。句中 "with purity higher than 99.9%" 作为定语修饰 "greatest production rates"。

2. The samples were prepared with automated 96-well solid-phase extraction. 译为：样品采用自动化 96 孔固相萃取制备。句中 "well" 翻译为 "孔" 或 "孔板"。

3. Lin investigated the effects of CSPs, cosolvents and flow rates on the separation of dihydromyricetin enantiomers, and the enantioresolution of 5.11 was achieved by using a high percentage of modifier in the mobile phase (CO_2/methanol 60∶40, *V/V*). 译为：Lin 研究了手性固定相、助溶剂和流速对二氢杨梅素异构体进行手性分离的影响，在流动相中使用高比例的调节剂时（CO_2 与甲醇的体积比为 60∶40），手性分离度可以达到 5.11。句中 "CO_2/methanol 60∶40" 是指 CO_2 与甲醇的体积比为 60∶40，*V* 为 volume 的缩写，即 CO_2 与甲醇的比例为体积比。

4. In the literature, SFC has been reported for the analysis of natural products including anthraquinones, triterpenoids, artemisinin and coumarins. 译为：据文献报道，SFC 可用于分析天然产物，包括蒽醌类、三萜类、青蒿提取物和香豆素类等。句中 "artemisinin" 可指 "青蒿素" 或 "青蒿提取物"，由于 "artemisinin" 前后的蒽醌类和香豆素类均为天然产物类型，并非单体，因此 "artemisinin" 在本句中建议翻译为 "青蒿提取物"。

Supplementary Parts

1. Medical and Pharmaceutical Terminology (7): Common Morphemes in English Terms for Pharmaceutical Analysis

Morpheme	Meaning	Example
a-	无, 非	aprotic solvent　非质子溶剂
alkal	碱	alkaloid　生物碱
amino	氨基	aminoglycoside　氨基糖苷
amper	安培, 电流	amperometric　电流测定的
aque	水	nonaqueous titration　非水滴定法
argent	银	argentometry　银量法
auto	自动	autoprotolysis constant　质子自递常数
aux	辅助	auxochrome　助色团

续表

Morpheme	Meaning	Example
brom	溴	bromimetry 溴量法
calor	热	calorimetry 量热法
chem	化学	chemometrics 化学计量学
chromato	颜色, 色谱	chromatography 色谱法
coul	库仑	coulometric titration 库仑滴定法
electr	电	electrophoresis 电泳
fluor	荧光	fluorometry 荧光分析法
grav	重	electrogravimetry 电重量法
holo	全	holographic grating 全息光栅
homo	相同, 均等	homolytic cleavage 均裂
iod	碘	iodimetry 碘量法
iso	相等	isoelectric focusing 等电聚焦
magnet	磁	electromagnetic spectrum 电磁波谱
photo	光	photodiode 光电二极管
spectr	看, 光	spectroscopy 光谱法
therm	热	thermospray 热喷雾
titri	滴定	titrimetric analysis 滴定分析法
volum	容量	volumetric analysis 容量分析法

(1) Decompose the following words and translate them into Chinese.

1) alkaloid _____

2) amperometric _____

3) argentometry _____

4) auxochrome _____

5) bromimetry _____

6) chromatography _____

7) electrophoresis _____

8) fluorometry _____

9) iodimetry _____

10) electromagnetic spectrum _____

11) spectroscopy _____

12) photodiode _____

(2) Word-matching.

1) calorimetry	A. 氨基糖苷
2) volumetric analysis	B. 非水滴定法
3) titrimetric analysis	C. 电重量法
4) chemometrics	D. 热喷雾
5) thermospray	E. 容量分析法
6) nonaqueous titration	F. 库仑滴定法

7) electrogravimetry		G. 全息光栅	
8) isoelectric focusing		H. 等电聚焦	
9) aminoglycoside		I. 化学计量学	
10) homolytic cleavage		J. 量热法	
11) holographic grating		K. 均裂	
12) coulometric titration		L. 滴定分析法	

2. English-Chinese Translation Skills: 药学英语翻译技巧 (3)：增、减词法

翻译时，为了对原文忠实，译文不能对原文意思进行任意增加或者减少，但这并不是说译文必须完全对等于原文，在文字上也不能有任何增减。实际上，由于英汉两种语言表达习惯存在差异，为了确切、充分地表达译文原义，或者使译文表达更加顺畅且符合汉语习惯，往往需要对译文进行文字增补或者省略。增词法主要指增加原文中无其词但有其意的一些词，绝不是无中生有地随意增词；减词法主要指原文中有些词在译文中可以省略，不必翻译出来。有些原文中因结构需要必不可少的词语，如冠词、代词、介词等，如果原原本本地译成汉语就会成为不必要的冗词，译文就会显得十分累赘，不符合汉语表达习惯。

例 1：The nutritional value of food is determined by chemical analysis for major components such as protein and carbohydrates and trace components such as vitamins and minerals. Indeed, even the calories in a food are often calculated from its chemical analysis.

参考译文：食品的营养价值是通过对其中蛋白质、碳水化合物等主要成分以及维生素、矿物质等微量成分的化学分析而得以确定。实际上，甚至食物的热量也经常通过化学分析的方法来计算。

说明：在上面例句中，the nutritional value of food 和 the calories in a food 两个词组的结构不同，但是翻译中介词 in 省略了，没有机械地译成"……中的"。原文中的两个 such as 也根据汉语表达需要省略了，没有直译出来。另外在翻译 are often calculated from its chemical analysis 时，原文在"化学分析"后增加了"……的方法"，使得译文表达更加具体。

例 2：Do not take aluminum-containing antacids at all while you are taking sucralfate. This combination increases aluminum absorption into the bloodstream.

参考译文：服用硫糖铝时禁用含铝抗酸药，二者联用会增加铝在血液中的吸收。

说明：这个例句来自药品说明书，在翻译 while you are taking sucralfate 时，考虑到主语 you 没有明确意义，要省略。

例 3：However, there are limited examples of success in developing biotherapeutic modalities for central nervous system (CNS) diseases in the drug development pipeline.

参考译文：然而，在药物研发过程中，鲜有生物治疗模式用于中枢神经系统疾病的成功案例。

说明：上面例句有两个 develop，意思都是"研发、开发"等，从整个句子的翻译来讲，省略 in developing biotherapeutic modalities 中的 develop，避免了重复也不妨碍整句意思。

翻译中增减词没有固定规律可言，主要还是出于译文表达需要，有时候在英文句子中没有什么省略，但是直接翻译成汉语，译文就不是很清楚，此时就必须根据汉语表达习惯适当增减词。

例 4：The basic experimental operation in titrimetric analysis is called titration. In titration, a solution of one reactant of accurately known concentration (the titrant, or standard solution) is added to a second solution of sample whose amount or concentration is to be determined. Titrant is added to the sample until the amount of titrant added is chemically equivalent to the amount of sample.

参考译文：滴定分析中基本的实验操作就是滴定。在滴定过程中，将已知准确浓度的反应物溶液

（滴定剂或标准溶液）加至另外一种反应物溶液中，也就是样品量或浓度待测定的样品溶液中。滴定剂不断地加入到样品溶液中，直到加入滴定剂的量与样品中待测物的量达到化学平衡。

　　说明：原文有三个小句。第二个小句中 in titration 被译成"在滴定过程中"，增加了"过程中"，其中"is added to a second solution of sample whose amount or concentration..."译文增加了"也就是"；第三小句中 Titrant is added to the sample until...，译文增加了"不断地"，与原文中的"until（直到）"呼应，以及在翻译 to the amount of sample 时，译文增加了"待测物的"，与前文"titrant added（加入滴定剂的）"相呼应。原文句子结构完整，意思明确，没有缺少什么词，但是汉语译文增加了一些词，这些增词都没有改变原文意义，也不显得啰唆，使译文表达更加通畅。

　　当然，这个例句中的第二句也涉及定语从句的翻译技巧，这在后面章节中另有讲解。

（翟兴英　陈　芸　乔玉玲　史志祥　龚长华）

Unit Eight

Natural Products

A natural product is a chemical compound or substance produced by a living organism—found in nature that usually has a pharmacological or biological activity for use in pharmaceutical drug discovery and drug design. A natural product can be considered as such even if it can be prepared by total synthesis.

Natural products may be extracted from tissues of terrestrial plants, marine organisms or microorganism fermentation broths. A crude (untreated) extract from any one of these sources typically contains novel, structurally diverse chemical compounds, which the natural environment is a rich source of.

Chemical diversity in nature is based on biological and geographical diversity, so researchers travel around the world obtaining samples to analyze and evaluate in drug discovery screens or bioassays. This effort to search for natural products is known as bioprospecting.

Pharmacognosy provides the tools to identify, select and process natural products destined for medicinal use. Usually, the natural product compound has some form of biological activity and that compound is known as the active principle—such a structure can act as a lead compound. Many of today's medicines are obtained directly from a natural source.

Moreover, some medicines are developed from a lead compound originally obtained from a natural source. This means the lead compound can be produced by total synthesis, or can be a starting point (precursor) for a semisynthetic compound, or can act as a template for a structurally different total synthetic compound. Because most biologically active natural product compounds are secondary metabolites with very complex structures.

天然产物是指由自然界的生物体产生的化合物或其他物质，通常具有一定的药理作用或生物活性，可用于药物发现和药物设计。尽管天然产物可以通过全合成来制备，上述定义仍然适用。

天然产物可以从陆生植物、海洋生物或微生物发酵液的组织中提取。来自上述任一来源的粗提取物通常含有新颖的、结构多样的化合物，自然环境是这些化合物的丰富来源。

在自然界中，化学多样性实质上取决于生物多样性和地理多样性，因此研究者们会在世界各地获取样本并在药物发现筛选或生物鉴定中加以分析和评价。这项寻找天然产物的工作称为生物勘探。

生药学提供了鉴别、筛选和优化药用天然产物的工具。通常，具有一定生物活性的天然产物，被称作活性成分，这种结构可用作先导化合物。目前许多药物可直接从自然资源中获取。

此外，有一些药物是以天然来源的先导化合物为基础研发而来。这意味着先导化合物可以通过全合成制备，或者可以作为半合成化合物的前体，抑或作为模板来合成结构截然不同的全合成化合物。由于大多数具有生物活性的天然产物是生物体的次级代谢产物，结构非常复杂。结构新颖是这些化合

This has an advantage in that they are extremely novel compounds but this complexity also makes many lead compounds' synthesis difficult and the compound usually has to be extracted from its natural source—a slow, expensive and inefficient process. As a result, there is usually an advantage in designing simpler analogues.	物的优势，但结构的复杂性也增加了全合成的难度，所以这些化合物通常是从其自然资源中提取——耗时、昂贵又低效。因此，设计结构更简单的类似物通常更具优势。

Text A
Drug Discovery and Natural Products

It may be argued that drug discovery is a recent concept that evolved from modern science during the 20th century, but this concept in reality dates back many centuries, and has its origins in nature. On many occasions, humans have turned to Mother Nature for cures, and discovered unique drug molecules. Thus, the term natural product has become almost **synonymous** with the concept of drug discovery. In modern drug discovery and development processes, natural products play an important role at the early stage of "lead" discovery, i.e. discovery of the active (determined by various **bioassays**) natural molecule, which itself or its structural analogues could be an ideal drug **candidate**.

Natural products have been enormous source of drugs and drug leads. It is estimated that 66.7 percent of the 1394 small-molecular new chemical entities (NCEs) introduced as drugs worldwide during 1981–2019 can be traced back to or were developed from natural products. These include unaltered natural products (71, 5.1%), natural product derivatives (356, 25.5%), and synthetic compounds with natural-product-derived **pharmacophores** (65, 4.7%) and synthetic compounds designed on the basis of knowledge gained from a natural product, i.e. a natural product **mimic** (272, 19.5%). Natural products have played a key role in drug discovery, especially for infectious diseases and cancer, about 70.6% of antibacterials and 33.5% of antitumor small-molecule NCEs are natural products or structural analogues of natural products. In other therapeutic areas, including cardiovascular diseases (for example, statins) and multiple sclerosis (for example, fingolimod), the contribution of natural products is also great.

Despite the impressive record and statistics regarding the success of natural products in drug discovery, "natural product drug discovery" has been neglected by many big pharmaceutical companies in the recent past. The declining popularity of natural products as a source of new drugs began in the 1990s, because of some practical factors, e.g. the apparent lack of compatibility of natural products with the modern **high throughput screening (HTS)** programs, where significant degrees of automation, robotics and computers are used, the complexity in the isolation and identification of natural products and the cost and time involved in the natural product "lead" discovery process.[1] Complexity in the chemistry of natural products, especially in the case of novel structural types, also became the rate-determining step in drug discovery programs. Attempts to discover new drug "leads" from natural sources have never stopped, despite being neglected by the pharmaceutical companies, but continued in academia and some semi-academic research organizations, where more traditional approaches to natural product drug discovery have been applied.

Neglected for years, natural product drug discovery appears to be drawing attention and immense interest again, and is on the verge of a comeback in the mainstream of drug discovery ventures. In recent years, a significant revival of interests in natural products as a potential source for new medicines has been observed among academics as well as several pharmaceutical companies. This extraordinary comeback of natural products in drug discovery research is mainly due to the following factors: combinatorial chemistry's promise to fill drug development pipelines with *de novo* synthetic small-molecular drug candidates is somewhat unsuccessful[2]; the practical difficulties of natural product drug discovery are being overcome by advances in separation and identification technologies and in the speed and sensitivity of structure elucidation and, finally, the unique and incomparable chemical diversity that natural products have to offer. Moreover, only a small fraction of the world's biodiversity has ever been investigated for bioactivity to date. For example, there are at least 250,000 species of higher plants that exist on this planet, but merely five to ten percent of these terrestrial plants have been investigated so far. In addition, re-investigation of previously investigated plants has continued to produce new bioactive compounds that have the potential for being developed as drugs. While several biologically active compounds have been found in marine organisms, e.g. antimicrobial compound cephalosporin C from marine organisms (*Cephalosporium acremonium* and *Streptomyces* spp.[3]) and antiviral compounds such as avarol and avarone from marine sponges, e.g. *Dysidea avara*, research in this area is still at the starting point. The following notes are the summary of the traditional as well as the modern drug discovery processes involving natural products.

Natural Product Drug Discovery: the Traditional Way

In the traditional, rather more academic, method of drug discovery from natural products, drug targets are exposed to crude extracts, and in the case of a hit, i.e. any evidence of activity, the extract is fractionated and the active compound is isolated and identified. Every step of fractionation and isolation is usually guided by bioassays, and the process is called bioassay-guided isolation. Sometimes, a straight forward natural product isolation route, irrespective of bioactivity, is also applied, which results in the isolation of a number of natural compounds (small compound library) suitable for undergoing any bioactivity screening. However, the process can be slow, ineffectual and labour intensive, and it does not guarantee that a "lead" from screening would be chemically workable or even patentable.

Natural Product Drug Discovery: the Modern Processes

Modern drug discovery approaches involve HTS, where, applying full automation and robotics, hundreds of molecules can be screened using several assays within a short time, and with very little amount of compounds. In order to incorporate natural products in the modern HTS programs, a natural product library (a collection of dereplicated natural products) needs to be built. Dereplication is the process by which one can eliminate recurrence or re-isolation of same or similar compounds from various extracts. A number of hyphenated techniques are used for dereplication, e.g. LC-PDA (liquid chromatography-photo-diode-array), LC-MS (liquid chromatography-mass spectrometry) and LC-NMR (liquid chromatography-nuclear magnetic resonance spectroscopy).

LC-HRMS can separate numerous isomers present in natural product extracts. Moreover, such combined methods might integrate HRMS and NMR, allowing the simultaneous use of the advantages of both techniques. NMR analysis of natural product extracts is simple and reproducible, and provides direct quantitative information and detailed structural information, although it has relatively low sensitivity, meaning that it generally enables profiling only of major constituents. The applications of NMR in natural product research are versatile and the technique is used both directly for metabolomics of unfractionated natural product extracts and for structural characterization of compounds and fractions obtained with appropriate separation methods. Most often LC-HRMS is the gold standard for qualitative and quantitative metabolite profiling and is most commonly applied in combination with LC. HRMS can also be used in the direct infusion mode (called DIMS), whereby samples are directly profiled by MS without a chromatography step, or in MS imaging (MSI), which enables determination of the spatial distribution of natural products within living organisms. HRMS enables routine acquisition of accurate molecular mass information, which together with appropriate heuristic filtering can provide unambiguous assignment of molecular formulae for hundreds to thousands of metabolites within a single extract over a dynamic range that may exceed five orders of magnitude.

To continue to exploit natural sources for drug candidates, the focus must be on exploiting newer approaches for natural product drug discovery. These approaches include the application of omic tools, gene technology, seeking novel sources of organisms from the environment, new screening technologies and improved processes of sample preparation for screening samples.

Metabolomics was developed as an approach to simultaneously analyse multiple metabolites in biological samples. Enabled by technological developments in chromatography and spectrometry, metabolomics was historically applied first in other research fields, such as biomedical and agricultural sciences. Advances in the analytical instrumentation used in natural product research, coupled with computational approaches that can generate plausible natural product analogue structures and their respective simulated spectra, have also enabled application of 'omics' approaches such as metabolomics in natural product-based drug discovery. Metabolomics can provide accurate information on the metabolite composition in natural product extracts, thus helping to prioritize natural products for isolation, to accelerate dereplication and to annotate unknown analogues and new natural product scaffolds. Moreover, metabolomics can detect differences between metabolite compositions in various physiological states of producing organisms and enable the generation of hypotheses to explain them, and can also provide extensive metabolite profiles to underpin phenotypic characterization at the molecular level. Both options are very useful in understanding the molecular mechanisms of action of natural products.

Advances in knowledge on biosynthetic pathways for natural products and in developing tools for analysing and manipulating genomes are further key drivers for modern natural product-based drug discovery. Two key characteristics enable the identification of biosynthetic genes in the genomes of the producing organisms. First, these genes are clustered in the genomes of bacteria and filamentous fungi. Second, many natural products are based on polyketide or peptide cores, and their biosynthetic pathways involve enzymes-polyketide synthases (PKSs) and nonribosomal peptide synthetases (NRPSs), respectively-that are encoded by large genes with highly conserved modules.[4]

'Genome mining' is based on searches for genes that are likely to govern biosynthesis of scaffold structures, and can be used to identify natural product biosynthetic gene clusters. Prioritization of gene clusters for further work is facilitated by advances in biosynthetic knowledge and predictive bioinformatics tools, which can provide hints about whether the metabolic products of the clusters have chemical scaffolds that are new or known, thereby supporting dereplication. Such predictive tools for gene cluster analysis can be applied in combination with spectroscopic techniques to accelerate the identification of natural products and determine the stereochemistry of metabolic products. Furthermore, to extend genome mining from a single genome to entire genera, microbiomes or strain collections, computational tools have been developed, such as BiG-SCAPE, which enables sequence similarity analysis of biosynthetic gene clusters, and CORASON, which uses a phylogenomic approach to elucidate evolutionary relationships between gene clusters.

In addition, the complex regulation of natural product biosynthesis in response to the environment means that the conditions under which producing organisms are cultivated can have a major impact on the chance of identifying novel natural products. Several strategies have been developed to improve the likelihood of identifying novel natural products compared with monoculture under standard laboratory conditions and to make 'uncultured' microorganisms grow in a simulated natural environment.

In conclusion, natural products remain a promising pool for the discovery of scaffolds with high structural diversity and various bioactivities that can be directly developed or used as starting points for optimization into novel drugs. While drug development overall continues to be challenged by high attrition rates, there are additional hurdles for natural products due to issues such as accessibility, sustainable supply and IP constraints. However, we believe that the scientific and technological advances discussed above provide a strong basis for natural product-based drug discovery to continue making major contributions to human health and longevity.

Word Study

1. avarol [əˈværɒl] *n.* 阿瓦醇
2. avarone [əvəˈrʌn] *n.* 阿瓦醌
3. bioassay [ˌbaɪəʊˈæseɪ] *n.* 生物检定,生物学鉴定法
4. biodiversity [ˌbaɪəʊdaɪˈvɜːsəti] *n.* 生物多样性
5. biosynthetic [biːəʊˈsɪnθetɪk] *adj.* 生物合成的
6. candidate [ˈkændɪdət] *n.* 候选人,候补者,应试者
7. cephalosporin [sefələʊˈspɔːrɪn] *n.* 头孢菌素
8. *Cephalosporium acremonium* 拉. 顶头孢霉菌
9. combinatorial [ˌkɒmbɪnəˈtɔːrɪəl] *adj.* 组合的,联合的
10. dereplication [deriːplɪˈkeɪʃn] *n.* 去重复化
11. *Dysidea avara* 拉. 贪婪倔海绵
12. high throughput screening (HTS) 高通量筛选
13. hyphenated [ˈhaɪfəneɪtɪd] *adj.* 带有连字符号的
14. LC-MS (liquid chromatography-mass spectrometry) *n.* 液相色谱 - 质谱联用
15. LC-NMR (liquid chromatography-nuclear magnetic resonance) *n.* 液相色谱 - 核磁共振联用
16. LC-PDA (liquid chromatography-photo-diode-array) *n.* 液相色谱二极管阵列
17. marine [məˈriːn] *adj.* 海产的
18. metabolomics [metæˈbɒləmɪks] *n.* 代谢组学
19. mimic [ˈmɪmɪk] *n.* 模仿,临摹,仿制品;*vt.* 模仿,模拟;*adj.* 模仿的
20. omics *n.* 组学,生物组学
21. patentable [ˈpeɪtəntəbl] *adj.* 可取得专利的
22. pharmacophore [ˈfɑːməkəfɔː] *n.* 药效团,药效基团,药效结构
23. pipeline [ˈpaɪplaɪn] *n.* 导管,流水线
24. polyketide [pɒˈlaɪkɪtaɪd] *n.* 聚酮,聚酮化合物,多聚乙酰
25. spectroscopy [spekˈtrɒskəpi] *n.* 光谱,光谱学

26. sponge [spʌndʒ] *n.* 海绵，海绵球，海绵动物

27. stereochemistry [stɪərɪəˈkemɪstrɪ] *n.* 立体化学

28. synonymous [sɪˈnɒnɪməs] *adj.* 同义的，暗示的

29. unfractionated [ʌnˈfrækʃnətɪd] *adj.* 未分级的

Notes

1. The declining popularity of natural products as a source of new drugs began in the 1990s, because of some practical factors, e.g. the apparent lack of compatibility of natural products with the modern high throughput screening (HTS) programs, where significant degrees of automation, robotics and computers are used, the complexity in the isolation and identification of natural products and the cost and time involved in the natural product "lead" discovery process. 译为：从 20 世纪 90 年代开始，天然产物作为新药来源的优势逐渐下降，这是因为一些实际因素，例如：天然产物与现代高通量筛选（HTS）技术存在明显的不兼容性，在现在的 HTS 程序中，自动化程度高，并使用机器人和计算机；而天然产物的分离和鉴定过程复杂烦琐，从天然产物发现先导化合物成本高、周期长。高通量筛选（high throughput screening, HTS）技术是指以分子水平和细胞水平的实验方法为基础，以微板形式作为实验工具载体，以自动化操作系统执行试验过程，以灵敏快速的检测仪器采集实验结果数据，以计算机分析处理实验数据，在同一时间检测数以千万计的样品，并以得到的相应数据库支持运转的技术体系，它具有微量、快速、灵敏和准确等特点。简言之，就是可以通过一次实验获得大量的信息，并从中找到有价值的信息。

2. Combinatorial chemistry's promise to fill drug development pipelines with *de novo* synthetic small-molecular drug candidates is somewhat unsuccessful. 译为：组合化学通过从头合成为药物开发提供大量小分子候选药物的预期并未充分实现。句中 "*de novo* synthetic" 为 "从头合成"，即生物体内用简单的前体物质合成生物分子的途径。包括脂肪酸的从头合成和核苷酸的从头合成。

3. sp. 是 speciales 的缩写，spp. 是 species pluralis 的缩写。pluralis 是 plural 的复数形式。此外，*Streptomyces* sp. 是指链霉菌属中的一个转化型，而 *Streptomyces* spp. 则泛指链霉菌属中的多个转化型。

4. Second, many natural products are based on polyketide or peptide cores, and their biosynthetic pathways involve enzymes—polyketide synthases (PKSs) and nonribosomal peptide synthetases (NRPSs), respectively—that are encoded by large genes with highly conserved modules. 译为：其次，许多天然产物基于聚酮核心或肽核心，它们的生物合成途径涉及的酶，聚酮合成酶（PKS）和非核糖体肽合成酶（NRPs），都由具有高度保守模块的大基因编码。句中 "polyketide synthases (PKSs) and nonribosomal peptide synthetases (NRPSs), respectively" 作为插入语，"that are encoded by large genes with highly conserved modules" 作为定语从句修饰 "enzymes"。

Exercises

1. Decide whether each of the following statements is true (T) or false (F) according to the passage.

(1) 90% to 95 % of terrestrial plants on this planet have not been investigated so far.

(2) In the traditional way, not every step of fractionation and isolation is usually guided by bioassays, and the process is called bioassay-guided isolation.

(3) Modern drug discovery approaches, applying full automation and robotics, hundreds of molecules can be screened using several assays within a short time, and with very little amount of compounds.

(4) LC-PDA (liquid chromatography-photo-diode-array detector), LC-MS (liquid chromatography-mass detector) and LC-NMR (liquid chromatography-nuclear magnetic resonance spectroscopy) are the hyphenated techniques used for dereplication.

(5) Metabolomics can't detect differences between metabolite compositions in various physiological states of producing organisms and disable the generation of hypotheses to explain them.

(6) In conclusion, natural products remain a promising pool for the discovery of scaffolds with high structural diversity and various bioactivities that can be directly developed or used as starting points for optimization into novel drugs.

2.   Questions for oral discussion.

(1) What were the practical factors responsible for the declining popularity of natural products as a source of new drugs in the 1990s?

(2) What is the difference between the traditional way and the modern processes in drug discovery from natural products?

(3) What are the new approaches for natural product drug discovery?

(4) What are two key characteristics that help to identify biosynthetic genes in the genomes of the producing organisms?

3.   Choose the best answer to each of the following questions.

(1) What is the meaning of "drug candidate"?
    A. purified isolate   B. total extract
    C. a new drug on market   D. a compound with some bioactivity

(2) Whose polarity in the following solvents is the weakest?
    A. Alcohol.   B. Ethyl acetate.
    C. Chloroform.   D. Acetone.

(3) Which of the following solvents will you select in order to extract most lipophilic ingredients from plants?
    A. Alcohol.   B. Butanol.
    C. Ethyl acetate.   D. Benzene.

(4) In normal phase partition chromatography, the stationary phase commonly used is _____.
    A. chloroform   B. water
    C. n-butanol   D. ethyl acetate

(5) In glycosidic linkage hydrolysis, which of the following is the easiest in different glycosidic atoms?
    A. Alcohol glycoside.   B. N
    C. Phenol glycosides.   D. S

(6) Generally, free alkaloids can easily dissolve in _____.
    A. methanol   B. alcohol
    C. diethyl ether   D. chloroform

(7) What is the full term for HTS?
    A. High Temperature Superconducting   B. Heat Transfer Salts
    C. High Throughput Screening   D. Heat-Treated Steel

(8) What category does simvastatin belong to?
    A. Lipid regulating agents.   B. Antineoplastic agents.
    C. Antibiotics of aminoglycosides.   D. Analgesics.

(9) What category does paclitaxel belong to?

  A. Lipid regulating agents.   B. Antineoplastic agents.

  C. Antibiotics of aminoglycosides.   D. Analgesics.

(10) What category does azithromycin belong to?

  A. Lipid regulating agents.   B. Antineoplastic agents.

  C. Antibiotics of macrolides.   D. Analgesics.

4. Match the words with the prefixes or suffixes according to the meaning(s).

1) angio-	A. pain
2) dermato-	B. heart
3) -algia	C. skin
4) -phobia	D. blood
5) cardio-	E. vessel
6) hemato-	F. inflammation
7) tachy-	G. fast
8) -itis	H. slow
9) brady-	I. fear
10) -cyte	J. cell

5. Translate the following sentences and paragraphs into Chinese.

(1) Attempts to discover new drug "leads" from natural sources have never stopped, despite being neglected by the pharmaceutical companies, but continued in academia and some semi-academic research organizations, where more traditional approaches to natural product drug discovery have been applied.

(2) The practical difficulties of natural product drug discovery are being overcome by advances in separation and identification technologies and in the speed and sensitivity of structure elucidation and, finally, the unique and incomparable chemical diversity that natural products have to offer.

(3) The applications of nuclear magnetic resonance spectroscopy (NMR) in natural product research are versatile and the technique is used both directly for metabolomics of unfractionated natural product extracts and for structural characterization of compounds and fractions obtained with appropriate separation methods.

(4) These approaches include the application of omic tools, gene technology, seeking novel sources of organisms from the environment, new screening technologies and improved processes of sample preparation for screening samples.

(5) In addition, the complex regulation of natural product biosynthesis in response to the environment means that the conditions under which producing organisms are cultivated can have a major impact on the chance of identifying novel natural products.

(6) Flavonoids are mainly water-soluble compounds. They can be extracted with 70% ethanol and remain in the aqueous layer, following partition of this extract with petroleum ether. Flavonoids are phenolic and hence change in colour when treated with base or with ammonia; thus they are easily detected on chromatograms or in solution. Flavonoids contain conjugated aromatic systems and thus show intense absorption bands in the UV and visible regions of the spectrum. Finally flavonoids are generally present in plants bound to sugar as glycosides and any one flavonoid aglycone may occur in a single

plant in several glycosidic combinations. For this reason, when analysing flavonoids, it is usually better to examine the aglycones present in hydrolysed plant extracts before considering the complexity of glycosides that may be present in the original extract.

(7) While in the recent past it was extremely difficult, time consuming and labour intensive to build such a library from purified natural products, with the advent of newer and improved technologies related to separation, isolation and identification of natural products the situation has improved remarkably. However, the best result can be obtained from a fully identified pure natural product library as it provides scientists with the opportunity to handle the 'lead' rapidly for further developmental work, e.g. total or partial synthesis, dealing with formulation factors, *in vivo* assays and clinical trials.

Value-Oriented Reflective Reading

K. K. Chen—Remington Medalist 1965

Ko Kuei Chen (K. K. Chen) is a graduate pharmacist who has pursued a long, illustrious career in the health sciences making significant contributions to knowledge especially through his work on the ephedrine alkaloids, toad poisons, digitalis glycosides, the treatment of cyanide poisoning Chinese drugs, alkaloids from the genus *Senecio*, and the newer synthetic drugs including analgesics.

Dr. Chen graduated from the Tsing Hua College in Peking, China in 1918 and, coming to the United States, he received his Bachelor of Science in pharmacy at the University of Wisconsin in 1920. Later, in 1923, he was awarded his Ph.D. in physiology and pharmacology by the University of Wisconsin. In 1927, Dr. Chen received his M.D degree from the Johns Hopkins University where he continued as an associate in pharmacology. In 1929 he joined the Eli Lilly Company as Director of Pharmacologic Research. He has been awarded honorary degrees by both the University of Wisconsin and the Philadelphia College of Pharmacy and Science.

In 1925, Dr. Chen, together with C. F. Schmidt, introduced the use of ephedrine into clinical medicine as the result of a Chinese pharmacist's assurance that Ma Huang (麻黄) was really a potent drug. Ephedrine had been previously isolated in a pure state by Nagai in 1887 and synthesized by him in 1911. It was Chen's classical studies, however, on the pharmacology, toxicology, chemistry, and clinical applications of ephedrine that finally led to its widespread use in Western medicine. Aided by a grant from the American Pharmaceutical Association Research Fund, he also demonstrated that the pupil dilating effect of cocaine, ephedrine and several related alkaloids is slight in Chinese and Black people, as contrasted with their effect in Caucasians.

Beginning in the early 1930's and continuing through the late 1950's, Dr. Chen perfected the treatment of cyanide poisoning. His technique was the use of amylnitrite by inhalation and the intravenous injection of sodium nitrite (10 ml of a 3% solution) followed by sodium thiosulfate (50 ml of a 25% solution). He also showed that ampuls of sodium nitrite and sodium thiosulfate remain stable for years if an antioxidant such as sodium sulfite is added. In cyanide poisoning, the cyanide prevents the respiratory enzyme, ferricytochrome oxidase, from transporting oxygen to the cells by forming a complex with it. Administration of amylnitrite or sodium nitrite causes the formation of methemoglobin from hemoglobin. Methemoglobin combines with the cyanide ion to from cyanmethemoglobin which has a low toxicity. Sodium thiosulfate, under the influence of the enzyme rhodanese, converts the cyanide to thiocyanate.

In addition, Dr. Chen has written extensively on the pharmacology and methods of evaluating a wide range of synthetic analgesics, pressor alkaloids, ergot alkaloids, cardiac glycosides, the cardiac action of toad poison, antimalarials, cardioactive steroids, hypoglycemic drugs, peptides, and sedatives and hypnotics. He has been a frequent contributor to the *Journal of the American Pharmaceutical Association* as well as to numerous biomedical, pharmacology and medical journals.

Throughout his long career, Dr. Chen has received a number of honors and has become a member of many professional and honorary organizations. During World War II, he served in the U.S. government Office of Science and Research Development. In 1956, he was named by the Department of State as an official delegate to the First General Assembly of the International Union of Physiological Science held in Brussels.

Author of more than 100 scientific articles, Dr. Chen is an outstanding example of an eminent scholar, a fruitful research worker, and a devoted teacher. Pharmacy honors itself when it honors such an outstanding pharmacist.

Questions for discussion:

1. How was ephedrine isolated and developed?
2. What is the significance of ephedrine in pharmaceutical research?
3. As a pharmaceutical student, what inspiration could we gain from K. K. Chen's experience?

Text B
How to Approach the Isolation of a Natural Product?

Introduction

It may seem a dreadful task, faced with a liter of fermentation broth a dark, viscous sludge—knowing that in there is one group of molecules that has to be separated from all the rest. Those molecules possibly represent only about 0.0001% or 1 ppm of the total biomass and are dispersed throughout the organism, possibly intimately bound up with other molecules. Like the proverbial needle in a haystack, you have to remove a lot of hay to be left with just the needle, without knowing what the needle looks like or where in the haystack it is.

1. What are Natural Products?

The term "natural product" is perhaps quite misleading. Strictly speaking, any biological molecule is a natural product, but the term is usually reserved for secondary metabolites, small molecules (mol wt < 1,500 amu approx) produced by an organism but those are not strictly necessary for the survival of the organism, unlike the more prevalent macromolecules such as proteins, nucleic acids, and polysaccharides that make up the basic machinery for the more fundamental processes of life.[1]

Secondary metabolites are a very broad group of metabolites, with no distinct boundaries, and grouped under no single unifying definition. Concepts of secondary metabolism include products of overflow metabolism as a result of nutrient limitation, or shunt metabolites produced during idiophase, defense mechanisms, regulator molecules, and so on.[2] Perhaps the most cogent theory of secondary metabolism has been put forward by Zahner, who described secondary metabolism as evolutionary "elbow room". If a secondary metabolite has no adverse effect on the producing organism at any levels of differentiation, **morphogenesis**, transport, regulation, or intermediary metabolism, it may be conserved for a relatively long period during which time it may come to confer a selective advantage. Secondary metabolism therefore provides a kind of testing ground where new metabolites have the opportunity, as it were, to exist without being eliminated, during which time they may find a role that will give an advantage to the producing organism. This is supported by the fact that secondary metabolites are often unique to a particular species or group of organisms and, while many act as **antifeedants**, sex attractants, or antibiotic agents, many have no apparent biological role. It is likely that all these concepts can play some part in understanding the production of the broad group of compounds that come under the heading of secondary metabolite.

Isolation of natural products differs from that of the more commonly occurring biological macromolecules because natural products are smaller and chemically more diverse than the relatively consistent proteins, nucleic acids and carbohydrates, and isolation methods must take this into account.[3]

2. The Aim of the **Extraction**

The two most fundamental questions that should be asked at the onset of an extraction are:

(1) What am I trying to isolate?

There are a number of possible targets of isolation:

a. An unknown compound responsible for a particular biological activity.

b. A certain compound known to be produced by a particular organism.

c. A group of compounds within an organism that are all related in some way, such as by a common structural feature.

d. All of the metabolites produced by one natural product source that are not produced by a different "control" source, e.g., two species of the same genus, or the same organism grown under different conditions.

e. A chemical dissection of an organism, in order to characterize all of its interesting metabolites, usually those secondary metabolites, confined to that organism, or group of organisms, and not universal in all living systems, such an inventory might be useful for chemical, ecological, or chemotaxonomic reasons, among others.

(2) Why am I trying to isolate it?

The second fundamental question concerns what one is trying ultimately to achieve, for defining the aims can minimize the work required. Reasons for the extraction might be:

a. To purify sufficient amount of a compound to characterize it partially or fully.

b. More specifically, to provide sufficient material to allow for confirmation or denial of a proposed structure. As in many cases this does not require mapping out a complete structure from scratch but perhaps simply comparison with a standard of known structure; it may require less material or only partially pure material. There is no point in removing minor impurities if they do not get in the way of ascertaining whether the compound is, or is not, compound X.

c. The generation/production of the maximum amount of a known compound so that it can be used for further work, such as more extensive biological testing. (Alternatively, it may be more efficient to chemically **synthesize** the compound; any natural product that is of serious interest, i.e., is required in large amounts, will be considered as a target for synthetic chemistry.)

3. Purity

With a clear idea of what one is trying to achieve, one can then question the required level of purity. This in turn might give some indication of the approach to be taken and the purification methods to be employed.

For example, if you are attempting to characterize fully a complex natural product that is present at a low **concentration** in an extract, you will probably want to produce a compound that is suitable for NMR. The purity needed is dependent on the nature of the compound and of the impurities, but to assign fully a complex structure, material of 95%–100% purity is generally required. If the compound is present at a high concentration in the starting material and there already exists a standard against which to compare it, structure confirmation can be carried out with less pure material and the purification will probably require fewer steps.

The importance of purity in natural products isolation has been highlighted by Ghisalberti, who described two papers that appeared at about the same time, both reporting the isolation from plants of ent-kauran-3-oxo-16,17-diol. In one paper, the compound has a **melting point** of 173–174 ℃ and $[\alpha]_D$–39.2° (CHCl$_3$); in the other, no melting point is reported, but the compound has an $[\alpha]_D$–73.1° (CHCl$_3$). Either the compounds are different or one is significantly less pure than the other.

If a natural product is required for biological testing, it is crucial to know at least the degree of purity and, preferably, the nature of the impurities. It is always possible that the impurities are giving rise to all or part of the biological activities in question. If a compound is to be used to generate pharmacological or **pharmacokinetic** data, it is usually important that the material be very pure (generally >99% pure), particularly if the impurities are analogs of the main compound and may themselves be biologically active.

In some cases, a sample needs only to be partially purified prior to obtaining sufficient structural information. For example, it may be possible to detect the absence of a certain structural feature in crude mixture– perhaps by absence of a particular ultraviolet (UV) maximum– and conclude that the mixture does not contain compound A. In other cases, such as X-ray **crystallography** studies, material will almost be certainly required in an extremely pure state, generally >99.9% pure.

It is worth bearing in mind that the relationship between the degrees of purity achieved in a natural product extraction, and the amount of work required to achieve this, is very approximately **exponential**. It is often relatively easy to start with a crude, complex mixture and eliminate more than half of what is not wanted, but it can be a painstaking **chore** to remove the minor impurities that will turn a 99.5% pure sample into one that is 99.9% pure. It is also probably true to say that this exponential relationship also often holds for the degree of purity achieved versus the yield of natural product. In the same way that no chemical reaction results in 100% yield, and no extraction step results in 100% recovery of the natural product. Compound will be lost at every stage; in many cases it may be that, to achieve very high levels of purity, it is necessary to sacrifice much of the desired material. In order to remove all the impurities it may be necessary to take only the cleanest "cuts" from a separation, thus losing much of the target material in the process (though these side fractions can often be reprocessed).

These factors may, of course, have some bearing on the level of purity deemed satisfactory, and it is useful to ask at each stage of the extraction, whether the natural product is sufficiently pure without any controversy.

At present, there are two main reasons why scientists extract natural products: to find out what they are and/or to carry out further experimental work using the purified compound. In the future, it may be easy to determine structures of compounds in complex mixtures; indeed, it is already possible to do this under some circumstances. Presently, most cases of structural determination of an unknown compound require that it be essentially pure. Likewise, to obtain valid biological or chemical data on a natural product usually requires that it be free from the other experimental variables present in the surrounding biological **matrix**.

Word Study

1. antifeedant [ˌæntɪfiːˈdænt] *n.* 拒食素
2. broth [brɒθ] *n.* 发酵液
3. chore [tʃɔː(r)] *n.* 家庭杂务，讨厌的或累人的工作
4. cogent [ˈkəʊdʒənt] *adj.* 强有力的，使人信服的
5. concentration [ˌkɒnsenˈtreɪʃən] *n.* 集中，专心，浓度
6. crystallography [ˌkrɪstəˈlɒɡrəfi] *n.* 结晶学，晶体学
7. exponential [ˌekspəˈnenʃl] *adj.* 指数的，幂的
8. extraction [ɪkˈstrækʃn] *n.* 提取，提炼，萃取
9. haystack [ˈheɪstæk] *n.* 草堆
10. idiophase [ˈɪdɪəfeɪz] *n.* 繁殖期，生殖期，分化期
11. isolation [ˌaɪsəˈleɪʃn] *n.* 隔离，孤立，分离
12. matrix [ˈmeɪtrɪks] *n.* 矩阵，发源地，基质，母体，子宫
13. melting point [ˈmeltɪŋ pɔint] 熔点
14. morphogenesis [ˌmɔːfəˈdʒenɪsɪs] *n.* [胚] 形态发生，形态形成
15. pharmacokinetic [fɑːməkəʊkaɪˈnetɪks] *n.* 药物代谢动力学
16. polysaccharides [ˈpɒlɪsækærɪdiːz] *n.* 多糖
17. shunt [ʃʌnt] *n.* 分流，转轨
18. sludge [slʌdʒ] *n.* 泥泞，淤泥，沉淀物
19. synthesize [ˈsɪnθəsaɪz] *v.* 合成，综合

Notes

1. Strictly speaking, any biological molecule is a natural product, but the term is usually reserved for secondary metabolites, small molecules (mol wt < 1,500 amu approx) produced by an organism but that are not strictly necessary for the survival of the organism, unlike the more prevalent macromolecules such as proteins, nucleic acids, and polysaccharides that make up the basic machinery for the more fundamental processes of life. 译为：严格来讲，任何生物分子均为天然产物，但该术语通常用于次级代谢物，即生物体产生的小分子（摩尔重量 <1 500 amu 左右）。这些小分子与构成生命重要过程的大分子物质（如蛋白质、核酸和多糖等）不同，它们不是生物体生存所必需的。句中 "mol wt" 为 "molecular weight" 的简写，即分子量；amu 为原子质量单位；approx 为 approximate(ly) 的简写，即大约。

2. Concepts of secondary metabolism include products of overflow metabolism as a result of nutrient limitation, or shunt metabolites produced during idiophase, defense mechanisms, regulator molecules, and so on. 译为：次级代谢的概念中包括因营养限制而产生的溢出代谢产物和在分化期、防御机制、分子调节等产生的分流代谢产物。overflow metabolism 指溢出代谢，shunt metabolites 指分流代谢物。代谢物质的流动过程是一种类似 "流体流动" 的过程，可以接受疏导、阻塞、分流、汇流等

"治理",也可能发生"干枯"和"溢出(泛滥)"现象。

3. Isolation of natural products differs from that of the more commonly occurring biological macromolecules because natural products are smaller and chemically more diverse than the relatively consistent proteins, nucleic acids and carbohydrates, and isolation methods must take this into account.
译为:天然产物的分离不同于更常见的生物大分子,因为天然产物与相对稳定的蛋白质、核酸和碳水化合物相比,分子量更小且更具化学多样性,所以分离方法也要将这些因素考虑在内。

Supplementary Parts

1. Medical and Pharmaceutical Terminology (8): Common Prefixes in Medical and Pharmaceutical English Terms

Prefixes	Meaning	Example
a-,an-	无,没有	amorphous 无定形的
ab-	从,离开	abarticular 非关节的,关节外的
ad-	向,靠近,到……上	adrenal 肾上腺的
allo-	异	allosome 异染色体
ana-	向上,重回到	anabolism 合成代谢
ante-	在前	anteflexion [医学]前屈(尤指子宫前屈)
anti-	反抗	antidote 解毒剂
auto-	自己	autotrophic 自造营养物质的,自给营养的
bi(n,s)-	两,加倍,二	biceps [解剖]二头肌,强健的筋肉
brady-	慢	bradycardia [医学]心动过缓
circum-	环行,围绕	circumduction 环转运动,环行,环转
co(n)-	与……在一起	cocarcinogenesis 助致癌作用
contra-	反,对抗	contraceptive 节育,避孕的
de-	从	deoxidation 脱氧
di-	二倍,加倍	diarthric 两关节的
dia-	通过	diathermy 透热疗法
dis	离开,分开	dislocation 脱位,脱臼
dys-	坏,痛的,困难	dysentery 痢疾
ecto-	外面,在外	ectoderm 外胚层
en-	内,在内	encephalic 脑的
endo-	内部	endocrine 内分泌
epi-	外面,上面,在上	epigastrium 上腹部
eu-	好,正常	euphoria 欣快,精神愉快
ex-	在之外,离开	excision 切除
extra-	在外面,超过	extracorporeal 体外的
hemi-	半	hemiparalysis 偏瘫
hetero-	异	heterogenous 异源的,异种的
homo-	同,等	homosexual 同性恋的
hyper-	超过,过多	hyperglycemia 高血糖
hypo-	低,少于正常	hypoglycemia 低血糖
in-	在内,进入	ingestion 摄入
in-	否定,不	incoagulability 不凝性
infra-	在下,低于	infracostal 肋下的

续表

Prefixes	Meaning	Example
inter-	在……之间	interventricular ［解剖］（心脏）室间的
intra-	在内	intravenous 静脉内的
iso-	同	isotope 同位素,放射性核素
macro-,megalo-	巨大	macroglossia 巨舌
micro-	微小	microscope 显微镜
multi-	多	multipara 经产妇
oligo-	少	oliguria 少尿
para-	旁,附着,异常	paranephric 肾旁的,肾上腺的
per-	通过	peroral 经过口的,口周围的
peri-	周围	perihepatitis 肝周炎
pluri-	多	plurimenorrhea ［医学］多次行经
poly-	多	polyuria 多尿症
post-	在后,在……后方	postnasal 鼻后的
pre-	在前,在……前方	premolar 前磨牙
pro-	在前,在……后方	prognosis 预后
pros-	到,靠近,动上	prosthetics 修复学,装补学
pseudo-	假	pseudomembrane 假膜
semi-	半	semisynthetic 半合成的
sub-	在下	subcutaneous 皮下的
super-	高于,超过	superlactation 泌乳过多
supra-	高于,超过	supracranial 颅上的
syn-	与,在一起,合成	synapse 突触
tachy-	快	tachycardia 心动过速
trans-	穿过,越	transabdominal 通过腹部的

2. English-Chinese Translation Skills: 药学英语翻译技巧 (4)：解包袱法

解包袱（unpacking）法一词最初由美国翻译理论家、语言学家尤金·A·奈达（Eugene A. Nida）提出。他建议译者在使用各种翻译技巧前,必须先将纠缠在一起的语义逻辑关系像解包袱一样解开,然后理顺。解包袱法是针对修饰语和被修饰语之间的语义关系不明而提出的一种策略性翻译方法,旨在挣脱形式上的修饰关系,根据语境去理解语义,它是理解乃至翻译的一个法宝。英汉两种语言词组性质基本相似,如名词性词组、动词性词组、形容词性词组等,但词组构成结构却不尽相同。如汉语中"食品商店"是卖食品的商店,"鞋帽商店"是卖鞋帽的商店,但是"儿童商店"是卖什么的商店呢？这些词组就像一个包袱,理解和翻译这些词组中词与词的关系就要一层层解开这个包袱。

在药学英语翻译中,正确"解包袱"还要了解药学英语语言特点以及药学基础知识。如：prepared sliced of Chinese crude drugs,根据正确的解包袱法,应该译成"中药饮片",而不是"中药备好的切片"。

例 1：The declining popularity of natural products as a source of new drugs began in the 1990s, because of some practical factors, e.g. the apparent lack of compatibility of natural products with the modern high-throughput screening (HTS) programs, where significant degrees of automation, robotics and computers are used, the complexity in the isolation and identification of natural products and the cost and time involved in the natural product "lead" discovery process.

参考译文：从 20 世纪 90 年代开始,因为一些实际原因,天然产物作为药物主要来源这一趋势明显开始下降,天然产物与现代高通量筛选（HTS）方法存在明显不兼容性,高通量筛选自动化程度高,大量使用机器人及计算机技术；在从天然产物发现"先导化合物"的过程中存在复杂的分离与鉴定以及经费和时间投入等方面的问题。

说明：翻译这段文章采用了"解包袱"法。原文中 the declining popularity of natural products 中的 popularity 就需要认真理解，这里的 popularity 不应该理解和翻译成"普及、流行"或者"通俗性、大众性"等，根据语境这里应该翻译成"趋势"。再如原文中 high throughput screening，从词组结构上看，throughput 修饰 screening，其基本意思是"吞吐量、吞吐率、生产量、生产能力"，但是对于专业技术名词词组翻译，解包袱时需要学科背景，随意解释和翻译会出现错译。High-throughput screening (HTS) 是近年来发展起来的药物筛选技术，具有微量、快速、灵敏和准确等特点，能在短时间内测试大量化合物的生物活性。根据专业性知识，high throughput screening 这个"包袱"可以成功解开，译成"高流通筛选"。另外，原文中 in the natural product "lead" discovery process，在理解和翻译时需要对"lead"进行仔细分析。这里的 lead 不是动词"领导、引导"等意思，而是形容词"领头的"，可以理解为"前期的"，药物化学中翻译成"先导的"，与文章涉及的"先导化合物"相呼应，具有隐喻意义。

例 2：A primary reason for the lack of application of biotheorapeutics to neuroscience <u>targets</u>, is that the blood-brain barrier (BBB) isolates and protects central nervous system (CNS) structures creating a unique <u>biochemically and immunologically</u> privileged environment.

参考译文：生物治疗药物较少应用在神经科学领域的首要原因是血脑屏障创造了一个独特的具有生化活性和免疫活性的特殊环境，隔离并保护了中枢神经系统。

说明：在上面例句中，理解和翻译 neuroscience targets 时，要对 target 进行分析。在医药英语中，target 意思是"靶"，如 targeted delivery drugs system（靶向给药系统）、target cell of immunologic reaction（免疫学反应靶细胞）等，neuroscience targets 中 target 采用了单词的基本意思，译成"靶向"。另外，a unique biochemically and immunologically privileged environment 中的两个副词 biochemically 和 immunologically，在理解和翻译时也需要解包袱，不能照字面翻译成"在生化和免疫方面"，而应该根据语言环境，进行词性转译，译成"具有生化活性和免疫活性的"，符合语义和汉语表达习惯。

（翟兴英　王　炜　乔玉玲　史志祥　龚长华）

Unit Nine

Biopharmaceuticals

Unit Nine
数字内容

The term "biopharmaceuticals" was coined in the 1980s and refers to pharmaceuticals produced in biotechnological processes using molecular biology methods. Thus, this group of products was distinguished from the broad category of biologics, which are pharmaceuticals produced using conventional biological methods.

Biopharmaceuticals consist of two groups, biosimilars and biobetters. "Biosimilars" refer to biological medical products containing a version of the active pharmaceutical ingredient found in previously registered reference biological medicinal products. Biobetters are biopharmaceuticals that have been structurally and/or functionally altered to achieve an improved or different clinical performance, compared to the approved reference products. Biopharmaceuticals have many advantages. For instance, they target only specific molecules, rarely causing the side effects associated with conventional small-molecule drugs. Additionally, compared with conventional drugs, biopharmaceuticals exhibit high specificity and activity. The application of biopharmaceuticals has facilitated the treatment of patients who respond poorly to traditional synthetic drugs.

Now, tremendous progress has been made in the research and development of biopharmaceuticals. Advances in manufacturing and processing revolutionized the production of biopharmaceuticals by using new technologies. Much has been learnt from the scientific and clinical experiences of these biological molecules. Further research and development of biopharmaceuticals continue to expand the opportunities to treat an ever increasing number of diseases, and intellectual property rights will remain a crucial incentive for such innovation. Biopharmaceutical drugs play a role in the discovery and development of biomarkers and will go hand in hand with

"生物药物"一词源于20世纪80年代,指的是利用分子生物学方法在生物技术过程中生产出来的药物。因此,这类产品有别于常见的生物制品,后者是使用传统生物学方法生产的药物。

生物药物包括两大类,生物仿制药(生物类似药)和改良型生物药物。"生物仿制药"是指包含有已注册对照生物医药产品中活性成分的生物医药产品。生物改良药是指在结构和/或功能上进行改变,以达到与已审批上市的参比制剂相比改善或具有不同临床性能的生物药品。生物药物有很多优势。例如,它们靶向运输特定的分子,很少如传统小分子药物一般引起不良反应。此外,与传统药物相比,生物药物具有较高的特异性和活性。生物药物的应用有利于对传统合成药物治疗效果不佳的患者。

目前,生物药物的研究和开发取得了巨大进展。新技术的应用促进了制造和加工技术的进步,从而使生物药物的生产产生了革新。这些生物分子在科学研究和临床应用中的经验使我们受益良多。对生物药物的进一步研究和开发将继续扩大在治疗疾病中的受益机会,而知识产权仍将是此类创新的关键激励因素。生物药物在生物标记物的发现和发展中也发挥着重要作用,并将与改善诊断、治疗和预防方法携手并进。新技术和新发现不断涌现,但

improved diagnostics, treatments and prevention methods. New technologies and discoveries are emerging, yet challenges remain. Identifying and validating new targets, the oral delivery of biopharmaceuticals, and improving the success rate of Phase Ⅲ clinical trials, remain to be addressed.

挑战依然存在。确定和验证新的靶点，解决生物药物口服递送问题，提高Ⅲ期临床试验成功率等都是需要解决和突破的难题。

Text A
Recent Progress in Biopharmaceutical Development

Biopharmaceuticals are an important and **integral** component of modern medicine that targets many chronic and acute disease areas with highly-specific treatments. Biopharmaceuticals derive primarily from human or animal sources and function as replacement therapies. The structures of biopharmaceuticals **mimic** those found within the body, thus they have a fewer side effects. Biopharmaceuticals have been proven to be effective in the treatment of diseases that had not been positively addressed by chemically-synthesized small molecule medicines. These complex medicines improve the quality of life of about 400 million patients worldwide, treating widespread diseases such as cancer and diabetes, **hepatitis** C, and chronic renal failure– as well as less common ones such as **haemophilia**, Fabry disease[1], growth deficiency, multiple sclerosis and Crohn's disease[2].

These medicines open new avenues for delivering cutting-edge treatments for numerous diseases and wide patient populations by acting on unique and diverse range of specific targets. Many patients are leading healthier lives as a result of biopharmaceuticals, often without realizing the source of these products. Biopharmaceuticals are made using living systems, which are more sensitive to change than the straight forward chemical synthesis process commonly used for small molecule medicines. The end product is therefore determined by a wide range of factors, which include the actual manufacturing process. Small changes in manufacturing can alter the final product, as biopharmaceuticals are composed of larger and more complex molecules which are difficult to characterize. The high complexity of this process requires precision, **conformance** to good manufacturing practices and defined specifications in order to maintain the safety and efficacy of the product over time.

1. Biopharmaceuticals versus synthetic drugs

Biopharmaceuticals differ from synthetic drugs in all respects. The differences between these two categories of drugs include the nature of the product, the source of the active agent, **bioequivalence** criteria, identity, structure, manufacturing methods, composition, dosing, formulation, handling, intellectual property rights, legal regulations, and marketing.

Biopharmaceuticals are produced in living cells, whereas synthetic drugs are the products of chemical processes. Most synthetic drugs are small molecules. In contrast, biopharmaceuticals are typically 100–1,000 times larger. The active pharmaceutical ingredient of such a drug may contain 2,000–25,000 atoms. Biopharmaceuticals are also structurally much more complex because of the formation of **polymeric** chains, which vary greatly in their structure.

Other characteristics of biopharmaceuticals that distinguish them from synthetic drugs are their sensitivity to degradation in the alimentary system and limited penetrability through the intestinal epithelium. As a result, they are typically administered parenterally via direct injection rather than orally. Biopharmaceuticals also require complex stabilization systems because of their temperature sensitivity.

Unlike synthetic drugs, biopharmaceuticals exhibit much more complex mechanisms of action. For example, interferon affects the expression of more than 40 genes. Such extensive complexity often makes it difficult to determine these pharmaceuticals' complete mechanisms of action.

2. Systems for manufacturing biopharmaceuticals

The active pharmaceutical ingredients in biopharmaceuticals include recombinant proteins[3] and nucleic acids. Currently, the vast majority of commercially available biopharmaceuticals contain recombinant proteins as their active pharmaceutical ingredient. These proteins are produced in prokaryotic systems or eukaryotic systems based on fungi, mammalian cells, insect cell lines, or plant expression system. The use of cell-free expression systems (in vitro systems), which greatly facilitates modifying synthesis conditions, has also been studied. The production of biopharmaceuticals in each of the aforementioned systems has advantages and drawbacks. For these reasons, many different expression systems are used based on the specific properties of a given recombinant protein.

Among the expression systems, mammalian cell lines are generally the preferred platform for manufacturing biopharmaceuticals. In recent years, a steady increase in the use of the expression system has been observed. This is because of the growing interest in the production of large, complex molecules that require specific posttranslational modifications that occur only in mammalian expression systems.

Nevertheless, bacteria remain the dominant expression system, facilitating the production of large quantities of active pharmaceutical ingredients used in biopharmaceuticals. According to the data provided by BioProcess Technology Consultants, in 2010, the total production of pure proteins as active pharmaceutical ingredients in biopharmaceuticals amounted to 26.4 tons. Of this, 68% were produced in bacterial systems and 32% in mammalian systems. The predominant group of proteins produced in bacteria comprised insulins, and the vast majority of those produced in mammalian systems were monoclonal antibodies[4].

3. Commonly-used biopharmaceuticals

3.1. Gene therapies

In addition to recombinant proteins, nucleic acids may also be biopharmaceuticals' active pharmaceutical ingredients. Most studies on gene therapy have focused on the induction or inhibition of cellular processes underlying diseases. Gene therapy is based on the introduction of genetic material into an organism or a patient, either directly or using viruses.

A breakthrough in the biopharmaceutical sector was the registration of a DNA-based drug (the first gene therapy). The first drug used in gene therapy (brand name Glybera) was approved for use in the European Union (EU) in 2012. This therapy compensates for the lipoprotein lipase deficiency found in rare hereditary disorders that leads to severe pancreatitis. Unfortunately, Glybera administration provides only temporary relief. Initially, the cost of a single treatment was estimated at $1.6 million. In 2015, this figure decreased to $1 million, yet this therapy remains the most expensive in the world. A few years earlier, in 2003, another drug used in human gene therapy, Gendicine, was approved in China for the treatment of head and neck **squamous cell carcinoma**. In 2011, Neovasculgen was registered in Russia as a first-in-class gene therapy drug for the treatment of **peripheral artery disease**.

In April 2016, European Medicines Agency (EMA) approved the first *ex vivo* stem cell gene therapy (Strimvelis) with indications to treat patients with **adenosine deaminase-deficient severe combined immunodeficiency**. Strimvelis consists of **autologous** gene-corrected **hematopoietic** stem cells and is prepared from the patient's own bone **marrow** hematopoietic stem cells, which are genetically modified using a **gamma-retroviral vector** to insert a functional copy of the adenosine deaminase gene.

Between 1989 and April 2017, 2,463 gene therapy clinical trials have been completed, are ongoing or have been approved worldwide. So far, most of them have been aimed at the treatment of cancer (64.4% of all gene therapy trials).

Recent research shows that the development of gene therapy can be accelerated by a new, revolutionary **genome** editing tool—clustered regularly interspaced short palindromic repeats (CRISPR[5]). It was successfully used for *in vitro* CRISPR-based genome editing to correct **defective** genotypes. Moreover, several studies have also shown that CRISPR therapies can be successfully **implemented** *in vivo*. There are currently two clinical trials involving CRISPR-Cas9[5] for targeted cancer therapies that have been approved in China and the United States. In 2017, another Chinese group plans to start three clinical trials of drugs developed using the CRISPR technique. These therapies target **bladder**, **prostate** and renal cell cancers. As CRISPR-based treatments have made enormous progress since their beginning only a few years ago, there is great hope that this tool will strongly accelerate the development of gene therapies. Nonetheless, more investigations are needed to fully **harness** the power of this technique, and the ethical issues involved must be fully considered."

3.2. Therapeutic antibodies

Monoclonal antibodies (mAbs) are the largest class of biopharmaceuticals and are currently utilized in therapies for cancer, inflammatory diseases, **cardiovascular** diseases, organ transplantations, infections, respiratory diseases, and **ophthalmologic** diseases. This group of biopharmaceuticals includes mAbs and **derivative** antibodies, such as **bispecific antibodies** (bsAbs), antibody-drug **conjugates** (ADC), **radiolabeled antibody conjugates**, **antigen-binding fragment (Fab)-fusion proteins**. The first monoclonal antibody-based biopharmaceutical was muromonab-CD3 (brand name Orthoclone OKT3), which is administered during acute kidney transplant rejection in 1986. As of March 2017, in the EU and the United States, a total of 71 monoclonal antibody-based drugs have been registered. Currently, fully human antibodies are growing as a proportion of mAbs in the clinic.

Most registered antibodies are **monospecific** antibodies that are capable of interacting with a single target. However, complex diseases, such as cancers or inflammatory disorders, are frequently **multifactorial** in character. In these cases, the inhibition of many different **pathogenic** factors and signaling pathways may enhance the therapeutic efficacy. For this purpose, bsAbs were designed. These antibodies are artificial proteins composed of **fragments** of two different monoclonal antibodies and thus bind to two different types of antigens. BsAbs are most commonly used in cancer **immunotherapy**, where they simultaneously bind to two targets, e.g., a tumor cell and **cytotoxic** cells. BsAbs efficiently stimulate the host immune system, facilitating the destruction of cancer cells. Currently, there are increased numbers of clinical trials being performed on novel, bsAb-based drugs. So far, there are three bsAb-based drugs approved in the world, including Catumaxomab targeting CD3 and EpCAM, blinatumomab targeting CD3 and CD19, and Emicizumab targeting FIX and FX.

Until now, most registered mAb-based drugs are used to treat cancers and autoimmune disorders. According to World Health Organization estimates, the number of new cancer cases will increase to 27 million in 2030 because of the growing number of elderly individuals. Taking into account these **epidemiological** data and the resulting huge demand for anticancer therapy, it is expected that anticancer drugs will be the leading group among all registered drugs. This is also confirmed by data on the number of mAbs that are entering clinical trials.

3.3. Vaccines

Subunit vaccines contain only defined antigens instead of whole pathogens, and, therefore, their application does not introduce the risk of infection. However, a major challenge for current subunit vaccine development is the fact that many new subunit vaccines are poorly **immunogenic** and **mobilize** insufficient immune responses for protective immunity. Therefore, effective adjuvants[6] are needed to enhance, direct, and maintain the immune response to vaccine antigens. New adjuvants are designed to not only **boost** immunological response but also to increase cross-protection against different strains or variants of the same pathogen. Several studies are also conducted on the **synergistic** effects of different adjuvants to identify new beneficial effects of vaccine efficiency.

Another crucial aspect of development of next-generation vaccines is the optimal presentation of the antigen to the immune system to achieve desirable immune response. In the quest for novel and effective presentation methods as well as delivery strategies, virus-like particles (VLPs) offer several promises. VLPs can **elicit** strong T and B cell immune responses because they contain repetitive displays of viral surface proteins that present **conformational** viral **epitopes**. VLPs are not infectious but have similar properties to **virions**, enabling them to be used as both particulate carriers and **adjuvants** in vaccine development. VLPs were successfully used in approved vaccines for hepatitis B and human **papillomavirus**.

Moreover, an important subject in biopharmaceutical development is the emergence of new technologies, which have the potential to revolutionize the vaccine field. These technologies include reverse vaccinology, structural vaccinology, and synthetic vaccines.

4.   The growth of biopharmaceuticals market

Currently, the industry consisting of the development, manufacturing, and marketing of biopharmaceuticals is a multibillion dollar industry. The common practice in market reports is to separately present information about vaccines and other biopharmaceuticals.

Vaccine research costs continue to grow. One of the major contributing factors to this growth is the use of state-of-the-art vaccine development techniques. On the other hand, society expectation is that a vaccine must be affordable for everyone. Because of that implied price cap, pharma industry generally regards vaccines as not the most profitable market **segment**. However, this **perception** of vaccine market is changing. In 2015, worldwide vaccination market generated 27.6 billion U.S. dollars and is projected to total around 39.0 billion U.S. dollars in 2022. The major factors contributing to the expected growth of the vaccines market include high **prevalence** of diseases, rising government and nongovernment funding for vaccine development, and increasing focus on **immunization** programs.

5.   Future prospects for biopharmaceuticals

In recent years, the biopharmaceutical market has been developing at a faster rate than the market for all drugs. According to analysts, this market will continue to grow.

The recently observed and anticipated steady increases in the sales of biopharmaceuticals are associated, among other factors, with the growth of the elderly population and the consequent increase in the number of chronic diseases, the growing number of diabetes and cancer patients, and an increase in the incidence of autoimmune diseases. Insight into the mechanisms underlying various medical conditions has facilitated the identification of specific factors and processes triggering the pathological changes. This has inspired continued research on the applicability of biopharmaceuticals in new clinical situations.

The confirmed efficacy of biopharmaceutical drugs and their acceptance as therapeutic solutions by doctors and patients all contribute to the growing demand for new biopharmaceuticals. One advantage of their application is that they offer targeted therapies rather than symptomatic treatment.

In many cases, they have facilitated the treatment of previously **incurable** diseases. The ability to produce proteins with properties superior to those of native proteins has played a major role in this regard. The growth rate of the biopharmaceuticals market may be significantly influenced by the development of molecular biology methods and their automation, increases in the knowledge about expression systems, and better understanding of the operational processes and technological factors related to the scale-up of recombinant protein production. The highly promising prospects of the biopharmaceutical market are related to breakthrough innovations, such as the development of immunotherapy, antibody-drug conjugates, and gene therapies.

Factors hindering the development of this market include the high costs of implementing the developed biopharmaceuticals. In the area of novel biopharmaceuticals, we may see a trend in the active pharmaceutical ingredients toward the enhancement of naturally found ones' therapeutic efficacies.[7] Considering the data on the preparations being currently tested in clinical trials, we can expect a steady increase in the numbers of newly registered mAbs and their dominant presence in the biopharmaceutical market. Because the patent protections of many of the best-selling biopharmaceuticals will **expire** soon, it appears logical to forecast the introduction of a significant number of **biosimilars**, which will be their equivalents.

Word Study

1. adenosine deaminase-deficient severe combined immunodeficiency 腺苷脱氨酶缺陷重症联合免疫缺陷

2. adjuvant ['ædʒuvənt] *n.* 佐剂, 佐药

3. aforementioned [əfɔː'menʃənd] *adj.* 上述的, 前文提及的

4. alimentary system [əli'mentərɪ 'sistəm] *n.* 消化系统

5. antigen-binding fragment (Fab)-fusion proteins *n.* 抗原结合片段（Fab）- 融合蛋白

6. autologous [ɒ'tɒləgəs] *adj.* 自体的, 自体同源的

7. bioequivalence [ˌbaɪəui'kwivələs] *n.* 生物等效性

8. biopharmaceutical [baɪəuˌfɑːmə'sjuːtikl] *n.* 生物药物; *adj.* 生物制药学的

9. biosimilars [ˌbaɪə'sɪmɪlə] *n.* 生物仿制药, 生物类似药

10. bispecific antibody [baɪ'spesɪfɪk 'æntɪˌbɒdɪ] *n.* 双特异性抗体

11. bladder ['blædə] *n.* 膀胱

12. boost [buːst] *v.* 增强, 使增长

13. cardiovascular [ˌkɑːdiəu'væskjələ(r)] *adj.* 心血管的

14. conformance [kən'fɔ:məns] *n.* 一致性，顺应性

15. conformational [,kɒnfɔ: 'meɪʃənəl] *adj.* 构象的

16. conjugate ['kɒndʒəgeɪt] *n.* 偶联物

17. cytotoxic [,saɪtə'tɒkəsɪk] *adj.* 细胞毒素的

18. defective [dɪ'fektɪv] *adj.* 有缺陷的

19. degradation [,degrə'deɪʃən] *n.* 降解

20. derivative [dɪ'rɪvətɪv] *adj.* 衍生的，派生的

21. elicit [ɪ'lɪsɪt] *v.* 引出，诱出

22. epidemiological [,epɪ,dɪmɪə'lɒdʒɪkəl] *adj.* 流行病学的

23. epithelium [,epɪ'θɪːlɪəm] *n.* 上皮，上皮细胞

24. epitope ['epɪtəup] *n.* ［免疫学］表位

25. eukaryotic [,juːkærɪ'ɒtɪk] *adj.* 真核的，真核生物的

26. expire [ɪk'spaɪə] *v.* 到期，失效

27. facilitate [fə'sɪlɪteɪt] *v.* 促进，使更容易

28. fragment ['frægmənt] *n.* 碎片，片段

29. fungi ['fʌŋgaɪ] *n.* 真菌

30. gamma-retroviral vector ['gaːmə ,retrə'vaɪrəl 'vektə] *n.* γ- 逆转录病毒载体

31. genome ['dʒiːnəum] *n.* 基因组

32. haemophilia [,hiːmə'fɪlɪə] *n.* 血友病

33. harness ['haːnɪs] *v.* 控制并利用

34. hematopoietic [,hemətəupɔɪ'iːtɪk] *adj.* 造血的，生血的

35. hepatitis [,hepə'taɪtɪs] *n.* 肝炎（hepatitis B: 乙型肝炎；hepatitis C: 丙型肝炎）

36. hereditary [hə'redɪt(ə)rɪ] *adj.* 遗传的

37. immunization [,ɪmjuːnaɪ'zeɪʃn] *n.* 免疫，免疫接种

38. immunogenic [ɪ,mjuːnəu'dʒenɪk] *adj.* 产生免疫反应的，免疫原性的

39. immunotherapy [ɪ,mjuːnəu'θerəpɪ] *n.* 免疫疗法

40. implement ['ɪmplɪmənt] *v.* 贯彻，实施

41. incurable [ɪn'kjuərəbl] *adj.* 不能治疗的，无法治愈的

42. insulin ['ɪnsjulɪn] *n.* 胰岛素

43. integral ['ɪntɪgrəl] *adj.* 完整的，构成整体所必需的

44. interferon [,ɪntə'fɪərɒn] *n.* ［生化］［药］干扰素

45. intestinal [ɪn'testɪnəl] *n.* 肠的

46. lipoprotein lipase deficiency ['lɪpəprəutiːn 'laɪpeɪz dɪ'fɪʃnsɪ] *n.* 脂蛋白脂肪酶缺乏

47. marrow ['mærəu] *n.* 骨髓，髓

48. mimic ['mɪmɪk] *v.* 模仿，模拟

49. mobilize ['məubə,laɪz] *v.* 动员，调动

50. monospecific [,mɒnəuspɪ'sɪfɪk] *adj.* 单特异性的

51. multifactorial [,mʌltɪfæk'tɔːrɪəl] *adj.* 多因素的

52. nucleic acid [njuː'kliːk 'æsid] *n.* 核酸

53. ophthalmologic [ɔf,θælmə'lɒdʒik] *adj.* 眼科学的

54. pancreatitis [,pænkrɪə'taɪtɪs] *n.* 胰腺炎

55. papillomavirus [,pæpɪ'ləumə,vaɪrəs] *n.* 乳头瘤病毒

56. parenterally [pə'rentərəlɪ] *adv.* 非肠道,不经肠道

57. pathogenic [ˌpæθə'dʒenɪk] *adj.* 致病的,病原的

58. penetrability [ˌpenɪtrə'bɪlɪtɪ] *n.* 穿透性,渗透性

59. perception [pə'sepʃn] *n.* 感知,认识

60. peripheral artery disease [pe'rɪfərəl 'ɑːtərɪ dɪ'ziːz] *n.* 外周动脉疾病

61. polymeric [ˌpɒlɪ'merɪk] *adj.* 聚合的,聚合体的

62. posttranslational [ˌpəʊsttræns'leɪʃənəl] *adj.* 翻译后的

63. predominant [prɪ'dɒmɪnənt] *adj.* 显著的,占主导地位的

64. prevalence ['prevələns] *n.* 流行,盛行

65. prokaryotic [prəʊˌkærɪ'ɒtɪk] *adj.* 原核的

66. prostate ['prɒsteɪt] *n.* 前列腺

67. radiolabeled antibody conjugate ['reɪdɪəʊ'leɪbəld 'æntɪˌbɒdɪ 'kɒndʒəgeɪt] *n.* 放射性标记抗体偶联物

68. recombinant [rɪ'kɒmbɪnənt] *adj.* (基因)重组的

69. segment ['segmənt] *n.* 部分,片段,(市场)细分的部分

70. squamous cell carcinoma ['skweɪməs sel ˌkɑːsɪ'nəʊmə] *n.* 鳞状细胞癌

71. stabilization [ˌsteɪbəlaɪ'zeɪʃn] *n.* 稳定,稳定化

72. subunit ['sʌbjuːnɪt] *n.* 亚组,亚单位

73. synergistic [ˌsɪnə'dʒɪstɪk] *adj.* 协同的,协作的

74. virion ['vaɪrɪən] *n.* 病毒粒子,病毒体

Notes

1. Fabry disease:法布里病。一种罕见的 X 连锁遗传性疾病,由于体内编码 α- 半乳糖苷酶 A 的基因突变,导致 α- 半乳糖苷酶 A 结构和功能异常,使其代谢产物三己糖神经酰胺(GL-3)和相关鞘糖脂在全身多个器官内大量堆积。

2. Crohn's disease:克罗恩病。一种慢性的全身性疾病,表现为胃肠道或消化道内炎症,发作时可引起持续性腹泻、腹痛和直肠出血。

3. Recombinant proteins: 重组蛋白,即通过重组 DNA 技术将两个或两个以上的 DNA 序列结合在一起表达得到的蛋白质。注意区分:重组 DNA 技术与体内自身发生的利用基因剪切将两段序列连接起来不一样,后者是细胞内调控基因表达的自有方式。

4. Monoclonal antibody:单克隆抗体。根据世界卫生组织 2021 年 11 月修订的单克隆抗体国际非专利名称(The WHO's International Nonproprietary Names, INN)命名规则,单克隆抗体的英文命名由前缀 + 亚词干 + 词干(后缀)组成。其中,前缀不做规定限制;词干与原有的统一词干 "-mab"(monoclonal antibody 的缩写)不同,根据抗体的类别分为了四类:

第一类:全长或抗体的 Fc 片段未经人工修饰改造的单克隆抗体,使用 "-tug"(unmodified immunoglobulin)为后缀词干。

第二类:利用抗体工程技术在抗体的 Fc 片段引入突变的单克隆抗体,使用 "-bart"(antibody artificial)为后缀词干。

第三类:双特异性或多特异性单克隆抗体,使用 "-mig"(multi-immunoglobulin)为后缀词干;

第四类:片段化抗体,使用 "-ment"(fragment)为后缀词干。

亚词干根据单克隆抗体所针对的疾病类型或作用机制进行选择。具体见下表。

Infix	Definition
-ami-	serum amyloid protein (SAP)/amyloidosis (pre-substem)
-ba-	bacterial
-ci-	cardiovascular
-de-	metabolic or endocrine pathways
-eni-	enzyme inhibition
-fung-	fungal
-gro-	skeletal muscle mass related growth factors and receptors
-ki-	cytokine and cytokine receptor
-ler-	allergen
-sto-	immunostimulatory
-pru-	immunosuppressive
-ne-	neural
-os-	bone
-ta-	tumor
-toxa-	toxin
-vet-	veterinary use
-vi-	viral

5. CRISPR 及 CRISPR-Cas9：CRISPR 全称为 clustered regularly interspaced short palindromic repeats（规律间隔成簇的短回文重复序列），是微生物基因组中存在的一些具有间隔重复特征的重复序列，具有免疫记忆和防御功能，可以作为微生物防御外源生物攻击的保护机制，一般直接用英文缩写 CRISPR 表示；Cas9 是一种可以识别特定序列的核酸酶。CRISPR-Cas9 表示一种基因编辑技术。所谓基因编辑，即利用核酸酶剪切和细胞自身具有的 DNA 损伤修复机制（一般为同源重组修复和非同源重组修复），直接在体内对基因组特定位置进行编辑的技术。

6. Adjuvant：佐剂，即添加到疫苗中可增强免疫反应强度和持久性的辅助试剂。免疫佐剂可以先于抗原或与抗原同时使用，能够非特异性地增强机体对抗原的特异性免疫应答反应，而自身不包含抗原性物质。

7. 在理解 "In the area of novel biopharmaceuticals, we may see a trend in the active pharmaceutical ingredients toward the enhancement of naturally found ones' therapeutic efficacies." 句子时，要注意两点：①本句的主要结构是：we see a trend in... toward... a trend toward...，意为"……的趋势"。②后半句中的 one's，指的是前文中的 ingredients，即 the enhancement of naturally found ingredients' therapeutic efficacies：增强天然发现成分的治疗效果。本句的意思是："在新型生物药物领域，我们可能会看到一种趋势，即活性药物成分会增强天然发现成分的治疗效果。"

Exercises

1. Decide whether each of the following statements is true (T) or false (F) according to the passage.

(1) Biopharmaceuticals are made using living systems more sensitive to change. Compared to synthetic drugs, they are composed of smaller and more complex molecules.

(2) The recombinant proteins as the active pharmaceutical ingredient are produced in prokaryotic systems, or eukaryotic systems or cell-free expression systems, and the specific properties of a given recombinant protein determines the use of different expression systems.

(3) The end products of biopharmaceuticals and synthetic drugs differ in all respects, such as the structure, identity, dosing, formulation, nature and manufacturing methods of the product, the source of the active

agent, etc. except in the bioequivalence criteria and legal regulations.

(4) Most registered antibodies are monospecific antibodies capable of interacting with a single target. In order to enhance a therapeutic efficacy, bsAbs composed of fragments of two monoclonal antibodies and thus binding to two types of antigens are designed to inhibit many different pathogenic factors and signaling pathways.

(5) Subunit vaccines contain only defined antigens instead of whole pathogens, and their application does not introduce the risk of infection, but some subunit vaccines are poorly immunogenic and mobilize insufficient immune responses for protective immunity.

(6) The growth of the elderly population and the increase in the number of chronic diseases, diabetes and cancers and autoimmune diseases contribute to the more sales of biopharmaceuticals, since they offer symptomatic treatment and targeted therapies.

2.　Questions for oral discussion.

(1) What are the differences between biopharmaceuticals and synthetic drugs?

(2) What are the major factors contributing to the expected growth of the vaccines market?

(3) What are the advantages and disadvantages of subunit vaccines?

(4) What's the future prospect for biopharmaceuticals?

3.　Choose the best answer to each of the following sentences.

(1) Which of the following is not the fact that explains why biopharmaceuticals have fewer side effects?

A. They can target many chronic and acute disease areas with highly-specific treatments.

B. They derive primarily from human or animal sources.

C. They structurally mimic those in living cells found within the body.

D. They exhibit high specificity and activity, targeting only specific molecules.

(2) Which of the following is not right according to the text?

A. Pharmaceuticals are produced in biotechnological processes using molecular biology methods.

B. Biologics are pharmaceuticals produced using conventional biological methods.

C. As replacement therapies, biopharmaceuticals are also effective in the treatment of conditions positively addressed by chemically-synthesized small molecule medicines.

D. Biopharmaceutical drugs contribute to the discovery and development of biomarkers, with the prospect of improved diagnostics, treatments and prevention methods.

(3) Which of the following statements is right according to the text?

A. Synthetic drugs are more sensitive than biopharmaceuticals to degradation in the alimentary system.

B. As the products of chemical process, synthetic drugs require complex stabilization system for their temperature sensitivity.

C. With their limited penetrability through the intestinal epithelium, biopharmaceuticals are typically administered parenterally via injection.

D. That interferon affects the expression of more than 40 genes indicates synthetic drug's more complex action mechanisms.

(4) As the active pharmaceutical ingredient, recombinant proteins can be produced in the following systems except _____.

A. prokaryotic system

B. mammalian cells

C. cell-free expression systems

D. bacterial expression system

(5) Among the drugs used in human gene therapy worldwide mentioned in the text, the first drug was

_____ in _____.

A. Gendicine; 2003   B. Glybera; 2012

C. Strimveils; 2016   D. Neovasculgen; 2011

(6) Because of many new subunit vaccines' poor immunogenicity, effective adjuvants are designed for the

following purposes except _____.

A. to mobilize sufficient immune responses for protective immunity

B. to enhance, direct, and maintain the immune response to vaccine antigens

C. to identify the beneficial effects of vaccine efficiency

D. to increase cross-protection against different strains or variants of the same pathogen

(7) Compared with monospecific antibodies with some clinical drawbacks, bsAbs were designed for the

following purposes but _____.

A. to focus on the interaction with the specific target for a better therapeutic efficacy

B. to be used in cancer immunotherapy targeting both the tumor cell and cytotoxic cells

C. to inhibit many different pathogenic factors and signaling pathways to enhance the therapeutic efficacy

D. to stimulate the host immune system facilitating the destruction of cancer cells

(8) Which of the following factors, according to the text, mostly leads to the growing of vaccine research

costs?

A. Social expectation that everyone could afford the vaccine.

B. The use of the newest and advanced vaccine development techniques.

C. Pharm industry's concern of the vaccine safety.

D. Public insistence of the vaccine's conformance to good manufacturing practices.

(9) According to the text, CRISPR-based treatments _____.

A. can be successfully implemented both *in vitro* and *in vivo*

B. can accelerate the development of the antibody research

C. are under clinical trials targeting bladder, prostate and renal cell cancers

D. need further investigations of their moral defect

(10) The confirmed efficacy of biopharmaceutical drugs contributes to the growing demand for new

biopharmaceuticals, whose application offers _____.

A. targeted therapies

B. symptomatic treatment

C. gene therapies

D. substitution therapy

4. Complete the following sentences with the correct form of the appropriate words given in the box.

edition, gene, prefer, innovate, optimize, modify, conjugate, address, recombine, reject, cell, regulate

(1) Currently, the vast majority of commercially available biopharmaceuticals contain _____ proteins

as their active pharmaceutical ingredient produced in prokaryotic systems, or eukaryotic systems based

on fungi etc.

(2) Mammalian express systems are the _____ platform for manufacturing biopharmaceuticals.

(3) One crucial aspect of developing next-generation vaccines is the _____ presentation of the antigen to the immune system to achieve desirable immune response.

(4) Recent research shows that CRISPR, a new, revolutionary genome _____ tool can speed up the development of gene therapy.

(5) Initially, bsAbs were generated via the chemical _____ of two different antibodies, producing a single molecule equipped with four antigen-binding regions.

(6) The first monoclonal antibody-based biopharmaceutical was Orthoclone OKT3 administered during acute kidney transplant _____ in 1980s.

(7) As our knowledge of disease increases, so does the potential of discovering and developing _____ medicines.

(8) Most studies on gene therapy have focused on the induction or inhibition of _____ processes underlying diseases.

(9) While most gene therapy trials have _____ cancer, a significant number of gene therapy trials have targeted rare inherited monogenic diseases.

(10) Gene therapy is based on the introduction of _____ material into an organism or a patient, either directly or using viruses.

5. Translate the following sentences and paragraphs into Chinese.

(1) Biopharmaceuticals represent some of the best accomplishments of modern science. These drugs are increasingly being used in practically all branches of medicine and have become one of the most effective clinical treatment modalities for a broad range of diseases, including cancers and metabolic disorders.

(2) DNA method has helped to produce biologically active proteins that do not exist in nature, such as chimeric, humanized or fully human monoclonal antibodies, or antibody-related proteins or other engineered biological medicines such as fusion proteins, using a range of different expression systems.

(3) Insulin plays a central role in regulating blood glucose levels, generally keeping it within narrow defined limits, irrespective of the nutritional status. Failure of the body to synthesize sufficient insulin results in the development of insulin dependent diabetes mellitus (IDDM), also known as type 1 diabetes.

(4) A vaccine contains a preparation of antigenic components derived from a pathogen. Normally, an initial dose administration is followed by subsequent administration of one or more repeat doses over an appropriate time scale serving to maximize the immunological response.

(5) Initially, bsAbs were generated via the chemical conjugation of two different antibodies, producing a single molecule equipped with four antigen-binding regions, with each of the fragment pairs binding a different molecule. Another approach to generating bsAbs is the fusion of two hybrids, producing antibodies with differing specificities.

(6) Research on molecular biology methods in vaccine development has discovered several promising results. There are a number of novel vaccines at various stages of the drug acceptance process, including vaccines against major infectious diseases such as HIV and tuberculosis, a universal flu vaccine, and vaccines against noninfectious diseases.

(7) The global vaccines market is segmented based on technology, type, disease indication, end-users, and regions. Based on increasing company investments, the highest growth rate in the vaccines market is expected to be registered in the conjugate vaccines segment.

Value-Oriented Reflective Reading

The Dawn of China Biopharma Innovation

China's biopharmaceutical ecosystem is experiencing a momentous shift from a formerly generics-focused play into one that nurtures innovation, with profound implications for patients and industry peers.

Innovation in Chinese biopharma is fast becoming a notable story, underscored by significant value creation on global capital markets. The market value of publicly listed biopharma innovation players from China across the Nasdaq, Hong Kong Stock Exchange (HKEX), and Shanghai Stock Exchange Science and Technology Innovation Board (STAR) has surged from $3 billion in 2016 to more than $380 billion in July 2021. Biotechnology companies originating in China accounted for $180 billion of that total. Public debuts for Chinese players have also accelerated, with 23 IPOs in 2020 alone. Indeed, Chinese biotechs are leading on IPO fundraising—seven out of the world's top ten largest biopharma IPOs from 2018 to 2020 originated from China.

Regulatory reforms, the emergence of bioclusters in areas such as the city of Suzhou, talent returning from overseas, and the opening of China's capital markets have all played a part in enabling Chinese biopharma to emerge on the global innovation stage.

To understand how China's biopharma innovation ecosystem is evolving and obtain a more nuanced understanding of the drivers behind its growth, McKinsey maintains the China Drug Innovation Index (CDII). First launched in 2016, the survey asks industry experts to gauge five dimensions that support healthy biopharma innovation: policy environment (split between regulatory reforms and market access policies), funding, research and development (R&D) capability, local innovation output, and integration with global markets. Participants rate China on a scale from 0 to 10, with 10 being the highest, and the United States serving as a benchmark with a score of 8.

Rapid regulatory reform has supported faster development and approvals

The regulatory environment subdimension showed the largest improvement, with the score advancing from 4.0 in 2016 to 6.2 in 2020. The speed and scale of the reform is quite unprecedented in China's history; a 2015 overhaul, with the goal to bring China's pharmaceutical regulations into line with international standards, had facilitated accession to the International Council for Harmonisation of Technical Requirements for Pharmaceuticals for Human Use by 2017. These steps enabled China's drug discovery and development ecosystem to integrate globally. Meanwhile, measures to accelerate new-drug reviews, including raising the number of staff at the Center for Drug Evaluation (CDE) from 150 in 2015 to 700-plus in 2018 (supplemented by over 600 external committee members), helped clear a backlog of 20,000 applications in two years, according to CDE data.

In parallel, China's National Medical Products Administration (NMPA) streamlined new-drug-approval procedures, beginning with the introduction of priority reviews in 2016. Based on NMPA data, the proportion of drugs under priority review increased from 14 percent in 2016 to 77 percent in 2019. In 2018, the NMPA added conditional approvals based on clinical trial data, and has since granted 34 conditional approvals, according to CDE data released at the 2021 Chinese Society of Clinical Oncology conference. In July 2020, Drug Registration Regulations introduced a new channel for breakthrough therapies, with over 70 drugs receiving the designation as of August 2021. These reforms helped energize a powerful innovation pipeline.

Innovation value-chain capabilities are steadily improving

Overseas returnees with decades of drug- development expertise and the booming growth of contract research organizations (CROs) and contract development and manufacturing organizations (CDMOs) helped lift the R&D score in 2020 to 5.5, a modest increase from 2016. The proliferation of CRO and CDMO infrastructure has helped to foster biotechnology innovation, allowing China to emerge as one of the leading providers of services in some subsegments. For example, WuXi AppTec and Pharmaron are now the world's largest providers of preclinical chemistry services. Our survey also highlights improvement in the clinical development and chemistry, manufacturing, and control (CMC) capabilities required to support ecosystem growth. That said, we still have gaps in academic research, drug discovery, and the infrastructure for technology transfer from academia to industry, according to the CDII.

Mapping the future of Chinese innovation: Three trends to watch

China's biopharma ecosystem is advancing in the right direction across the CDII, showing incremental improvements in most of the areas necessary to foster innovation. These advances are ushering China's biopharma industry into a new phase characterized by three major trends: faster drug development, deeper differentiation, and the ambition to make an impact on the global innovation landscape.

China-based biopharmas have historically pursued a fast-follower strategy, developing a risk-balanced portfolio heavily weighted in favor of clinically validated targets pioneered overseas. More recently, many players are shortening the time lag with global leaders targeting the same mechanism of action (MoA) while turning toward early-stage, nonclinically validated MoA.

Investment by Chinese biotechs in innovation and differentiation is bearing fruit. For instance, Junshi Biosciences is developing an anti-BTLA mAb with first-in-class potential, while I-Mab's anti-CD47 mAb has best-in-class potential due to an elevated safety profile that lowers red blood cell binding.

Chinese biopharmas are exploring options to go global and secure the full value of their innovations. As a result, one could expect more international partnerships that encompass overseas clinical trials and aim to develop and commercialize innovative drugs discovered in China for patients in US and European markets. As a corollary, Chinese biopharma innovations are gaining regulatory recognition worldwide.

Questions for discussion:

1. What can show the significant value creation on global capital markets of China's innovation in biopharma?

2. What are the major trends of China's innovation in its biopharma ecosystem?

3. What have been the major parts of regulatory reforms in China? Why do you think they have been effective in promoting China's development of its biopharma industry?

Text B
mRNA Vaccines for Infectious Diseases:
Principles, Delivery, and Clinical Translation

Vaccination is the most effective public health intervention for preventing the spread of infectious diseases. Successful vaccination campaigns eradicated life-threatening diseases such as **smallpox**, and the World Health Organization estimates that vaccines prevent two to three million deaths every year from

tetanus, **pertussis**, influenza, and **measles**. Despite their evident success, however, conventional vaccines do not effectively tackle pathogens such as hepatitis C and human immunodeficiency virus (HIV), which evade **immune surveillance**. Furthermore, they require regular modification to address rapidly mutating pathogens, such as the influenza virus.

mRNA vaccines were conceived more than three decades ago in the hope of generating safe and versatile vaccines that are easy to produce[1]. Unlike some viral vaccines, mRNA does not integrate into the genome, obviating concerns about insertional mutagenesis. mRNA vaccines can be manufactured in a cell-free manner, allowing rapid, scalable, and cost-effective production. Moreover, a single mRNA vaccine can encode multiple antigens, strengthening the immune response against resilient pathogens and enabling the targeting of multiple microbes or viral variants with a single formulation. However, mRNA was not pursued as a therapeutic because of concerns about its stability, poor efficacy and excessive **immunostimulation**. Fortunately, over the past decade, by determining mRNA pharmacology, developing effective delivery vehicles, and controlling mRNA **immunogenicity**, interest in clinical applications of mRNA has renewed.

1. Principles of mRNA design and synthesis

mRNA vaccines comprise synthetic mRNA molecules that direct the production of the antigen that will generate an immune response. *In vitro*-transcribed mRNA mimics the structure of endogenous mRNA, with 5'-cap, 5'-untranslated region (UTR), an open reading frame that encodes the antigen, 3'-UTR, and a poly(A) tail. The mRNA is synthetically produced and formulated into vaccines: (1) Once the genome of a pathogen has been sequenced, a sequence for the target antigen is designed and inserted into a plasmid DNA construct. (2) Plasmid DNA is transcribed into mRNA by **bacteriophage** polymerases *in vitro* and mRNA transcripts are purified by high performance liquid chromatography (HPLC) to remove contaminants and reactants. (3) Purified mRNA is mixed with lipids in a microfluidic mixer to form lipid **nanoparticles**. Rapid mixing causes the lipids to **encapsulate** mRNA instantaneously and precipitate as self-assembled nanoparticles. (4) The nanoparticle solution is dialysed or filtered to remove non-aqueous solvents and any unencapsulated mRNA and the filtered mRNA vaccine solution is stored in sterilized vials.

All native mRNAs include modified **nucleosides**, the immune system has evolved to recognize unmodified single-stranded RNA, which is a hallmark of viral infection. Basing on that, the mRNA sequence typically incorporates modified nucleosides, such as **pseudouridine**, N1-methylpseudouridine or other nucleoside analogues. The use of modified nucleosides, particularly modified uridine, prevents recognition by pattern recognition receptors[2], enabling sufficient levels of translation to produce prophylactic amounts of protein. Another strategy to avoid detection by pattern recognition receptors uses sequence engineering and codon optimization to deplete uridines by boosting the GC content of the vaccine mRNA.

2. Delivery vehicles for mRNA vaccines

Because mRNA is large (10^4–10^6 Da) and negatively charged, it cannot pass through the **anionic lipid bilayer** of cell membranes. Moreover, inside the body, it is engulfed by cells of the innate immune system and degraded by nucleases. Various techniques, including **electroporation**, gene guns and *ex vivo* transfection can intracellularly deliver mRNA in a dish. *In vivo* application, however, requires the use of mRNA delivery vehicles that transfect immune cells without causing toxicity or unwanted immunogenicity. Fortunately, several innovative materials-based solutions have been developed for this purpose. For example, lipid nanoparticles encapsulate mRNA in their core. They consist of four components: **ionizable** lipids, such as DLin-MC3-DMA42, SM-102, ALC-0315, A18-Iso5-2DC18, and 306Oi10; **cholesterol** or its variants, β-sitostero and 20α-**hydroxycholesterol**; helper lipids, such as DSPC and DOPE; and PEGylated lipids, such as ALC-0159 and PEG-DMG. Polymers that form polymer-mRNA complexes are also useful mRNA delivery vehicles. Squalene-based cationic **nanoemulsions** also deliver mRNA. These nanoemulsions consist of an oily squalene core stabilized by a lipid shell that adsorbs mRNA onto its surface.

In addition to lipid and polymer-based vehicles, peptides can also deliver mRNA into cells, thanks to the cationic or **amphipathic** amine groups (for example, arginine) in their backbone and side chains that **electrostatically** bind to mRNA and form nanocomplexes. For example, a fusogenic cell-penetrating peptide containing repetitive arginine-alanine-leucine-alanine (RALA) **motifs** changes conformation at **endosomal** pH, facilitating pore formation in the membrane and endosomal escape. RALA delivers mRNA to dendritic cells (professional antigen-presenting cells of the immune system) to elicit T cell-mediated immunity.

3. Progress with mRNA vaccines for infectious diseases

Vaccines for infectious diseases are currently the most advanced application for mRNA therapeutics. Most mRNA vaccines currently in preclinical trials and in clinical use are administered as a bolus injection into the skin, muscle, or subcutaneous space, where they are taken up by immune or non-immune cells and translated into antigens that are displayed to T and B cells. Both the mRNA and the delivery vehicle enhance the immunogenicity and efficacy of mRNA vaccines.

By the end of 2019, fifteen mRNA vaccine candidates against infectious diseases had entered clinical trials, with none in phase Ⅲ trials. At that time, it was thought that it would be at least another 5–6 years before an mRNA vaccine would obtain regulatory approval.

Influenza viruses

Influenza viruses are responsible for an estimated 290,000–650,000 deaths annually worldwide. Current vaccines target the virus **haemagglutinin** protein, which facilitates viral entry. However, the virus mutates rapidly, causing antigenic drift that requires yearly review and modification of the haemagglutinin antigen component of the vaccines. Conventional influenza vaccines, which are inactivated influenza viruses grown in chicken eggs, are subject to long production times and purification difficulties. There is a real need, therefore, for alternative antigen targets and production methods. Synthetic mRNAs transcribed *in vitro* can meet this need and ensure rapid vaccine production in the event that an entirely new influenza strain[3] emerges.

There has also been work towards a universal influenza vaccine that would not require yearly modification. Such a vaccine would confer immunity against several influenza strains (heterologous immunity) and subtypes (**heterosubtypic** immunity). In the first demonstration of an effective mRNA vaccine against influenza in 2012, three intradermal injections of 80 μg RNActive-mRNA encoding haemagglutinin from the PR8 H1N1 strain induced homologous and **heterologous** immunity against H1N1 and H5N1 strains, respectively, and protected the mice against a lethal viral dose. Since then, several delivery vehicles, alternative mRNA technologies, and alternative antigen targets have been evaluated for mRNA-based influenza vaccines.

Notably, the conserved stalk region of haemagglutinin, which is not prone to mutation, has recently emerged as a novel universal vaccine target. A primer-booster regimen of an LNP-based mRNA vaccine encoding the conserved haemagglutinin stalk from the Cal09 H1N1 strain produced a stalk-specific antibody response in mice, ferrets and rabbits. The broadly protective antibodies conferred homologous immunity against Cal09 H1N1, heterologous immunity against PR8 H1N1 and heterosubtypic immunity against H5N1 in mice and protected them against a lethal viral challenge.

In two separate phase I trials in 2016, Moderna evaluated two influenza candidates. These vaccines were dosed via two intramuscular injections of LNPs encapsulating nucleoside-modified[4] mRNA expressing full-length haemagglutinin from H10N8 and H7N9. Both produced excellent **seroconversion** and **seroprotection**. Adverse effects were limited to pain at the injection site, redness, muscle pain, joint pain, headache, fatigue and chills/common-cold-like symptoms, indicating that the vaccine is safe and well tolerated.

Zika viruses

Zika virus infection was first identified in 1947, and patients infected with *Zika* are often **asymptomatic** or experience mild symptoms such as fever, rash, and muscle pain. However, *Zika* emerged as a global health crisis during the 2015–2016 epidemic in the Americas when the virus caused severe fetal **neuroma** formations and fetal death during pregnancy. Fortunately, all *Zika* infections are caused by a single **serotype**, suggesting that vaccinating against an antigen from any strain could protect against all *Zika* strains. The membrane and envelope protein (prM-E) is a common antigen choice for mRNA vaccines against *Zika*, as neutralizing antibodies[5] against prM-E can prevent viral fusion.

One study showed that a single 30 μg or 50 μg dose of an LNP-encapsulated nucleoside-modified prM-E mRNA protected mice and **rhesus macaques**, respectively, from a *Zika* challenge. Of note, the **neutralizing antibody titres** generated by the mRNA vaccine were 50–100 times higher than those induced by purified inactivated virus and DNA vaccines in mice, and 50 times higher than a 1 mg DNA vaccine in macaques.

Importantly, poorly designed *Zika* virus vaccines can increase the infectiousness of the ***Dengue virus***. *Dengue virus* is from the same viral family as *Zika*, and their envelope proteins share 54%–59% overlapping amino acid sequence. Therefore, it is possible that the envelope protein antigen encoded by a *Zika* vaccine spurs the production of antibodies that are cross-reactive with the dengue envelope protein. In the event of a subsequent *Dengue virus* infection, antibody-dependent enhancement can occur in which the suboptimal anti-*Zika* antibodies bind to the *Dengue virus*. This binding enhances the entry of the virus into host cells and exacerbates dengue symptoms. Moderna collaborated with Washington University School of Medicine to deliver a modified prM-E mRNA containing a mutated fusion loop epitope in the E protein. Two 10 μg doses of the LNP-encapsulated modified mRNA delivered 21 days apart protected mice from a *Zika* challenge and diminished the production of dengue-enhancing antibodies. These encouraging preclinical results prompted a phase I trial, and interim results suggest that the vaccine—mRNA-1893— induces 94%–100% seroconversion in 10 μg and 30 μg dose groups and is well tolerated.

Human immunodeficiency virus (HIV)

Globally, HIV currently affects 38 million people and is projected to affect up to 42 million people by 2030. In 2020 alone, there were 1.5 million new infections and 680,000 deaths. Despite 30 years of research, no effective vaccine has been developed, primarily owing to the remarkable antigenic diversity of the HIV envelope protein and the dense 'glycan shield' that conceals crucial envelope protein epitopes. Several preclinical studies have delivered mRNA vaccines encoding HIV proteins using multiple delivery vehicles, including cationic nanoemulsions, DOTAP/DOPE liposomes, polymers, and ionizable LNPs, but they have had varied success. These studies suggest that novel antigens are necessary to effectively target HIV in addition to potent delivery vehicles.

A novel vaccination strategy against HIV is to isolate broadly neutralizing mAbs from infected individuals who neutralize several HIV strains. Notably, the broadly neutralizing mAbs, VRC01, have recently gained attention thanks to their ability to neutralize 98% of HIV strains and prevent transmission of antibody-sensitive strains with 75.4% efficacy. In one study, a single 0.7 mg/kg intravenous injection of an LNP-encapsulated, nucleoside-modified mRNA expressing VRC01, produced similar antibody concentrations to those typically achieved by injecting a 10–20 mg/kg dose of mAb protein. Importantly, a single dose protected mice from intravenous challenge with HIV-1.

Respiratory syncytial virus

Respiratory syncytial virus (RSV) is the leading cause of acute lower respiratory infection globally. Annually, it is responsible for an estimated 60,000 deaths in children under the age of 5 and more than 14,000 deaths in people over 65 years of age. Although the burden of RSV is well recognized, 40 years of vaccine development have not yet produced an approved RSV vaccine owing to numerous challenges. In 1968, for example, a formalin-inactivated RSV vaccine candidate caused vaccine-associated enhanced disease (VAED) in children. This response triggered excessive **eosinophil** and **neutrophil** infiltration in the lungs, resulting in severe **bronchiolitis** or pneumonia in 80% of the vaccinated children and two fatalities. Although the exact mechanisms of VAED remain unclear, the formation of non-neutralizing antibodies and a T helper 2 (TH2)-skewed T cell response marked by upregulation of **cytokines** such as IL-4, IL-5 and IL-13 have been implicated.

Current RSV vaccine candidates focus on targeting the highly conserved F protein, which facilitates viral fusion. Although some candidates have failed clinical trials owing to insufficient neutralizing antibody titres, newfound structural insights into F protein conformation have revealed that vaccinating against the prefusion conformation elicits superior neutralizing antibody response. This discovery will hopefully improve future vaccine design. Fortunately, mRNA vaccines can be designed to encode stabilized F protein conformations by engineering the coding sequence. In preclinical studies, mRNA vaccines encoding either the native RSV F protein or the stabilized prefusion conformation were successfully delivered using cationic nanoemulsions and LNPs without any observed instances of VAED.

Moderna is evaluating three single-dose vaccine candidates encoding the prefusion F protein: mRNA-1172 (Merck's proprietary LNPs) and mRNA-1777 (Moderna's proprietary LNPs) for adults, as well as mRNA-1345 (Moderna's proprietary LNPs) for children. In phase I clinical trials, mRNA-1777 elicited a robust humoral response with RSV neutralizing antibodies, a CD4$^+$ T cell response to RSV F peptides and no serious adverse events. The sequence of mRNA-1345 has been further engineered and codon-optimized to enhance translation and immunogenicity relative to mRNA-1777. Interim phase I data suggest that a 100 μg dose of mRNA-1345 produces approximately eightfold higher neutralizing antibody titres than mRNA-1777 one month after vaccination. Ultimately, Moderna aims to integrate mRNA-1345 with its pediatric human metapneumovirus/parainfluenza virus type 3 (hMPV/PIV3) candidate mRNA-1653 and vaccinate children against three distinct pathogens with a single formulation.

Plasmodium

Although the vast majority of mRNA vaccines under development are for protection from viruses, there are also efforts to prevent other infectious diseases. Malaria, which is caused by unicellular eukaryotic parasites of the genus *Plasmodium*, is at the top of that list owing to its incidence and lethality. Annually, malaria afflicts more than 200 million people and kills more than 400,000 patients worldwide. Antimalarial vaccine production has been difficult owing to the lack of surface antigens and complex life cycle of *Plasmodium*. Fortunately, the interrogation of the body's natural immune response to *Plasmodium* infection has identified potential non-surface antigen targets.

For example, the *Plasmodium*-secreted cytokine, **macrophage** migrating inhibitory factor (PMIF), has been shown to prevent T cells from developing long-term memory. Following this discovery, a vaccine was created from a squalene-based cationic nanoemulsion loaded with self-amplifying mRNA encoding PMIF. Two 15 µg primer–booster doses improved helper T cell development and elicited anti-*Plasmodium* IgG antibodies and memory T cell responses. Moreover, adoptive transfer of T cells from vaccinated mice protected unvaccinated mice from *Plasmodium sporozoites*.

4. Outlook

Decades of progress in mRNA design and nucleic acid delivery technology, together with the discovery of novel antigen targets have made mRNA vaccines an extraordinary tool for combating emerging pandemics and existing infectious diseases. The first two mRNA vaccines have elevated LNPs and RNA therapy from small-market products for niche diseases to a prophylactic treatment deployed successfully in large swathes of the population. The resultant abundance of positive safety and efficacy data, together with a proven path to regulatory approval, leave us optimistic that mRNA therapeutics will transform modern medicine's approach to vaccination, cancer immunotherapy, protein replacement therapy and beyond.

Word Study

1. amphipathic [ˌæmfɪˈpæθɪk] *adj.* 两性分子的,两亲的
2. anionic [ænaɪˈɒnɪk] *adj.* 阴离子的
3. asymptomatic [ˌeɪsɪmptəˈmætɪk] *adj.* 无症状的
4. bacteriophage [bækˈtɪərɪəˌfeɪdʒ] *n.* 噬菌体
5. bronchiolitis [ˌbrɒŋkɪəʊˈlaɪtɪs] *n.* 支气管炎
6. cholesterol [kəˈlestərɒl] *n.* 胆固醇
7. cytokine [ˈsaɪtəʊˌkaɪn] *n.* 细胞因子
8. dengue virus [ˈdeŋɡɪ ˈvaɪrəs] *n.* 登革病毒
9. electroporation [ɪˌlektrəpɒˈreɪʃn] *n.* 电穿孔
10. electrostatically [ɪˌlektrəˈstætɪkəlɪ] *adv.* 静电地
11. encapsulate [ɪnˈkæpsjuleɪt] *v.* 用胶囊（或囊状物）装,封装
12. endosomal [enˈdɒsəməl] *adj.*（细胞）核内体的
13. eosinophil [ˌiːəʊˈsɪnəˌfɪl] *n.* 嗜曙红细胞,嗜酸性细胞
14. haemagglutinin [ˌhiːməˈgluːtɪnɪn] *n.* 血凝素,血细胞凝集素
15. heterologous [ˌhetəˈrɒləɡəs] *adj.* 异种的,不同的,不等的,异质的
16. heterosubtypic [ˌhetərəˈsʌbtɪpɪk] *adj.* 异源亚型的

17. hydroxycholesterol [haɪˌdrɒksɪkəˈlestəˌrɒl] *n.* 羟基胆固醇, 羟胆固醇

18. immune surveillance [ɪˈmjuːn səˈveɪləns] *n.* 免疫监视 (监管)

19. immunogenicity [ˌɪmjuːnəudʒɪˈnɪsɪti] *n.* 免疫原性

20. immunostimulation [ˌɪmjuːnəustɪmjuˈleɪʃn] *n.* 免疫刺激

21. ionizable [ˌaɪəˈnaɪzəbl] *adj.* 可离子化的

22. lipid bilayer [ˈlɪpɪd baɪˈleɪə] *n.* 脂质双分子层

23. macrophage [ˈmækrəfeɪdʒ] *n.* 巨噬细胞

24. measles [ˈmiːzlz] *n.* 麻疹

25. motif [məuˈtiːf] *n.* 基序

26. nanoemulsion [ˌnænəlˈmʌlʃən] *n.* 纳米乳

27. nanoparticle [ˈnænəupɑːtɪkl] *n.* 纳米粒

28. neuroma [njuˈrəumə] *n.* 神经瘤

29. neutralizing antibody [ˈnjuːtrəlaɪzɪŋ ˈæntɪˌbɒdɪ] *n.* 中和抗体

30. neutrophil [ˈnjuːtrəˌfɪl] *n.* 中性粒细胞

31. nucleoside [ˈnjuːklɪəsaɪd] *n.* [生化]核苷

32. pertussis [pəˈtʌsɪs] *n.* 百日咳

33. plasmodium [plæzˈməudɪəm] *n.* 疟原虫, 变形体, 原形体

34. pseudouridine [ˌsjuːdəuˈjuərɪdiːn] *n.* [生化]假尿嘧啶

35. respiratory syncytial virus [ˈrespərətərɪ sɪnˈsaɪʃəl ˈvaɪrəs] *n.* 呼吸道合胞体病毒

36. rhesus macaque [ˈriːsəs məˈkɑːk] *n.* 恒河猴

37. seroconversion [ˌsɪərəukənˈvəːʒən] *n.* [免疫][生化]血清转化

38. seroprotection [ˌsɪərəuprəˈtekʃn] *n.* 血清保护

39. serotype [ˈsɪərətaɪp] *n.* 血清型

40. smallpox [ˈsmɔːlpɒks] *n.* 天花

41. tetanus [ˈtetənəs] *n.* 破伤风

42. titre [ˈtaɪtə] *n.* 滴度

43. Zika virus [ˈzaɪkə ˈvaɪrəs] *n.* 寨卡病毒

Notes

1. 疫苗基础知识: 以往的传统疫苗, 采用的是灭活 / 减活的病原体, 或者人工合成的病原体蛋白质外壳。将它们注射到体内时, 这些外来物会被机体免疫系统所识别, 从而生产针对它们的抗体, 还有记忆 B 细胞。mRNA 疫苗的原理则是直接往细胞里输送能够合成病原体蛋白质外壳的 mRNA, 细胞就可以照着制作出同样的蛋白质外壳作为抗原来激发机体产生对应的免疫反应, 从而产生抗体。

2. Pattern recognition receptors: 模式识别受体, 这是一种结合于免疫细胞细胞膜上或在细胞质内的蛋白家族, 可以识别微生物的关键部位 (如细菌的多糖、核酸、多肽、肽聚糖、脂蛋白等结构, 以及病毒的核酸等), 从而激发机体产生免疫效应。mRNA 疫苗在进入细胞后会被细胞内的模式识别受体所识别, 与所产生的抗原一起激活免疫系统。

3. Strain: 同种病原微生物不同来源的品系即为一个 strain, 对于细菌可译为 "菌株", 对于病毒可译为 "毒株"。病原微生物发生变异时产生一个变异株, 如新型冠状病毒的变异株奥密克戎, 则为 "Omicron variant"。不同的微生物品系在传染性、致病性、免疫应答等方面均存在差异, 因此疫苗开发时必须要针对多种品系进行验证。如在本文中出现了流感的不同变异株 "PR8 H1N1" "Ca109 H1N1" 等。

4. Nucleoside-modified：mRNA 属于核糖核酸，其基本组成成分是核糖核苷（nucleoside）和磷酸，为避免 mRNA 疫苗进入细胞后被核酸酶识别并水解从而无法产生效应，同时也为了提高 mRNA 疫苗的稳定性及生产效率。目前多需要对构成 mRNA 疫苗的核糖核苷进行化学修饰（chemical modification）。

5. Neutralizing antibody：中和抗体，指在细胞内产生的可以结合病原体或抗原，从而阻止其感染细胞的抗体。这是评价疫苗效力的重要指标之一，一般用中和滴度（neutralization titres）衡量。

Supplementary Parts

1. Medical and Pharmaceutical Terminology (9): Common Suffixes in Medical and Pharmaceutical English Terms

Suffixes	Meaning	Example
-ac	……的	cardiac 心脏的
-al	……的	bronchial 支气管的
-algia	痛	arthralgia 关节痛
-ar	……的	tonsillar 扁桃体的
-arctia	狭窄	bronchiarctia 支气管狭窄
-ary	……的	ciliary 睫状的
-blast	未分化的原始胚细胞	hemocytoblast 成血细胞，原血细胞
-cele	突出、疝气	thyrocele 甲状腺肿
-centesis	外科穿刺吸液	amniocentesis 羊膜腔穿刺术
-cide	杀，割	germicide 杀菌剂
-clysis	洗	bronchoclysis 支气管灌洗
-cyte	细胞	leukocyte 白细胞
-eal	……的	esophageal 食管的
-ectasia, -ectasis	扩张，膨胀	nephrectasia 肾扩张
-ectomy	切除	appendectomy 阑尾切除术
-emia	血的情况	leukemia 白血病
-form,-oid	形，样	filiform 线形的
-gram	记录，图	radiogram 放射照片
-graphy,-graph	记录	electrocardiography 心电描记术
-ia	条件，情况	anemia 贫血
-iatry,-iatrics	常用于医学分支	podiatry 足医术
-ic	……的	hepatic 肝的
-ist	专家，学者	dermatologist 皮肤病专家
-itis	炎症	hepatitis 肝炎
-ium	部分与整体关系，与……有关；部位	pericardium 心包
-lith	结石	cholelith 胆结石
-logist	学者和治疗者	urologist 泌尿专家
-logy	学科	pharmacology 药理学
-lysis	溶解	hemolysis 溶血
-malacia	软化症	osteomalacia 骨软化
-meter	测量用器具	thermometer 温度计
-metry	测量	pelvimetry 骨盆测量

续表

Suffixes	Meaning	Example
-myces	霉菌	streptomyces 链霉菌
-odynia	痛	cardiodynia 心痛
-oid	类似,像	cystoid 囊样的
-oma	肿胀,肿瘤	sarcoma 肉瘤
-opsy	观	autopsy 尸检
-or(er)	工作者(指人或工具,物)	incisor 切牙,门齿
-osis	异常或病理情况	sclerosis 硬化症
-ous	……的	mucous 黏液的
-pathy	病,病理情况	ophthalmopathy 眼病
-penia	不足,缺少	leukocytopenia 白细胞减少
-pexy	固定,缝于……处	hepatopexy 肝固定手术
-phil	嗜	eosinophil 嗜酸性粒细胞
-phob	惧怕	hydrophobia 恐水症
-plasty	外科整形或修补	osteoplasty 骨成形术
-plegia	麻痹,瘫痪	thermoplegia 热射病,中暑
-ptosis	落下	nephroptosis 肾下垂
-rrhagia	大量流出,出血	gastrorrhagia 胃出血
-rrhaphy	缝合术	herniorrhaphy 疝缝补术
-rrhea	流出,分泌	diarrhea 腹泻
-rrhexis	破裂	hepatorrhexis 肝破裂
-sclerosis	硬化	arteriosclerosis 动脉硬化
-scope	检查用器具	ophthalmoscope 检眼镜
-scopy	检查,视诊	cystoscopy 膀胱镜检查
-some	体	chromosome 染色体
-stasis	停止,制止	bacteriostasis 制菌作用
-stenosis	变窄,狭窄	arteriostenosis 动脉狭窄
-stomy	开口或吻合	gastrostomy 胃造口术
-tome	切割用器具	arthrotome 关节刀
-tomy	切,切开	craniotomy 开颅术、颅骨切开术
-uria	尿的情况	hematuria 血尿
-y	情况,动作,过程	splenomegaly 脾大

(1) Fill in the blanks with the missing word root, prefix or suffix.

1) _____articular   非关节的,关节外的

2) _____renal   肾上腺的

3) _____ceps   二头肌

4) broncho_____   支气管灌洗

5) leuk_____   白血病

6) _____paralysis   偏瘫

7) _____glycemia   高血糖

8) chole_____   胆结石

9) cardi_____   心痛

10) hepato_____   肝固定手术

11) osteo_____　骨成形术

12) _____synthetic　半合成的

13) arthr_____　关节痛

14) bronchi_____　支气管狭窄

15) _____cardia　心动过缓

16) append_____　阑尾切除术

17) hepat_____　肝炎

18) _____glossia　巨舌

19) strepto_____　链霉菌属

20) leukocyto_____　白细胞减少

21) _____uria　多尿症

22) hepato_____　肝破裂

23) cysto_____　膀胱镜检查

24) arterio_____　动脉狭窄

(2) Word-matching 1.

1) anabolism		A. 热射病
2) hypoglycemia		B. 心动过速
3) encephalic		C. 肾旁的
4) incoagulability		D. 合成代谢
5) tachycardia		E. 脑的
6) paranephric		F. 修复学
7) chromosome		G. 甲状腺肿
8) thermoplegia		H. 羊膜腔穿刺术
9) prosthetics		I. 低血糖
10) bacteriostasis		J. 制菌作用
11) thyrocele		K. 染色体
12) amniocentesis		L. 不凝性

(3) Word-matching 2.

1) antidote		A. 支气管的
2) deoxidation		B. 肉瘤
3) tonsillar		C. 解毒剂
4) endocrine		D. 外胚层
5) ophthalmopathy		E. 关节刀
6) sarcoma		F. 脾大
7) bronchial		G. 动脉硬化
8) ectoderm		H. 内分泌
9) infracostal		I. 肋下的
10) splenomegaly		J. 眼病
11) arthrotome		K. 扁桃体的
12) arteriosclerosis		L. 脱氧

2. English-Chinese Translation Skills: 药学英语翻译技巧 (5)：长句、复杂句翻译法

英语语言强调 "形合"（hypotactic），结构严密, 句子成分逻辑关系强, 长句、复杂句较多; 汉语语

言强调"意合"（paratactic），结构松散，句子成分的逻辑关系蕴含在词语当中，句式相对简单。药学英语中句式较长、逻辑关系复杂、附加成分多的长句较为常见，其中往往大量使用连词、介词、非谓语动词等。除此之外，药学英语复杂句子也可能由多个抽象名词、多个动词短语表现多层意义，或者为了结构平衡，还会出现倒装句子结构。但是无论句子多么长、句式多么复杂，翻译时要抓住主谓（宾）这个核心，理清各成分之间逻辑关系，就可以化繁为简，一目了然。

药学英语长句、复杂句翻译可以采用切分法。所谓切分法，就是翻译时根据句子成分逻辑关系，将长句、复杂句切分成几个意义相对独立的小句。切分长句、复杂句是一种常用的翻译方法，可以使原文错综复杂的逻辑关系用简单的小句子表述出来。

例1：Controlled drug delivery improves bioavailability by preventing premature degradation and enhancing uptake, maintains drug concentration within the therapeutic window by controlling the drug release rate, and reduces side effects by targeting to disease site and target cells.

参考译文：控制药物传递，可以防止药物过早降解和加强药物摄取从而提高生物利用度，可以控制药物释放速率而使药物浓度维持在治疗窗范围内，可以靶向疾病位点和目标细胞从而减少不良反应。

说明：从句子结构看，上面例句不算很复杂，其主要结构是：Controlled drug delivery improves...，maintains...，and reduces... 每个谓语动词后面又都接了一个 by+*v*-ing 短语。翻译这样句子，可以直接使用切分法，还要注意每个切分后小句表达前后连贯。参考译文在拆分后的小句前增加了"可以"，使原文中的三个动词短语连成一体。

例2：To ensure that a drug meets the requirements of safety, identity and strength, and meets the quality and purity characteristics that it purports or is represented to possess, the methods used in, or the facilities or controls used for, its manufacture, processing, packing or holding have to conform to or be operated or administered in conformity with current GMP regulations.

参考译文：为了确保一种药物达到安全性、同一性和浓度的要求，并且达到它所说明的或被描述应具备的质量和纯度特性，使用的方法或设施，或者采用的控制方法、生产、加工、包装或贮藏必须符合现行的 GMP 规范，或者在现行的 GMP 规范下进行经营和管理。

说明：上面例句结构相对比较复杂。翻译时，首先要分析清楚句子主要成分以及各成分之间的逻辑关系，然后再将复杂句子结构拆分，用简洁语言表达出来。原英文句子主要结构是：主语是 the methods, or the facilities or controls, its manufacture, processing, packing or holding，谓语是 have to conform to or be operated or administered。在名词 the methods 后面有一个动词过去分词 used in 作定语，在名词 the facilities or controls 后面有一个动词过去分词 used for 作定语，在谓语结构后面有一个介词短语。主语之前的动词不定式 To ensure that a drug meets the requirements of safety, identity and strength, and meets the quality and purity characteristics that it purports or is represented to possess 作状语，这个状语又有三层结构，首先动词 ensure 后接以 that 引导的宾语从句，这是第一层结构；在 that 引导的从句中，主语是 a drug，后接两个"meets+ 名词"并列谓语，这是第二层；在第二个谓语 meets 后面的宾语 the quality and purity characteristics 后面又有一个定语从句 that it purports or is represented to possess，这是第三层结构。

参考译文保持了原文基本结构：状语 + 主句。状语部分的翻译没有拆分，定语从句 that it purports or is represented to possess 正常调整到名词 the quality and purity characteristics 前面；在翻译谓语部分时，采用了拆分法，将连动谓语 conform to or be operated or administered 拆分为两个小句，并且根据表达需要重复了 current GMP regulations。

用切分法翻译药学英语长句、复杂句，不是随意对原句子进行拆分，不能改变原文中句子成分逻辑关系，而且切分后汉语表达要顺畅自然。

（付爱玲　欧田苗　龚长华　史志祥　龚长华）

Unit Ten

Clinical Pharmacy

Clinical pharmacy is a health science discipline in which pharmacists provide patient care that optimizes medication therapy and promotes health, wellness, and disease prevention. Change the traditional focus of pharmacy education from "medicine" to "people". The practice of clinical pharmacy embraces the philosophy of pharmaceutical care: it blends a caring orientation with specialized therapeutic knowledge, experience, and judgment for the purpose of ensuring optimal patient outcomes. As a discipline, clinical pharmacy also has an obligation to contribute to the generation of new knowledge that advances health and quality of life.

Within the system of healthcare, clinical pharmacists are experts in the therapeutic use of medications. They routinely provide medication therapy evaluations and recommendations to patients and healthcare professionals. Clinical pharmacists are a primary source of scientifically valid information and advice regarding the safe, appropriate, and cost-effective use of medications.

临床药学是一门有关健康科学的学科,该学科主要内容是药师为患者提供药学服务,包括优化药物治疗、促进健康、保健及预防疾病。把过去传统的药学教育重点由"药"转向"人"。临床药学的实践涵盖药学服务的理念,它将服务定位与专业治疗知识、经验、判断相结合,旨在确保患者最佳的治疗效果。作为一门学科,临床药学还有责任促进产生新的医疗知识,以提高健康水平和生活质量。

在医疗卫生保健系统中,临床药师是药物治疗使用领域的专家。他们定期向患者和医疗卫生保健人员提供药物治疗评价和建议。在安全、适当、经济用药这一过程中,临床药师是获取科学有效信息和建议的主要来源。

Text A
Patients, Pharmacists and Practice

About the patient

Patients' values, beliefs, and concepts of health drive their interactions with health professionals. Patients seek care while holding diverse and varied values about what is important in terms of their own health. To be responsive to the patient-perceived needs, pharmacists must learn what the patient's concepts of health are. While medical care in the United States for the most part follows Western medicine principles that **compartmentalize** the body and mind, **cognition** and emotion, and spirituality, patients hold a mixture of beliefs about what constitutes health. Zahra et al. (2015) studied lay people's perceptions of health and factors affecting health across 29 countries. People belonging to different backgrounds had different perceptions regarding determinants of health. The highest percentage of people agreed that environment was the determinant of health, which was consistent with the scientific view of increased burden of diseases

165

caused by environmental factors. Lay perspectives on health were found to be composed of three qualities: **wholeness**, **pragmatism**, and individualism.

Wholeness is related to health as a **holistic** phenomenon where a person lives according to one's personal values. Absence of disease is not enough when the whole life situation is considered. Family welfare is part of health wholeness. Pragmatism explains health as a relative phenomenon based on what is reasonable to expect, given age, medical conditions, and social situation. In this way, health is not necessarily freedom from disease or loss of functional abilities. Other positive values in life can compensate for different types of losses. Most people are realistic in their life expectations. Finally, individualism relates to health as a highly personal phenomenon. The perception of health depends on who you are as a person.

The World Health Organization offers a generally accepted definition of health as "health is a state of complete physical, mental, and social well-being and not merely the absence of disease or **infirmity**". This definition promoted for the first time that, in addition to physical and mental health, social welfare is an integral component of the overall health, because health is closely linked to the social environment and living and working conditions. This definition of health supports the concept of health that is consistent with patient-centered care delivery and is often adopted for use because it is patient-centric in its concept.

About the pharmacist

Pharmacist role and responsibilities

Pharmacists today are considered the leading expert on all forms of drugs and treatments, holding that social position for centuries. Pharmacy has evolved in response to social need and cultural change. In the 1990s a major shift from a focus on the pharmaceutical product, then a disease or condition-centered practice, to expanding clinically oriented patient care services with the ultimate adoption of the term "pharmaceutical care".

Pharmacists unique training and expertise in the appropriate use of medications is applied to individual patients resulting in reduced harm and injury from adverse events, improved safety, and optimized medication use resulting in improved health outcomes. This has been achieved through caring for the patient through guiding **optimal** medication use with the patient; the patients' caretakers; other health professionals serving the patient; and optimizing the dispensing, distribution, monitoring and education of the patient being served.

Patient-centered care pharmacy practice

In 2014 further **consensus**-building occurred across the leadership of the national pharmacy associations to describe the patient care process for pharmacists that is followed for delivering patient care in any setting. The outcome from this effort is a comprehensive approach to patient-centered care entitled the Pharmacists' Patient Care Process. The care process uses principles of evidence-based practice to collect, assess, plan, implement, monitor, and evaluate in order to adjust the plan for each person.

The critical role that medication management plays in treating chronic diseases requires integration of pharmacists into chronic-care delivery to improve health outcomes. Studies of pharmacists providing MTM[1] (Medication Therapy Management) services to improve therapeutic outcomes indicate that such services improve outcomes and reduce costs. When pharmacists provide care, it is the individualized patient-centered care plan that keeps the pharmacist, the patient, and other care providers on track and informed about progress and change.

Practice settings

Where pharmacists practice

Pharmacists practice settings range from having physical walls to occupying **virtual** places. Regardless, provision of patient centered care requires that the individual pharmacist patient relationship is recognized and supported through the practice setting. The structure of the environment can maximize the comfort for patients and assurance that privacy and personal health concerns are respected and protected. Restructuring the pharmacy workplace has been occurring in more recent years to support the patient-centered practice approach of pharmacists.

Practice infrastructure needs

Pharmacists need a physical and technical environment that supports efficient and expert practice. A private, **confidential** area for communicating with patients, performing physical assessments including skin, eye, ear, throat and other examinations, and documenting care are essential. Pharmacists need healthcare equipment to support the performance of physical assessment and should expect that such equipment is available in the workplace.

Documentation using electronic health records and/or eCare Plan software

Pharmacists need documentation tools that support on going care of their patients as they follow the pharmacists' patient care process and support integration and coordination efforts with other health professionals on a patient's care team. Within health systems environments, such as hospitals and **ambulatory** clinics, pharmacists typically document within the Electronic Health Record (EHR[2]) accessed by all care providers in the system. However, within community-based pharmacies, eCare Plan software is now emerging that supports practical documentation of pharmacists and supports transmission of information to other providers to keep them informed and interactive with changes.

The Pharmacist eCare Plan (PeCP) is an **interoperable** standard that allows for pharmacy technology providers to have a common method of exchanging information. Like the EHR, this is a pharmacist generated record of specific pharmacy clinical data. The PeCP is modeled after the Health Level Seven International (HL7) care plan standard and identifies problems using the Systematized Nomenclature of Medicine codes (SNOMED) consistent with EHRs and supporting electronic interchange; slightly modified to support the pharmacist's focus on medication use optimization, planning, and follow-up. HL7 provides a framework for the exchange, integration, sharing, and retrieval of electronic health information. When a product meets HL7 standards, it has demonstrated that the information for exchange is packaged and communicated from one party to another successfully using the language, structure, and data types for seamless integration between systems. HL7 is the most commonly used standards set in the world. Clinical terms in the PeCP are represented by SNOMED codes; a language that represents groups of clinical terms enabling health care information to be exchanged globally for the benefit of patients and health care providers and systems.

This PeCP standard is adoptable by multiple technology **vendors**, uses technology already in the pharmacy workflow at the choice of the pharmacy, and has standardized data formats to support quality assurance and **interoperability** to support data exchange and care coordination. By having pharmacists share medication-related services documentation with the patients, other providers and payers, payers can obtain the needed information to support value-based payment models and compensate pharmacists for clinical care services. Some of the commercial vendor products presently on the market include

AssureCare, BestRx Pharmacy Software, DocsInk, DocStation, Pharmetika, PioneerRx Pharmacy Software, Prescribe Wellness, QS/1, and Strand, to name a few.

Team care

Team-based care produces timely and individualized care, empowers patients, and facilitates communication and coordination among team members. When pharmacists are functioning within a health care team, outcomes improve related to preventing or managing chronic diseases (e.g., blood pressure, blood glucose, cholesterol, obesity, smoking cessation) and adherence.

In 2011 the chief pharmacist officer of the US Public Health Service authored a report highlighting the efficacy of pharmacists in advanced practice roles and advocated for intensified utilization of pharmacists in alleviating our nation's imminent primary care-provider crisis. The report was endorsed and supported by surgeon general, Vice Admiral Dr. Regina Benjamin, who recommended that health leadership and policy-makers optimize the pharmacist's role through implementation of collaborative practice models; recognition of pharmacists as providers, clinicians, and essential members of the health care team; and exploration of additional compensation models to support pharmacists in these expanded roles.

Interprofessional models

Collaborative practice models

A patient's health information must be generated by an interprofessional patient-centered approach. Opportunities for strengthening the pharmacist's role in existing programs and policies include ensuring that the pharmacist's contribution is identified in state and national HIEs[3] (Health Information Exchange), expanding the pharmacist's role in the adoption and meaningful use of the EHR through the use of the pharmacist's EHR functional profile, and ensuring that pharmacists are involved in the bidirectional exchange of clinical information.

Collaborative practice agreements

Under CPAs[4] (Collaborative Practice Agreements), pharmacists work in collaboration with physicians and primary care clinicians to help patients, particularly those with chronic conditions, manage, and optimize their medication regimens. On July 6, 2016, "the Collaborative Practice Workgroup, convened by the National Alliance of State Pharmacy Associations (NASPA), developed recommendations for what elements of pharmacist collaborative practice authority should appropriately be defined under state law and regulation and what elements are best left to be determined between pharmacists and other practitioners when developing their specific collaborative practice arrangement". The National Association of Boards of Pharmacy defined elements that should be part of CPAs. Those elements are:

1. Identification of the practitioner (s) and pharmacist (s) who are parties to the Agreement and types of decisions the pharmacist is allowed to make.

2. A method for the practitioner to monitor compliance with the Agreement and clinical outcomes and to intercede when necessary.

3. A description of the Continuous Quality Improvement Program used to evaluate the effectiveness of patient care and ensure positive patient outcomes.

4. A provision that allows the practitioner to override a Collaborative Practice decision made by the pharmacist whenever he or she deems it necessary or appropriate.

5. A provision that allows either party to cancel the Agreement by written notification.

6. An effective date.

7. Signatures of all collaborating pharmacists and practitioners who are party to the agreement, as well as dates of signing (Pharmacy Health Information Technology Collaborative, 2018; American College of Clinical Pharmacy, 2015).

Word Study

1. adherence [əd'hɪərəns] *n.* 坚持
2. ambulatory ['æmbjələtəri] *adj.* 可移动的
3. bidirectional [ˌbaɪdə'rekʃənl] *adj.* 双向的
4. cognition [kɒɡ'nɪʃn] *n.* 认知
5. compartmentalize [ˌkɒmpɑː't'mentəlaɪz] *v.* 划分
6. confidential [ˌkɒnfɪ'denʃl] *adj.* 秘密的
7. consensus [kən'sensəs] *n.* 共识
8. convene [kən'viːn] *v.* 召集
9. empower [ɪm'paʊə(r)] *v.* 授权
10. holistic [həʊ'lɪstɪk] *adj.* 全面的
11. infirmity [ɪn'fɜːməti] *n.* 体弱
12. interoperability ['ɪntərɒpərə'bɪlətɪ] *n.* 互用性，互操作性
13. interoperable [ˌɪntər'ɒpərəbl] *adj.* 互用的
14. optimal ['ɒptɪməl] *adj.* 最适宜的
15. override [ˌəʊvə'raɪd] *v.* 否定，推翻
16. practitioner [præk'tɪʃənə(r)] *n.*（尤指医学或法律界的）从业人员
17. pragmatism ['præɡmətɪzəm] *n.* 实用主义
18. utilization [ˌjuːtəlaɪ'zeɪʃn] *n.* 利用
19. vendor ['vendə(r)] *n.* 供应商
20. virtual ['vɜːtʃuəl] *adj.* 事实上的，虚拟的
21. wholeness [həʊlnəs] *n.* 完整性

Notes

1. "MTM" 的全称是 "Medication Therapy Management"。药物治疗管理服务是优化患者个体药物治疗效果独特的一组服务。MTM 的核心要素适用于包括慢病管理在内的复杂处方的优化工作以及直接面向患者服务的药学门诊，提供了良好的工作模式。美国 MTM 培训主要由美国药师协会负责。

2. "EHR" 的全称由 "Electronic Health Record" 的首字母组成。是基于一个特定系统的电子化病人记录，该系统提供用户访问完整准确的数据、警示、提示和临床决策支持系统的能力。

3. "HIE" 的全称是 "Health Information Exchange"。医疗信息交换战略规划确立了三个主要目标：为每个人创建一份健康档案；改进医疗业务运营；利用数据促进投资和政策决策。

4. "CPAs" 的全称是 "Collaborative Practice Agreements"。美国药师合作实践协议需要临床医师对患者做出诊断后将患者介绍给签约药师，药师根据协议为患者提供药物治疗管理服务，药师的行为受临床医师监督与管理。

Exercise

1.   Decide whether each of the following statements is true (T) or false (F) according to the passage.

(1) Pragmatism defines health as a phenomenon based on reasonable expectations, given age, medical conditions and social conditions.

(2) The health of an individual is the absence of disease or infirmity.

(3) "Pharmaceutical care" is a disease-centered care service.

(4) Medication Therapy Management (MTM) improves outcomes but increases the cost of treatment.

(5) Both PeCP and EHR are pharmacy-specific clinical data records completed in part by pharmacists.

(6) Pharmacists play an important role in preventing or managing chronic diseases.

2.   Questions for oral discussion.

(1) Why do people from different backgrounds hold different views on the determinants of health?

(2) What expertise should pharmacists have to reduce harm from adverse events?

(3) Why do pharmacists need documentation tools to support the continuous care for their patients?

(4) Who are the team-based members working with the pharmacist and how can they facilitate communication and coordination among themselves?

3.   Choose the best answer to each of the following questions.

(1) The job responsibilities of a pharmacist do not include _____.

   A. assisting clinicians in drug selection and rational drug use

   B. carrying out pharmacy information and consulting services

   C. undertaking hospital clinical pharmacy education and training pharmacists, physicians, and community physicians

   D. participating in disease diagnosis

(2) Which of the following can be the qualify/qualities of non-professional perspectives on health?

   A. Holistic.   B. Pragmatic.

   C. Individualistic.   D. All of the above.

(3) Which of the following is wrong about the World Health Organization's definition of health?

   A. No disease or infirmity.   B. Being socially well-adjusted.

   C. Mental health.   D. Physical health.

(4) The main job of a pharmacist is to focus on the services of _____.

   A. pharmaceutical product   B. disease

   C. condition   D. patient care

(5) Utilization of computer system to facilitate prescription processing becomes _____.

   A. impossible   B. universal

   C. possible in some states   D. possible in the near future

(6) Pharmacists can improve health outcomes by instructing patients in the medication process, all except _____.

   A. reduce adverse events   B. improve security

   C. avoid complaints   D. optimize drug use

(7) Scope of practice settings for pharmacists _____.

   A. carries out within physical walls   B. gradually changes to a virtual position

   C. violates the dignity of the patient   D. reduces patient comfort

(8) The medical information established by medical institutions with the help of computers and database systems to record the patient's morbidity, changes in the condition and the process of diagnosis and treatment is called _____ .

    A. electronic health record   B. course record

    C. medical file   D. health file

(9) The HL7 standard is mainly used for _____ .

    A. exchange of medical information   B. communication of test results

    C. image result communication   D. disease code

(10) As of 2011, the US emphasized the role of pharmacists in advanced practice, including _____ .

    A. implementing a collaborative practice model

    B. recognizing pharmacists as key members of the healthcare team

    C. exploring additional compensation modes

    D. all of the above

4. Match the words with the Chinese versions.

1) responsive		A. 可移动的
2) compartmentalize		B. 互用性
3) perspective		C. 制药的
4) pharmaceutical		D. 停止
5) ambulatory		E. 命名法
6) nomenclature		F. 否定
7) interoperability		G. 反应热烈的,热情的
8) cessation		H. 背书,赞同,支持
9) endorse		I. 观点,景观
10) override		J. 划分

5. Translate the following sentences and paragraphs into Chinese.

(1) While medical care in the United States for the most part follows Western medicine principles that compartmentalize the body and mind, cognition and emotion, and spirituality, patients hold a mixture of beliefs about what constitutes health.

(2) This definition of health supports the concept of health that is consistent with patient-centered care delivery and is often adopted for use because it is patient-centric in its concept.

(3) In the 1990s a major shift from a focus on the pharmaceutical product, then a disease or condition-centered practice, to expanding clinically oriented patient care services with the ultimate adoption of the term "pharmaceutical care".

(4) Pharmacists unique training and expertise in the appropriate use of medications is applied to individual patients resulting in reduced harm and injury from adverse events, improved safety, and optimized medication use resulting in improved health outcomes.

(5) Pharmacists need a physical and technical environment that supports efficient and expert practice. A private, confidential area for communicating with patients, performing physical assessments including skin, eye, ear, throat and other examinations, and documenting care are essential.

(6) Within health systems environments, such as hospitals and ambulatory clinics, pharmacists typically document within the Electronic Health Record (EHR) accessed by all care providers in the system. However, within community-based pharmacies, eCare Plan software is now emerging that supports

practical documentation of pharmacists and supports transmission of information to other providers to keep them informed and interactive with changes.

(7) This Pharmacist eCare Plan (PeCP) standard is adoptable by multiple technology vendors, uses technology already in the pharmacy workflow at the choice of the pharmacy, and has standardized data formats to support quality assurance and interoperability to support data exchange and care coordination. By having pharmacists share medication-related services documentation with the patients, other providers and payers, payers can obtain the needed information to support value-based payment models and compensate pharmacists for clinical care services.

Value-Oriented Reflective Reading

Tenets of Professionalism for Pharmacy Students

As a pharmacy practitioner, acquiring knowledge and competence is an essential component of a student's education during pharmacy school, yet developing professional attitudes and behaviors is just as critical to delivering quality patient care. The American College of Clinical Pharmacy National StuNet Advisory Committee has developed the "Tenets of Professionalism for Pharmacy Students", which outlines the essential attitudes and behaviors that signify professionalism and that should be developed and practiced by all students. The following tenets reinforce the expectations that the health care system and patients hold for pharmacy students, as well as the expectations of the schools of pharmacy and the profession at large in educating and molding future practitioners.

Altruism

Make an unselfish commitment to serve the best interests of the patient above your own

Pharmacy students must recognize that the patient is the top priority in all health care decisions. The patient's well-being should come before anything else, such as ability to pay, managerial opinions, or self-interests. Students must actively listen, be patient, and be compassionate when interacting with patients to establish and maintain mutual trust.

Honesty and Integrity

Display honesty and integrity in all that you do

Professional pharmacy students are responsible for their actions in all settings. Proper classroom behavior and personal integrity maintain academic honesty in the classroom. Preserving patient confidentiality can uphold professional integrity in experiential settings.

Respect for Others

Treat others as you would want to be treated

Every human being deserves to be treated with respect. In simple terms, respect for others means holding high regard for others' feelings, needs, thoughts, and opinions. Respecting others is an essential part of professionalism. Pharmacy students should consistently demonstrate respect for others, whether they are patients, peers, faculty, preceptors, or other health care providers.

Professional Presence

Instill trust through professional presence

Pharmacy students must conduct themselves in a professional manner in both professional and personal settings. Students have an obligation to establish trusting relationships with patients, peers, and other health care providers. Therefore, a professional attitude and appearance should be maintained in any setting where one represents the pharmacy profession.

Professional Stewardship

Actively participate and engage in school, organizations, and other worthwhile endeavors in the profession of pharmacy

The power of active participation both inside and outside the classroom will help students develop as future pharmacists and as individuals. Pharmacy students can be engaged in established organizations and begin taking on challenges to contribute positively to the profession.

Dedication and Commitment to Excellence

Strive for excellence and assume responsibility for your learning and professional development

Pharmacy students must acquire the core knowledge and skills of the profession. In the academic environment, individuals must accept and embrace ultimate responsibility for their learning and self-development. With modern medicine advancing at an exponential rate, pharmacy students should aspire to be lifelong learners constantly seeking to improve their knowledge and skills.

Questions for discussion:

1. What should a pharmacy student give top priority to when treating a patient?

2. Being a pharmacy student, if you have a different view toward a patient's regimen, what should you do and how could you communicate with your fellows and the patient?

3. Please talk with your classmates on how to keep yourself updated and what you should learn after graduation with the rapid development of healthcare technology.

Text B
Standards of Practice for Clinical Pharmacists: The Time Has Come

This document sets forth American College of Clinical Pharmacy's[1] expectations for clinical pharmacists within the United States and countries around the world where clinical pharmacy is emerging. It is also intended to serve as a reference for those designing and assessing clinical pharmacy education and training programs. In addition to articulating the clinical pharmacist's process of care and documentation, the eight standards below **address** the clinical pharmacist's involvement in **collaborative**, team-based practice and privileging; professional development and maintenance of **competence**; **professionalism** and ethics; research and scholarship; and other professional responsibilities. The standards define for the public, health professionals, and policy-makers what they can and should expect of clinical pharmacists.

1. Qualifications

Clinical pharmacists are practitioners who provide comprehensive medication management and related care for patients in all health care settings. They are licensed pharmacists with specialized advanced education and training who possess the clinical competencies necessary to practice in team-based, direct patient care environments. Accredited residency training or equivalent post-licensure experience is required for entry into direct patient care practice. Board certification is also required once the clinical pharmacist meets the eligibility criteria specified by the Board of Pharmacy Specialties (BPS).

2. Process of Care

Clinical pharmacists work in collaboration with other providers to deliver comprehensive medication management that optimizes patient outcomes. Care is coordinated among providers and across systems of care as patients transition in and out of various settings.

The clinical pharmacist's process of care comprises the following components.

A. Assessment of the patient

The clinical pharmacist assesses medication related needs by:

● Reviewing the medical record using a problem-oriented framework (e.g., interpreting and analyzing subjective and objective information) to determine the clinical status of the patient.

● Meeting with the patient/caregivers to obtain and document a complete medication history to identify all of the patient's current medications (including regimens and administration routes), medication-taking behaviors, adherence, allergies, and attitudes and experiences with medication therapy.

● Obtaining, organizing, and interpreting patient data.

● Prioritizing patient problems and medication-related needs.

B. Evaluation of medication therapy

The clinical pharmacist identifies strategies to optimize medication therapy by:

● Assessing, with other members of the health care team, the appropriateness of current medications on the basis of health conditions, indication, and the therapeutic goals of each medication.

● Evaluating the effectiveness, safety, and affordability of each medication.

● Assessing medication-taking behaviors and adherence to each medication.

● Identifying medication-related problems and evaluating collaboratively with other members of the health care team the need for intervention.

C. Development and implementation of a plan of care

The clinical pharmacist develops and implements, collaboratively with the patient and his/her health care providers, a plan for optimizing medication therapy by:

● Reviewing the patient's active medical problem list to inform and guide the development of an individualized assessment and plan for optimizing medication therapy.

● Formulating a comprehensive medication management assessment and plan in collaboration with the health care team and implementing this plan to achieve patient-specific outcomes.

● Educating the patient/caregivers (both verbally and in writing) to ensure understanding of the care plan, to optimize adherence, and to improve therapeutic outcomes.

● Establishing patient-specific measurable parameters and time frames for monitoring and follow-up in collaboration with other members of the health care team.

D. Follow-up evaluation and medication monitoring

The clinical pharmacist performs follow-up evaluations in collaboration with other members of the health care team to continually assess patient outcomes by:

● Coordinating with other providers to ensure that patient follow-up and future **encounters** are aligned with the patient's medical and medication-related needs.

● Revisiting the medical record to obtain updates on the clinical status of the patient and then meeting with the patient/caregivers to obtain an updated medication history to identify, assess, and document any new medication-related needs or problems.

● Conducting ongoing assessments and refining the plan of care to optimize medication therapy and ensure that individual goals are achieved.

● Monitoring, modifying, documenting, and managing the plan of care in collaboration with the patient/caregivers and his/her other health care providers.

3. Documentation

Clinical pharmacists document directly in the patient's medical record the medication-related assessment and plan of care to optimize patient outcomes. This documentation should be compliant with the accepted standards for documentation (and billing, where applicable) within the health system, health care facility, outpatient practice, or pharmacy in which one works. Where applicable, accepted standards must be considered as they relate to the use of electronic health records (EHRs), health information technology and exchange systems, and e-prescribing.

The following components of the encounter are essential to include in the documentation, which may be communicated in the form of a traditional <u>SOAP</u>[2] (subjective data, objective data, assessment, plan) note or other framework consistent with the standards of documentation within the practice setting.

A. Medication history

● A brief summary of the patient's past medication use and related health problems as an introduction to the documentation that will follow.

● A list of all current medications that includes information regarding actual use, adherence, and attitudes toward therapy.

● A list of medication-related allergies and any adverse drug events that may affect prescribing and monitoring or preclude the future use of a medication.

B. Active problem list with assessment of each problem

● A list of current health conditions and supporting data for the status of each condition, emphasizing associated medications and medication-related problems that may have an impact on desired goals.

● A list of any additional medication-related problems or other medical issues that may be unrelated to current health conditions.

C. Plan of care to optimize medication therapy and improve patient outcomes

● The specific medication therapy plan that has been or will be implemented collaboratively by the health care team, including drug, dose, route, frequency, and relevant monitoring parameters.

● The collaborative plan for follow-up evaluation and monitoring as well as future visits.

4. Collaborative, Team-Based Practice and Privileging

Clinical pharmacists work with other health professionals as members of the health care team to provide high-quality, coordinated, patient-centered care. They establish written collaborative drug therapy management (CDTM[3]) agreements with individual physicians, medical groups, or health systems and/or hold formally granted clinical **privileges** from the medical staff or credentialing system of the organization in which they practice. These privileging processes, together with the applicable state pharmacy practice act, confer certain authorities, responsibilities, and accountabilities to the clinical pharmacist as a member of the health care team and contribute to the enhanced efficiency and effectiveness of team-based care.

5. Professional Development and Maintenance of Competence

Clinical pharmacists maintain competence in clinical problem-solving, judgment, and decision-making; communication and education; medical information evaluation and management; management of patient populations; and a broad range of therapeutic knowledge domains. Clinical pharmacists maintain competency through:

A. Certification and maintenance of certification in the appropriate specialty relevant to their practice, including those specialties recognized by the Board of Pharmacy Specialties (BPS[4]) or other nationally recognized multiprofessional certifications;

B. Consistent participation in continuing professional development (CPD)[5] activities that enhance direct patient care practice abilities;

C. Maintenance of active licensure, including required continuing pharmacy education activities, through the appropriate state board(s) of pharmacy.

Clinical pharmacists also pursue professional and career development by participating in formal and informal activities that enhance research and scholarship, teaching, leadership, and/or management.

6. Professionalism and Ethics

Clinical pharmacists have a **covenantal**, "**fiducial**" relationship with their patients. This relationship relies on the trust placed in the clinical pharmacist by the patient and the **commitment** of the clinical pharmacist to act in the best interest of individual patients and patient populations, within the context of legal and ethical parameters. Clinical pharmacists exhibit the traits of professionalism: responsibility, commitment to excellence, respect for others, honesty and integrity, and care and compassion. They subscribe to the pharmacy profession's **code of ethics** and adhere to all pharmacist-related legal and ethical standards.

7. Research and Scholarship

Clinical pharmacists support and participate in research and scholarship to advance human health and health care by developing research questions; conducting or participating in clinical, translational, and health services research; contributing to the evolving literature in evidence-based pharmacotherapy; and/or disseminating and applying research findings that influence the quality of patient care.

8. Other Responsibilities

Clinical pharmacists serve as direct patient care providers, but they may also serve as educators, researchers, clinical **preceptors**/mentors, administrators, managers, policy developers, and consultants. As the clinical pharmacy discipline grows, it must continue to familiarize more patients, families, caregivers, other health professionals, payers/insurers, health care administrators, students, and trainees with the full range of clinical pharmacists' responsibilities.

Word Study

1. address [ə'dres] *v.* 说明，讲述
2. code of ethics *n.* 道德规范
3. collaborative [kə'læbərətɪv] *adj.* 合作的
4. commitment [kə'mɪtmənt] *n.* 承诺，保证
5. competence ['kɒmpɪtəns] *n.* 能力，胜任
6. covenantal [kʌvə'næntl] *adj.* 盟约的
7. eligibility [ˌelɪdʒə'bɪləti] *n.* 合格，资格
8. encounter [ɪn'kaʊntər] *n.* 接触，见面
9. fiducial [fɪ'djuːʃəl] *adj.* 信托的
10. implement ['ɪmplɪmənt] *v.* 实施
11. preceptor [prɪ'septə] *n.* 指导教师
12. privilege ['prɪvəlɪdʒ] *n.* 特权
13. professionalism [prə'feʃənəlɪzəm] *n.* 职业精神
14. residency ['rezɪdənsi] *n.* 住院医生实习期

Notes

1. "American College of Clinical Pharmacy"（美国临床药学学会）的简称为"ACCP"。这是一个以职业发展和相关临床药学科学研究并重的学会，官方网站为 http://www.accp.com。目前在全美有19个不同的分会，为临床药师教育培训、资源共享以及新理念推广提供平台。
2. "SOAP"由"subjective data, objective data, assessment, plan"的首字母组成。这是临床药师进行临床药历书写过程中的四个核心要素，包括有关患者的主观信息、客观信息、病情评价和治疗计划。
3. "CDTM"的全称是"collaborative drug therapy management"（以合作共享为基础建立的药物治疗管理方案）。在这一新理念倡导下，临床药师成为治疗团队中的一部分，以自身的优势，与临床医生及不同临床部门共同合作，提供更高质量的以患者为中心的医疗服务。
4. "BPS"的全称"Board of Pharmacy Specialties"（药学专业委员会）。自20世纪70年代以来，在美国临床药师相继出现了专业的细化，例如核药学、营养药学、药物治疗学、肿瘤药学等不同的分支，这些分支都是由不同方向的药学专业委员会来管理的。
5. "continuing professional development (CPD)"的意思是继续职业教育，是针对临床药师在临床实践工作中专业知识的更新完善，可通过不定期的授课、讲座、培训等形式多样的方式进行。

Supplementary Parts

1. Medical and Pharmaceutical Terminology (10): Common Morphemes of Numbers in Medical & Pharmaceutical English Terms

Number	Greek & Latin Morphemes	Number	Greek & Latin Morphemes
1/2	hemi-, semi-	5	pento-, quinque-
1	mono-, haplo-, uni-	6	hexa-, sex(i)-
2	di-, bi-, duo-, bis-	7	hepta-, septi-
3	tri-, triplo-, ter-	8	octa-
4	quarto-, tetra-, quadri-	9	nona-, novem-

续表

Number	Greek & Latin Morphemes	Number	Greek & Latin Morphemes
10	deca-, decem-	40	tetraconta
11	undeca, hendeca	50	pentaconta
12	dodeca	60	hexaconta
13	trideca	70	heptaconta
14	tetradeca	80	octaconta
15	pentadeca	90	enneaconta
16	hexadeca	10^{18}	exa- (E)
17	heptadeca	10^{15}	peta- (P)
18	octadeca	10^{12}	tera- (T)
19	nonadeca	10^{9}	giga- (G)
20	eicosa	10^{6}	mega- (M)
21	heneicosa	10^{3}	kilo- (k)
22	docosa	10^{2}	hecto- (h)
23	tricosa	10^{1}	deca- (da)
24	tetracosa	10^{-1}	deci- (d)
25	pentacosa	10^{-2}	centi- (c)
26	hexacosa	10^{-3}	milli- (m)
27	heptacosa	10^{-6}	micro- (μ)
28	octacosa	10^{-9}	nano- (n)
29	nonacosa	10^{-12}	pico- (p)
30	triaconta	10^{-15}	femto- (f)
31	hentriaconta	10^{-18}	atto- (a)

2. English-Chinese Translation Skills: 药学英语翻译技巧 (6)：被动句翻译

　　药学英语中大量使用被动结构，以动作对象作为主语，将动作发出者隐退，强调过程和结果。翻译被动句时，可根据句子整体结构、使用语境以及汉语表达习惯，采用恰当的方法。一般说来，药学英语被动句翻译可以有以下三种方法：①将被动句译成汉语的主动句；②将被动句译成汉语的无主句；③将被动句译成汉语的被动句。

　　（1）将被动句译成汉语的主动句：英语中被动结构常用 in、by 等介词将动作发出者表示出来，将英文句子被动结构翻译成汉语主动结构，是一种常见的翻译策略。如下。

　　例 1：A good number of the products found in a grocery or drug store are regulated by the FDA.

　　参考译文：许多在食品店和药店中可以找到的产品都由 FDA 管理。

　　有时候英语原句中动作发出者没有出现，将被动句翻译成主动句时，可以根据具体情况加上一个主语。如下。

　　例 2：Significant efforts through genomic approaches have been dedicated towards the identification of novel protein interactions as promising therapeutic targets for indications such as Alzheimer's disease, Parkinson's disease and neuropsychiatric disorders.

　　参考译文：科学家针对识别新型蛋白质相互作用的基因组学方法做出了大量研究工作，这些新型蛋白质相互作用可为如阿尔兹海默病、帕金森病、神经精神紊乱等疾病提供较有希望的治疗方法。

　　说明：上面例句是一个简单句，主句是被动结构，主语是 significant efforts through genomic approaches，译文根据上下文增加了主语"科学家"，将原被动句改成了主动句，并且利用重复 novel protein interactions，将原句拆分成两个小句，表达顺畅自然。

（2）将被动句译成汉语的无主句

例3：A drug such as neomycin will not be absorbed when given orally and will appear in the feces unchanged.

参考译文：像新霉素这类药物口服不吸收，原形在粪便中排出。

说明：此例句中有两个被动结构，分别出现在谓语部分和时间状语从句中，译文很好地理解原句成分的结构关系，将被动结构用主动式表述出来。

例4：Many fundamental biological processes, such as regulation of blood pressure, learning and memory, defence against microorganisms and tumors are now known to be dependent upon the formation of metal nitrosyl complexes.

参考译文：现在已经知道，诸如血压的调节、学习和记忆、微生物及肿瘤的预防等许多基本生物过程都依赖于金属亚硝基络合物的形成。

说明：根据英语和汉语语言表达习惯，例句中原文被动结构在翻译成汉语时变成了主动结构，在原被动结构无法准确确定动作发出者的情况下，可以用无主句陈述。

英语中有一种结构，比如 It has been established that... 在翻译成汉语时往往都译成无主句。

例5：It has been pretty well established that the increase in strains of bacteria resistant to an antibiotic correlates directly with the duration and extent of use of that antibiotic in a given location.

参考译文：现在已经确定在一些地区抗生素广泛和长期的使用与细菌耐药性增加有直接的相互关系。

类似这样的英语结构还有：it is reported..., It has been accepted that..., It is estimated that...，等等。有时候，这样的结构还可以加个主语，译成"人们……"。

（3）将被动句译成汉语的被动句：有时候，出于表达效果需要，英语中被动句也被译成汉语被动句。如下。

例6：Medications for food producing animals, often mixed with feeds, are closely monitored because remaining drug residues in the animal tissue are ultimately consumed at dinner tables.

参考译文：食用动物使用的药物经常和饲料混合在一起，也是受到严密监督的，因为在动物组织中的药物残留物最终会在餐桌上被吃掉。

说明：原文中有两个被动结构 are closely monitored 和 are consumed 出现在主句和从句中，译文用"受到……""被……"等保留了它们的被动结构，分别译成"受到严密监督""被吃掉"，突显了被动动作，更好地表述了原文的意思。

（唐　漫　杜伟杰　易　玲　史志祥　龚长华）

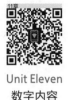

Unit Eleven
数字内容

Unit Eleven

Drug Regulation

Drug laws and regulations aim to regulate all activities pertaining to drug R&D, manufacture, distribution, use and surveillance. They function to ensure drug quality, safeguard the safety and efficacy of medications and crack down the manufacture and sale of adulterants and counterfeits. Different categories of laws and regulations are required upon manufacturers, distributors, non-clinical safety evaluation research institutions and clinical trial institutions. The main categories can be summarized as: laws and regulations for drug R&D, such as GLP and GCP; laws and regulations for drug manufacture, such as GMP; laws and regulations for drug distribution, such as GSP; and laws and regulations for medication use and pharmaceutical administration, such as the *Controlled Substances Act*.

药事法规旨在规范与药品研发、生产、经营、使用和监测相关的所有活动，对于保证药品质量，保障药品安全性和有效性，打击制售假冒药品发挥着重要作用。不同类别法律法规适用于不同对象，包括药品生产企业、经营企业、药品临床前安全性评价研究机构和临床试验机构。药事法规主要可分为以下类别：药品研发领域法律法规，例如《药物非临床研究质量管理规范》（GLP）与《药物临床试验质量管理规范》（GCP）；药品生产领域法律法规，例如《药品生产质量管理规范》（GMP）；药品流通领域法律法规，如《药品经营质量管理规范》（GSP）；以及药物使用及药品管理领域法律法规，例如《管制物质法案》（美国）。

Text A
Good Manufacturing Practices (GMP)

GMP[1] is probably the most widespread quality system followed across the pharmaceutical industry as a whole. GMP **compliance** is a requirement within the R&D environment for the manufacture and testing of clinical trial materials (both drug product and API[2]) and for commercial manufacture and testing of these materials for human and animal consumption. R&D facilities performing these operations may be subject to audit for compliance to GMP; commercial facilities will be audited by the appropriate regulatory authority, possibly without prior warning.

1. USA/GMP Regulations

The Federal Food, Drugs and Cosmetics Act (FD&C Act)[3] states that all drugs shall be manufactured, processed and packaged in accordance with current good manufacturing practice. No distinction is drawn between the manufacture of drug products (secondary manufacture) and the manufacture of APIs (primary manufacture). It is also noted in the **preamble** to the FD&C Act that the act applies to all drugs for human use, and this therefore includes the requirement for both APIs and drug products manufactured for clinical trials to be manufactured according to Current Good Manufacturing Practice (cGMP)[4].

The requirements for compliance to cGMP are laid down in the following *Code of Federal Regulations* (21CFR)[5]:

Part 210 Current Good Manufacturing Practice in manufacturing, processing, packing or holding of drugs;

Part 211 Current Good Manufacturing Practice for finished pharmaceuticals.

It must be noted that the US regulations refer to current GMP. The regulations as detailed in 21CFR parts 210 and 211, give the pharmaceutical manufacturer plenty of scope to interpret the requirements appropriately for his specific facility and process, but in doing this, the regulations require the manufacturer to adopt best current practice. The **onus** is placed upon the manufacturer to keep current with what the industry is doing (best practice), with what the current interpretations of the regulations are, and what the US FDA's expectations are.

Although the FD&C Act requires all drugs (products and APIs) to be manufactured to cGMP, the regulations 21CFR parts 210 and 211 are only mandatory for the manufacture of drug products and not APIs. In the past, the onus has been on the pharmaceutical industry to interpret these requirements with respect to the manufacture of APIs. FDA has published guidelines in the form of guides for FDA inspectors, to assist industry to meet compliance to cGMP and to place their interpretation on cGMP requirements for APIs and a number of other key areas such as impurities in new drugs, allowable solvent **residues** and stability testing. Guides issued by International Council for Harmonisation of Technical Requirements for Pharmaceuticals for Human Use (ICH)[6] have now supplemented most of these guidelines and these, along with other FDA guidelines, will be discussed in more detail later.

These regulations and guidelines may not always be appropriate for the manufacture of clinical trial materials. Although most of the regulations are reasonably applicable in an R&D drug product environment, they may become inappropriate where attempts are made to apply them to the early manufacture of clinical APIs within an R&D environment. It is only with the issue of the ICH, *Harmonized Tripartite Guideline ICH Q7 A—Good Manufacturing Practice Guide for Active Pharmaceutical Ingredients* in November 2000, that the worldwide pharmaceutical industry finally received detailed guidance for manufacture of APIs for both commercial and R&D purposes.

If one looks at the major headings of 21CFR part 211, the similarity with other quality systems becomes apparent. The following areas of these regulations that will be most important for a pharmaceutical analyst will be:

Organization and personnel—this includes the requirement to have a Quality Control (QC) unit having responsibility and authority to approve and reject all starting materials, drug product containers, **closures**, in-process materials, packaging materials, labeling and drug products and the authority to review production records to assure that no errors have occurred or, if errors have occurred, that they have been fully investigated. Further requirements cover laboratory facilities and the responsibility of the quality unit for approving or rejecting all materials, specifications and procedures.[7] The responsibilities of the quality unit must be described in written procedures.

Laboratory controls—this part covers mainly **calibration** of equipment, testing and release procedures, stability testing, reserve samples, laboratory animals and penicillin **contamination**.

Records and reports—this part describes the key records that require to be retained. These include starting materials and container/closure records, labeling records, production records, production record review, laboratory records, distribution records and complaint files.

These requirements can be further compared with the ICH guidelines for API manufacture later when discussing worldwide harmonization.

In conclusion, the USA cGMP regulations apply to interstate commerce within the USA and to any facility worldwide, that exports pharmaceutical materials (drug products, APIs, or components of these products) to the USA or, wishes to perform clinical trials in the USA. These facilities are open to inspection for cGMP compliance by US FDA inspectors and for those facilities found to be in non-compliance with these requirements the material will be deemed **adulterated** with respect to identity, **strength**, quality, and purity. Products from these facilities will be refused entry for sell or use within the USA. Data from these facilities may not be accepted in support of regulatory filings.

2. EU/UK GMP Requirements

Two European directives lay down the principles and guidelines for GMP in the EU, one for medicinal products for human use and the other for veterinary products. These directives have been incorporated in the national law of member states. The European Commission has issued nine volumes of *The Rules Governing Medicinal Products in the EU*. The latest edition was issued in 1998. Volume four covers GMP for medicinal products for human and veterinary use. These are now used as a basis for inspection by the various national regulatory authorities, e.g. Medicines and Healthcare Products Regulatory Agency (MHRA)[8] in the UK.

If one looks at the requirement of the EU GMP rule, the similarity with 21 CFR part 211 is clear, as is the consistency with other quality systems.

3. USA/EU GMP Differences

Historically, there have been distinct and fundamental differences between USA regulation and EU/UK requirements for GMP. As discussed previously, the US required all drugs to be made to GMP requirements and performed inspections throughout the world in support of these requirements. In the UK, only drug products and biological manufacturers (not APIs, except some specified antibiotics) were inspected by the regulatory authority for compliance to GMP. Other EU countries, such as France and Italy, did require audits of API manufacturers, but the requirements and standards varied widely throughout the EU.

Although drug product manufacturers have always been audited by the UK authorities, the UK GMP guideline (*The Orange Guide*[9]) was not mandatory and did not have the force of law. The original *European Directive* defined a medicinal product as "Any substance or combination of substances presented for treating or preventing disease in human beings or animals." This applied to finished pharmaceutical dosage forms (drug products) only.

There are fundamental differences between a drug product and API that makes the application of many GMP drug product requirements difficult or inappropriate. An API is normally prepared by chemical processes that involve purification at each stage of manufacture, and early raw materials and processing stages may not have much influence over the quality of the final API. Impurities that are present in the final API will not be removed and will still be present in the manufactured drug product. However, if the **morphic** form of the API is changed through unassessed changes in the API manufacture, this could have a considerable effect on the bioavailability of the drug product. To use the API based on end-product testing, as previously discussed, is not in keeping with the principles of quality assurance (QA).

Historically, in the UK and Europe, there has been no legal requirement to manufacture drug products or APIs to GMP for use in clinical trials (<u>investigational medicinal products, IMPs</u>[10]). This has always been a requirement under the USA FD&C Act.

The situation in the EU with respect to APIs and IMPs is now changing with the requirement for consistent standards throughout the EU and the wish to harmonize inspection standards and other regulatory requirements with other countries. The lack of GMP controls for APIs and IMPs has been seen as a major barrier to harmonization with the USA. Harmonization with the US through a *Mutual Recognition Agreement* (MRA) is seen as a big saving of inspection resources to both the EU and the USA, through mutual acceptance of facility inspection reports.

Word Study

1. adulterate [ə'dʌltəreɪt] *v.* 掺假
2. calibration [ˌkælɪ'breɪʃn] *n.* 标定,校准
3. closure ['kləʊʒə(r)] *n.* 密封件
4. compliance [kəm'plaɪəns] *n.* 遵守,合规性
5. contamination [kənˌtæmɪ'neɪʃn] *n.* 污染
6. morphic ['mɔːfɪk] *adj.* 形态(上)的
7. onus ['əʊnəs] *n.* 义务,职责,责任
8. preamble [priˈæmbl] *n.* 前文,序文,前言
9. residue ['rezɪdjuː] *n.* 残渣,残留
10. strength [streŋθ] *n.* 规格

Notes

1. GMP（Good Manufacture Practices）:药品生产质量管理规范,要求制药、食品等生产企业应具备良好的生产设备、合理的生产过程、完善的质量管理和严格的监测系统,确保最终产品质量符合法规要求。GMP 标志由世界卫生组织于 1975 年正式公布。

2. API:active pharmaceutical ingredient 活性药物成分,即法规中通常所说的原料药。

3. *The Federal Food, Drugs and Cosmetics Act* (FD&C Act):美国联邦食品、药品、化妆品法案。A set of laws passed by Congress in 1938 giving authority to the U.S. Food and Drug Administration (FDA) to oversee the safety of food, drugs, and cosmetics.

4. cGMP（Current Good Manufacture Practices）:动态药品生产质量管理规范,也译为现行药品生产管理规范,要求在产品生产和物流的全过程都必须验证。cGMP 是目前美国、日本、欧洲等国家和地区执行的 GMP 规范,也被称作 "国际 GMP 规范"。所谓动态药品生产管理规范,就是强调现场管理（current）,生产现场的 cGMP 合规性检查所遵循的是国际协调会议（ICH）所制定的原料药 cGMP 规范,即 ICH Q7A。

5. *Code of Federal Regulations* (21CFR):CFR 是 Code of Federal Regulations 的简称,中文译为《联邦法规编纂》。它是美国联邦政府机构制定和修订法规的官方出版物。CFR 由各个联邦政府部门和机构根据它们所管理的领域和职能,制定或修改规定其活动的规范性文件。CFR 是联邦法规的最终授权,并反映了联邦政府在各个领域的行为准则。目前,CFR 共分为 50 卷,涵盖了各个领域的规程,其中第 21 卷涉及食品及药品,21CFR 为食品及药品方面的法规。

6. ICH（International Council for Harmonisation of Technical Requirements for Pharmaceuticals for

Human Use）：国际人用药品注册技术协调会。ICH 是一个将监管当局和制药业的人员召集在一起讨论药品的科学和技术问题，并制定 ICH 指导原则的非营利性国际组织。自 1990 年成立以来，ICH 不断发展，以应对制药业的日益全球化，同时 ICH 指南被越来越多的监管机构所采用。2018 年 6 月 7 日，在日本神户举行的国际人用药品注册技术协调会（ICH）2018 年第一次大会上，中国国家药品监督管理局当选为 ICH 管理委员会成员。

7. Further requirements cover laboratory facilities and the responsibility of the quality unit for approving or rejecting all materials, specifications and procedures. 译为：更进一步的要求包括实验室设施，以及质量部门批准或拒收所有物料、质量标准和规程的职责。

8. Medicines and Healthcare Products Regulatory Agency (MHRA)：（英国）药品和健康产品管理局（MHRA）为英国卫生部下属的执行政府机构，保证药物和医疗器械的安全和有效。同时也与英国血液服务组织及卫生机构合作，监管血液及血液制品，保证血液质量和安全。

9. *The Orange Guide*：橙色指南，指英国 GMP 指南（*UK Guidance on Good Manufacturing Practice*），因其封面是橙色而得名。

10. investigational medicinal products, IMPs：临床试验用药物，注意 "investigational" 一词的使用。

Exercises

1. Decide whether each of the following statements is true (T) or false (F) according to the passage.

(1) GMP compliance is a requirement only for the manufacture of drug products.

(2) According to FD&C Act, only drug products shall be manufactured in accordance with cGMP.

(3) ICH Q7 A is a worldwide guidance for the manufacture of drug products for both commercial and R&D purposes.

(4) Same as that in the USA, all drug products are inspected by the regulatory authority for compliance to GMP in the UK.

(5) Impurities in the final API will be removed because it will influence the quality of drug products.

(6) Each stage of API production will significantly influence the quality of final API.

2. Questions for oral discussion.

(1) Please state briefly the scope that GMP is applied to.

(2) Please discuss the development of regulations and guidelines in the USA for the manufacturing of APIs.

(3) Please describe the differences between the US and EU GMP regulations.

(4) Why is the use of API based on end-product testing not keeping with the principles of quality assurance?

3. Choose the best answer to each of the following questions.

(1) GMP aims to regulate activities in the _____ of drugs.

　　A. manufacturing　　　　　　　　　　　B. distribution

　　C. clinical trials　　　　　　　　　　　　D. non-clinical trials

(2) GMP compliance is a requirement for the manufacture of _____.

　　A. APIs　　　　　　　　　　　　　　　B. investigational medicinal products

　　C. drug products　　　　　　　　　　　D. all of the above

(3) GMP compliance requirement is stated in _____.

　　A. FD&C Act　　　　　　　　　　　　　B. QC

　　C. ICH　　　　　　　　　　　　　　　　D. MRA

(4) Which of the following is not appropriate for the interpretation of the word "current"?

A. Keeping current with the best practice of pharmaceutical industry.

B. Keeping current with the interpretations of the regulations.

C. Keeping current with FDA's expectations.

D. Keeping current with the requirements of patients.

(5) ICH Q7 A is a guideline for the manufacture of _____.

A. drug products   B. APIs

C. raw materials   D. biologics

(6) The cGMP of the US applies to all the following except _____.

A. interstate commerce within the USA

B. any facility worldwide which exports pharmaceutical material to the USA

C. any facility that wishes to import pharmaceutical material from the USA

D. any facility that wishes to perform clinical trials in the USA

(7) _____ is the drug regulatory agency in the UK.

A. FDA   B. MHRA

C. EMA   D. CFDA

(8) Which of the following statements about the US and the UK requirements on GMP is NOT true?

A. The US requires all drugs should be manufactured according to GMP requirements.

B. The UK only inspects drug products and biological manufacturers.

C. The UK GMP is mandatory.

D. The US GMP has the force of law.

(9) The UK authorities might not require _____ to be audited for compliance to GMP.

A. drug products   B. biological manufacturers

C. APIs   D. some specified antibiotics

(10) "Starting material" includes _____.

A. raw material   B. excipients

C. both A and B   D. packaging material

4. Please choose appropriate word from a list of word bank to complete the following sentences

> compliance; FD&C Act; ICH Q7A; non-clinical; impurities; bioavailability; mandatory; current; investigational; APIs

(1) That all drugs shall be manufactured in accordance with cGMP is specified in _____.

(2) It is only with the issue of _____ that the pharmaceutical industry finally received the guidance for the manufacture of APIs.

(3) _____ GMP is a series of regulations must be adhered to by pharmaceutical industry in the US.

(4) GLP is a practice regulating activities in _____ process.

(5) _____ present in final API will not be removed.

(6) In the UK, GMP guideline was not _____ and only manufacturers of drug products, not _____, were inspected to comply with GMP.

(7) If there is a change in the morphic form of API, a considerable effect on _____ will be the result.

(8) GMP _____ is also required within the R&D environment for the manufacture and testing of _____ medicinal products.

5. Translate the following sentences and paragraphs into Chinese.

(1) GMP compliance is a requirement within the R&D environment for the manufacture and testing of clinical trial materials (both drug product and API) and for commercial manufacture and testing of these materials.

(2) It is only with the issue of ICH Q7 A that the worldwide pharmaceutical industry finally received detailed guidance for manufacture of APIs for both commercial and R&D purposes.

(3) Any facility that wishes to perform clinical trials in the US should be inspected for GMP compliance.

(4) QC unit has the responsibility and authority to approve and reject all starting materials, drug product containers, closures, in-process materials, packaging materials, labeling and drug products.

(5) Harmonization with the US through a Mutual Recognition Agreement (MRA) is seen as a big saving of inspection resources to both the EU and the USA, through mutual acceptance of API facility inspection reports.

(6) There have been distinct and fundamental differences between USA regulation and EU/UK requirements for GMP. The US required all drugs to be made to GMP requirements and performed inspections throughout the world in support of these requirements. In the UK, only drug products and biological manufacturers (not APIs. except some specified antibiotics) were inspected by the regulatory authority for compliance to GMP.

(7) An API is normally prepared by chemical processes and even if purification is involved at each stage of manufacture, impurities in APIs cannot be removed thoroughly. Therefore, trace impurities are allowed to be present in drug product to a limited extent. If the morphic form of the API is changed through unassessed changes in the API manufacture, this could have a considerable effect on the bioavailability of the drug product.

Value-Oriented Reflective Reading

New Rules in Pipeline to Overhaul e-Healthcare

China's new rules on internet healthcare are expected to benefit internet hospitals and foster the healthy and sustainable development of the sector, industry experts said. The comments came after the National Health Commission issued draft rules last month, imposing tighter regulation over China's fast-growing internet healthcare industry.

The rules propose that medical institutions should have special departments to manage the medical quality, medical safety, pharmaceutical care and information technology of Internet diagnosis and treatment, and establish corresponding management systems, including but not limited to the legal practice self-examination system of medical institutions, medical quality and safety management system related to internet diagnosis and treatment, patient safety adverse event reporting system, medical staff training and assessment system, patient informed consent system, prescription management system, electronic medical record management system, information system use management system, etc.

Internet diagnosis and treatment implements the real name system. Patients are obliged to provide real identity certificates and basic information to medical institutions, and shall not fake others for treatment. Physicians are required to authenticate their real identity before providing consultation to ensure real-person services. Using substitutes, or artificial intelligence software, will not be allowed for such services anymore.

Leveraging online consultations on internet healthcare platforms to sell prescription drugs will be prohibited. The rules proposed the personal income of healthcare workers must not be linked to income from drugs and medical examinations, and doctors must not designate locations to purchase drugs and consumables.

"This is the first detailed document launched for internet healthcare since 2018. It raised specific requirements for various links in internet healthcare, including institutions, personnel, business and safety. It also banned behaviors such as AI-enabled drug prescriptions and drug rebates. The draft rules imposed stricter supervision over the industry," said Zhang Xiaoxu, a research fellow at online healthcare website VCBeat.

The release of the draft rules generated widespread interest in the Chinese healthcare industry, and has been well-received among insiders. The move is seen as beneficial to the development of the internet healthcare industry, especially for some large digital medical platforms that engage in strictly online medical services.

Liao Jieyuan, founder of China's leading digital medical service platform WeDoctor, believes the move released a clear signal that online medical consultations should be of the same quality as those provided by brick-and-mortar institutions, reflecting China's determination to develop digital medical services essential for standardized development and market expansion of internet healthcare.

The booming online healthcare industry has become an integral part of China's medical system. Imposing stricter regulations on the industry, the document raised a lot of requirements for increasing the quality of medical services, and is dedicated to promoting the development of internet healthcare in a safer, more standardized manner.

Although currently internet healthcare services are only offered during follow-up visits, with the broader application of technologies such as 5G, AI, big data and cloud computing, it is expected that internet healthcare will be applied in more scenarios.

Note:

Oct 27, 2021, the National Health Commission issued a public announcement on the *Detailed Rules for the Supervision of Internet Diagnosis and Treatment (Draft for Comments)*. The draft proposes that medical institutions should have special departments to manage the medical quality, medical safety, pharmaceutical care and information technology of Internet diagnosis and treatment, and establish corresponding management systems, including but not limited to the legal practice self-examination system of medical institutions, medical quality and safety management system related to Internet diagnosis and treatment, patient safety adverse event reporting system, medical staff training and assessment system, patient informed consent system, prescription management system, electronic medical record management system, information system use management system, etc. Internet diagnosis and treatment implements the real name system. Patients are obliged to provide real identity certificates and basic information to medical institutions, and shall not fake others for treatment.

Questions for discussion:

1. How will the new rules ensure the rights of patients?

2. Why do we say that the new measures are beneficial to the development of the Internet healthcare industry?

3. What are your comments on beefing up the supervision of digital medical service?

Text B
Recent Regulatory Trends in Pharmaceutical Manufacturing and Their Impact on the Industry

1. Introduction

The pharmaceutical industry is one of the most regulated manufacturing environments. Since the first implementation of good manufacturing practices (GMP) by the WHO in the 1960s, to the implementation of PIC/S[1] GMP guide in 1970s, and the later implementation of the EU GMP Guide in 1989, these rules and regulations have been under constant refinement and adaptation. Nowadays, GxP[2] is implemented in all aspects of pharmaceutical manufacturing. This covers technical aspects such as manufacturing of active pharmaceutical ingredients (API) or drug substances, ranging from classic chemical synthesis of small molecules to biomolecules like antibodies, drug product manufacturing, to device manufacturing. In addition, the guidelines also cover aspects such as packaging and distribution of medicines, outsourcing activities, documentation as well as data governance and quality risk management.

In Switzerland, the 'Arzneimittel-Bewilligungsverordnung, AMBV'[3] from 2001 lists in parallel the PIC/S GMP Guide and the EU GMP Guide as guiding documents for the pharmaceutical industry, both of which are under constant review and revision. In contrast to the opinion that these regulations pose a significant burden to the industry and restrict innovation and flexibility, these rules often induce the development of new, innovative technologies and more scientific approaches to guarantee the quality and supply security of medicines.

In the following article, we would like to highlight this drive to innovation and science by reviewing three recent up-dates on the GMP expectations to industry. We will discuss the requirements and their impact on the pharmaceutical industry with the examples from the production of small molecule active pharmaceutical ingredients (APIs). The first example is the implementation of ICH Q3D[4] 'Guideline for elemental impurities'. Second is the EU-GMP Guideline Part III Chapter 'Guideline on setting health based exposure limits for use in risk identification in the manufacture of different medicinal products in shared facilities' from 01. June 2015, and third are the new guidelines to data **integrity** such as 'PIC/S 041-1 Good Practices for Data Management and Integrity in regulated GMP/GDP environments'.

2. Elemental Impurities According to the new Guideline ICH Q3D and USP[5] <232>: A (R)evolution

The determination of elemental impurities in pharmaceutical products such as residual metals from catalytic reactions or production process-related equipment **aberrations** is one of the oldest quality control activities performed in the industry. In order to assess the evolution vs. revolution of the implementation of ICH Q3D, one has to understand what the historic procedure to determine elemental impurities was and where we are today. For more than 100 years, the elemental **impurity** profile of a pharmaceutical product was principally assessed by wet chemical and **colorimetric** limit tests, i.e. according to the formerly valid

European Pharmacopoeia (EP)[6] Heavy Metals chapter 2.4.8 and United States Pharmacopeial Convention (USP) General Chapter <231> 'Heavy Metals'. However, these wet chemistry procedures are not element-specific and even highly variable in the response/sensitivity of the elements and therefore do not deliver the quality and specificity **commensurate** with the risks attributed to these process impurities.

Over the past years, industry **consortia**, pharmacopoeias, and regulators developed a more effective approach to the control of elemental impurities, leading to a replacement of existing wet chemical and colorimetric tests, EP 2.4.8 and USP <231>. The USP, in parallel with the International Council for Harmonization of Technical Requirements for Pharmaceuticals for Human Use (ICH), has published new standards for measuring and controlling inorganic impurities in pharmaceuticals and their ingredients. The new approach is used for the assessment and control of elemental impurities in the final drug product on the basis of risk management principles as outlined in ICH Q9. The ICH method is defined in the '*Guideline for Elemental Impurities*' (Q3D), which has been in effect since June 2016 for new marketing authorization applications and was implemented in December 2017 for previously authorized medicinal products. Several Health Authorities have aligned their specific chapters to the content of ICH Q3D, such as the new USP General Chapters <232> (Elemental Impurities-Limits) and <233> (Elemental Impurities-Procedures), which were implemented in January 2018. Now we employ state of the art ICP/MS instruments where critical elemental impurities can be controlled down to 50 ppb further reducing the risk for the patient.

In essence, the ICH Q3D consists of three parts: ⅰ) the evaluation of **toxicity** data for potential elemental impurities, ⅱ) the establishment of a **permitted daily exposure** (i.e. limits) for each element of toxicological concern and ⅲ) application of a risk-based approach to control elemental impurities in drug products (usually done in risk assessments). Thus, the control of elemental impurities in pharmaceuticals transits from a routine testing of concentrations in components to controls based on risk and permitted daily exposures.

The evaluation of element- and route-specific toxicological data resulted in permitted daily exposures (PDEs). The PDE is a limit for an elemental impurity in a pharmaceutical product per daily consumption and is dependent on oral, **parenteral** and **inhalational** routes of administration. These limits are defined in the ICH and USP chapters and a detailed summary of the deduction of PDEs is given in an appendix to ICH Q3D. Based on their toxicity (PDE) and likelihood of occurrence in the drug product, the elements included in ICH Q3D were divided into three classes. Class 1 consists of the elements As, Cd, Hg, and Pb which are highly toxic to humans and consequently should have limited or no use in the manufacture of pharmaceuticals. Class 2 elements are considered as route-dependent human toxicants and are further divided in two sub-classes (2A and 2B) based on their relative likelihood of occurrence in the drug product. The class 2A elements are: Co, Ni, and V and, due to the high likelihood of occurrence, should always be evaluated in a risk assessment. Class 2B elements include: Ag, Au, Ir, Os, Pd, Pt, Rh, Ru, Se, and Tl and have reduced risk of occurrence and can only be included if intentionally added to the process. In class 3 are elements with a relatively low toxicity by the oral route of administration (high PDEs, generally >500 g/day) but it could be necessary to consider those in the risk assessment for inhalation and parenteral routes of administration. Elements that are not included in class 3 are elements with low inherent toxicity.

While USP <232> and ICH Q3D apply to all drug products, there is broad industry and regulatory agreement that very few drug products will require routine release testing. However, all products require a documented risk assessment, as defined by ICH Q3D and from this an appropriate control strategy should be deducted that justifies if levels of elemental impurities require additional controls not inherent in the existing control process. The risk assessment should be science-based and connect safety considerations for patients with an understanding of the risk in the product and its manufacturing process. These documents should scientifically justify why elemental impurities testing is not required for the final drug product or define what testing or additional controls need to be added in order to ensure that elemental impurities in the drug product will not exceed the PDE. This justification should specifically address each of the ICH Q3D-defined potential sources of elemental impurities: ⅰ) drug substance, ⅱ) **excipients**, ⅲ) facilities & utilities, ⅳ) manufacturing equipment and ⅴ) container closure system (the packaging used for drug products and APIs).

3. Implementation of the <u>EMA</u>[7] Guideline on Setting Health-based Exposure Limits

Another guideline impacting the pharmaceutical industry over the last years was the introduction of <u>health-based exposure limits (HBEL)</u>[8], or permitted daily exposure limits (PDEs), respectively, which had a major impact on cleaning **validation** processes in the pharmaceutical industry.

In 2014, the European Medicine Agency (EMA) published a guideline on setting health-based exposure limits that was made effective in June 2015. This guideline introduced PDEs as a "substance-specific dose that is unlikely to cause adverse effects if an individual is exposed at or below this dose every day for a lifetime" and is based on toxicological and pharmacological data to ensure safety of human patients. PDEs provide a scientifically justified approach based upon toxicological and pharmacological data to establish **carryover limits** for active pharmaceutical substances (APIs) in shared pharmaceutical production facilities. Previously, carry-over limits were established by applying default limits such as 1/1000 of the minimal daily dose (0.001 MinDD), 10 ppm concentration limit as well as a visual clean **criteria**.

While the PDE approach can be considered conservative, there are still objections to the use of PDEs from pharmaceutical industrial groups and some authorities. The EMA Q&A draft document to the guideline demonstrated the difficulties in overcoming traditional limit setting, which resulted in the re-establishment of the 0.001 MinDD limit. For this reason, a pharmaceutical working group was formed in 2017 comprising of toxicology, manufacturing, quality and GMP inspectors to give clear recommendations on limit- setting based upon PDEs. According to the risk management principles in ICH Q9 "The level of effort, formality and documentation of the quality risk management process should be commensurate with the level of risk". PDEs can be used to identify the highest risk for cross-contamination not only for finished products (APIs) but also for intermediate products and starting material products where dose information is not available but cross-contamination is still a risk.

Also the wider acceptance of health-based exposure limits has encouraged suppliers of cleaning agents to provide PDEs for their products (e.g. **detergents**). Due to the inherent low toxicity of the cleaning agents, the carryover limits are less conservative. Although the scientific approach of applying PDEs justifies higher carryover limits, this does not mean that equipment can be left 'dirty' as cleaning limits are only one part of the risk management. The cleaning validation process as specified under GMP guidelines also takes into account criteria such as visually clean, margin of safety, process knowledge, constant improvements and ongoing verification. Even if higher cleaning limits are allowed, meeting the general visual clean requirement may be the most stringent criteria as observable residue levels are usually very low. However the higher limits for cleaning agents and detergents have allowed a wider use of cleaning aids which enables the reduction of solvents for a more environmentally friendly and economic cleaning process in chemical production.

4. Data Integrity Aspects in the Pharmaceutical Industry

One of the more recent focus areas of health authority inspections is the topic of data integrity. Though the control of data is not a new concept in the GMP regulated environment and already part of several GMP regulations, the focus of the documentation aspect of manufacturing processes and analytical work was changed by several publications of health authorities in recent years. In the past there was a strong focus on equipment qualification and the way electronic data is generated and processed in the application as well as where and how it is stored. With the new interpretation of data integrity requirements there is a broader focus on the overall process of data handling and the data lifecycle process from data creation, processing, review, reporting and **retention**. Thus, the key data integrity question is: "Do I have my data and the data flow under control, from first data generation until the retention of the last data record at the end of my process?"

Therefore, several health authorities or inspecting bodies started to publish dedicated rules and regulations. Three key documents that impacted the industry significantly are, ⅰ) the 'MHRA *GMP Data Integrity Definitions and Guidance for Industry* document in March 2015', ⅱ) the PIC/S Pharmaceutical Inspection Convention/Pharmaceutical Inspection Co-Operation Scheme Draft guidance '*Good Practices For Data Management and Integrity in Regulated GMP/GDP Environments*' from August 2016 and ⅲ) the USFDA '*Guidance on Data Integrity*'. All these documents guide and mandate the industry to establish well-controlled systems to ensure data integrity throughout the complete manufacturing/analytical process as well as the life cycle of a product from development to fade out of the production.

4.1 Get a Grasp of the Data Integrity Basics

One of the key aspects of data integrity is the ALCOA (+) principle. ALCOA is an acronym for: attributable, legible, contemporaneous, original and accurate. It has been widely associated with data quality at the FDA and describes the critical attributes to data integrity and documentation. The (+) stands for complete, consistent, enduring and available. These additional terms are based on a European Medicines Agency Guideline Eudralex, Volume 4, chapter 4 as well as the aforementioned PIC/s draft guidance '*Good Practices for Data Management and Integrity in Regulated GMP/GDP Environments*'. In the following we would like to describe the impact of this expectation to an industry from either the lab or manufacturing side.

- Attributable: Data is expected to be traceable to its primary source and attributable to the individual who observed and recorded it. For electronic data this can be achieved with thorough user access management, audit trail and e-signature.

- Legible: All data recorded must be human-readable and permanent throughout the data lifecycle. This also includes metadata such as audit trail.

- Contemporaneous (at the same time): Information is recorded at the time when the activity is carried out, at the time of data generation and in chronological order. Within an electronic system, the audit trail record ensures this by creating timestamps for all data entry and modification.

- Original: The information must be accessible and preserved in its original form as it was created the first time.

- Accurate: Data and records should be free from errors, complete, truthful and reflective of the observation. There must be sufficient information to recreate the chain of events without any **ambiguity**.

These data integrity expectations significantly impact the way data are documented and managed, specifically for processes where data are captured and transferred between paper-based and electronic systems. These so-called hybrid systems usually pose the biggest risk to data transcription, data storage, the ALCOA principles and therefore to the overall data integrity principles.

4.2   Understanding the Data Processes and the Related Risks

To understand and manage the data integrity risk of e.g. **discrepancies** between paper and electronic data or undetected data manipulation we implemented a rigorous data process mapping exercise to identify and mitigate data integrity risks. The main objectives of data mapping are to systematically describe and understand:

- the process, different steps and individual activities,
- the related data flow through systems and equipment,
- the overall data lifecycle (generation, storage / archival, **retrieval**, destruction) using a standardized procedure with process- and dataflow diagrams, FMEA risk analysis and resulting action plan.

With this approach it was possible to identify weaknesses in manual data recording (people and business process flows) and in data processing and storage in the systems or equipment (data flows). Based on these findings either procedural controls or significant investments into technical solutions, such as new computer systems (and more sophisticated software versions) were put in place to reduce such data integrity risks to an acceptable level or eliminate it completely.

5. Conclusion

New regulations or adaptions to existing guidelines pose a challenge to our daily routines and disrupt our current processes. This requires continuous adaptations to the way we work. On the other hand, the drive for new processes on the basis of thorough scientific principles also fosters innovation and continuously improves the quality of our products to benefit of patients around the world.

Word Study

1. aberration [ˌæbəˈreɪʃn] *n.* 误差、偏差
2. ambiguity [ˌæmbɪˈgjuːəti] *n.* 模棱两可，含糊不清
3. carryover limit 残留限度
4. colorimetric [ˌkʌlərɪˈmetrɪk] *adj.* 比色分析的，色度的
5. commensurate [kəˈmenʃərət] *adj.* 相称的
6. consortium [kənˈsɔːtɪəm]（［复］consortia [kənˈsɔrʃə]）*n.* 联合，协会，联盟
7. criterion [kraɪˈtɪərɪən]（［复］criteria [kraɪˈtɪərɪə]）*n.* 标准
8. detergent [dɪˈtɜːdʒənt] *n.* 洗涤剂，清洁剂
9. discrepancy [dɪsˈkrepənsi] *n.* 差异，不符
10. excipient [ɪkˈsɪpɪənt] *n.* 赋形剂，辅料
11. impurity [ɪmˈpjʊərəti] *n.* 杂质，不纯
12. inhalational [ˌɪnhəˈleɪʃnəl] *adj.* 吸入的
13. integrity [ɪnˈtegrəti] *n.* 完整，完全
14. parenteral [pəˈrentərəl] *adj.* 不经肠道的，注射用药物的
15. permitted daily exposure 每日允许暴露量
16. pharmacopoeia [ˌfɑːməkəˈpiːə] *n.* 药典

17. retention [rɪ'tenʃn] *n.* 保留,存放
18. retrieval [rɪ'tri:vl] *n.* 检索,提取
19. toxicity [tɒk'sɪsəti] *n.* 毒性,毒效
20. validation [ˌvælɪ'deɪʃn] *n.* 验证

Notes

1. PIC/S(Pharmaceutical Inspection Convention and Pharmaceutical Inspection Co-operation Scheme):国际药品认证合作组织,成立于 1995 年,前身是 1970 年成立的药品审查合作组织(Pharmaceutical Inspection Convention,简称 PIC)。其任务是引导协调化的 GMP 规范和药品领域质量体系检查领域在国际层面上的发展、实施和维护。2021 年 4 月 26 日,PIC/S 发布了其新版的 GMP 指南 PE 009-15。

2. GxP(good x practice):指药品质量管理相关的各法规,如 GMP(good manufacture practice 药品生产质量管理规范)、GSP(good supply practice 药品经营质量管理规范)、GLP(good laboratory practice 药物非临床研究质量管理规范)等。

3. AMBV(*Arzneimittel-Bewilligungsverordnung*):源自德语,即 *Ordinance for the Authorization of Pharmaceuticals*(《药品授权条例》),瑞士联邦委员会于 2001 年 10 月 17 日颁布的关于药品许可的法令。

4. ICH Q3D:ICH Q3D 元素杂质指南,于 2014 年 12 月发布,已纳入欧盟和美国的药典,并于 2018 年 1 月开始实施,《中国药典》(2020 年版)也收录了此部分内容。Q 指 quality,Q3 指南包括 Q3A、Q3B、Q3C、Q3D。ICH Q3A 指导原则将杂质分为有机杂质、无机杂质和残留溶剂;Q3A 和 Q3B 主要针对有机杂质;Q3C 主要针对残留溶剂;Q3D 对无机杂质中的金属提出分类要求。Q3D 主要由三部分构成:评估潜在元素杂质的毒性数据;确定每一种有毒元素的每日允许暴露量(PDE);运用 ICH Q9 质量风险管理指导原则来评估和控制药品中的元素杂质。

5. USP(*United States Pharmacopeia*):《美国药典》。*U.S. Pharmacopeia/National Formulary*《美国药典/国家处方集》(简称 USP/NF)是由美国政府所属的美国药典委员会(The United States Pharmacopeial Convention)编辑出版。《美国药典》是美国政府对药品质量标准和检定方法作出的技术规定,也是药品生产、使用、管理、检验的法律依据。NF 收载了《美国药典》(USP)尚未收入的新药和新制剂。

6. EP(*European Pharmacopeia*):《欧洲药典》,为欧洲药品质量检测的唯一指导文献,由欧盟药品质量管理局(EDQM)负责出版和发行。所有药品和药用底物的生产厂家在欧盟范围内推销和使用的过程中,必须遵循欧洲药典的质量标准。

7. EMA(European Medicines Agency):欧盟医药管理局,是欧盟药品评估机构,负责泛欧洲范围的药品审批。成立于 1995 年,总部设于英国伦敦,2004 年之前称作欧洲药品评估局(European Agency for the Evaluation of Medicinal Products)。

8. HBEL(hcalth-based exposure limits):健康暴露限度,EMA 于 2014 年 11 月发布了"Guideline on setting health based exposure limits for use in risk identification in the manufacturc of different medicinal products in shared facilities(在公共设施中生产不同药品使用风险辨识建立健康暴露限度指南)"。2015 年 1 月,修订了 EU GMP 第 3 章和第 5 章,更新了预防交叉污染的章节,这些修订于 2015 年 3 月 1 日生效。

Supplementary Parts

1. Medical and Pharmaceutical Terminology (11): Irregular Singular and Plural Forms of Greek & Latin Endings in Nouns

Singular	Plural	Example (Singular)	Example (Plural)	Meaning
-a	-ae	antenna	antennae	触角, 天线
		aqua	aquae	水（剂）
		conjunctiva	conjunctivae	结膜
		cornea	corneae	角膜
		mucosa	mucosae	黏膜
		formula	formulae	公式
-is	-es	analysis	analyses	分析
		dermatosis	dermatoses	皮肤病
		diagnosis	diagnoses	诊断
		hydrolysis	hydrolyses	水解
		paralysis	paralyses	麻痹
-ix	-ices	appendix	appendices	阑尾, 附录
		cervix	cervices	颈
-ex,	-ices	cortex	cortices	皮质
-ax	-aces	thorax	thoraces	胸
-ma	-mata	carcinoma	carcinomata	癌
		fibroma	fibromata	纤维瘤
-um	-a	bacterium	bacteria	细菌
		cerebrum	cerebra	大脑
		myocardium	myocardia	心肌
		spectrum	spectra	光谱
-us	-i	fungus	fungi	真菌
		bacillus	bacilli	杆菌
		focus	foci	病灶
-on	-a	phenomenon	phenomena	现象
		protozoon	protozoa	原虫

Write down the plural forms of the following words.

1) formula _____

2) analysis _____

3) appendix _____

4) thorax _____

5) fibroma _____

6) cerebrum _____

7) bacillus _____

8) phenomenon _____

2. English-Chinese Translation Skills: 药学英语翻译技巧 (7)：定语从句翻译

　　定语从句在句子结构中属于次要成分，但在语言表达功能上却占有重要地位。药学英语中大量使用定语从句，有长有短，结构有繁有简，对先行词的限制有强有弱，起着补充说明作用。汉语中的定语成分，包括定语从句都是在所修饰名词之前，少有结构复杂、描述性强的定语从句用在名词前面。因此翻译英语定语从句时，不能一律把它们译成前置定语。药学英语英译汉中，定语从句有时候不一定译成定语,根据实际情况还可以译成表示目的、让步、条件等状语。从技巧上看,翻译定语从句可以采用拆分法、转译法等。

例1:This review summarizes these studies with an emphasis on major natural antioxidants found in three categories of plant-based foods (fruits, vegetables and legume) and mechanisms that these antioxidants may use in promoting cardio-health.

参考译文:本文对这些实验进行了综述性总结,并着重强调了植物性食物即水果、蔬菜、豆类中发现的三种主要天然抗氧剂,以及这些抗氧剂促进心血管健康的作用机制。

说明:例句中 mechanisms 后面有一个定语从句,译文直接根据汉语表达习惯将定语从句前置,这种处理法是英汉语翻译中常见的方法,符合英汉两种语言特点。但是在药学英语翻译中,大多数定语从句的翻译要视具体情况而定。

例2:Green tea is a widely consumed beverage that has attracted more attention in the recent years due to its health benefits like antioxidant, antimicrobial, anticarcinogenic and anti-inflammatory properties.

参考译文:由于具有抗氧化、抗菌、抗癌和抗炎等特性,绿茶饮料近年来受到人们越来越多的关注,是一种广泛消费的饮品。

说明:例句原文主句是 Green tea is a widely consumed beverage,在 beverage 后面有一个 that 引导的定语从句。译文根据实际情况,没有将定语从句提前到名词之前做前置定语,而是将定语从句分拆开来,单独成句,与主句并列,从整体看,并没有改变原句意思,符合汉语表达习惯。

一般来讲,翻译非限定性定语从句时要用拆分法,但要注意被拆分小句与原来主句之间顺序,而且往往要重复被修饰的名词。如下。

例3:Inhaled insulin, which could replace shots for millions of people with diabetes, won approval Friday from the Food and Drug Administration, making it the first new form of insulin since the hormone was discovered nearly 90 years ago.

参考译文:吸入胰岛素可以代替成百万糖尿病患者所采用的注射方式,它在星期五获得了(美国)食品药品管理局的许可,这使它成为发现该激素近90年以来第一种新形式的胰岛素。

说明:例句原文中,which 引导的非限定性定语从句修饰前面 inhaled insulin。译文采用了拆分法将定语从句和主句分译成两个小句,根据原文的意思,将定语从句小句放在前面,并将原主句的主语用"它"表示,译文顺畅自然,符合汉语言表达习惯。但有的时候非限定性定语从句采用拆分法翻译时,表达效果不是很好,这个时候可以将非限定性定语从句糅合到主句当中,增加主句信息容量,如下。

例4:Pharmacognosy is a study of drugs that originate in the plant and animal kingdoms.

参考译文:生药学研究的是源自动、植物界的药物。

在有些情况下,英语中定语从句可以翻译成汉语中状语从句,但转译从句功能前提是不能改变原句意义,并且要符合汉语言表达习惯。如下。

例5:When some of the structures and functions of the body deviate from the norm to the point where the ability to maintain homeostasis is destroyed or threatened or where the individual can no longer meet environmental challenges, disease is said to exist.

参考译文:当机体的某些结构和功能偏离正常值,维护内环境的能力受到破坏或受到威胁时,或者是个体再也不能面对环境的挑战时,就可以说患病了。

说明:例句中 to the point 后面有两个 where 引导的定语从句,表示程度,但细致分析原文结构和意思,这里的定语从句具有表示时间的意思,因此译文将两个 where 引导的定语从句处理成时间状语从句,跟前面 when 引导的时间状语从句并列,没有改变原文意思,也使译文自然流畅。

(张朝慧　郭　昊　史志祥　龚长华　陈　菁)

Unit Twelve

Pharmacopoeia

Pharmacopoeia is an official compendium containing drug standard and specifications in a country. Pharmacopoeia is usually compiled and implemented under the supervision of the health administration department of the country and the international pharmacopoeia is compiled under the negotiation of the publicly recognized organizations and countries. Setting drug standards plays a crucial role in regulating the drug quality, ensuring the quality and safety of medication and guaranteeing the people's health. Drug standard is the most important component in drug modern production and the quality regulation, and is also the statutory basis jointly followed by the departments of drug production, drug supply and drug use and the supervision and management departments. Drug standard usually includes official name, description, identification, purity test, content (potency or activity) assay, dosage, strength, storage and preparation etc. Some important pharmacopoeias include *United States Pharmacopoeia/National Formulary, British Pharmacopoeia, European Pharmacopoeia, Japanese Pharmacopoeia* and *Pharmacopoeia of the People's Republic of China* or *the Chinese Pharmacopoeia.*

药典是一个国家记载药品标准、检测项目的法典，一般由国家卫生行政部门主持编纂、颁布实施，国际性药典则由公认的国际组织及有关国家协商编订。制定药品标准对加强药品质量的监督管理、保证质量、保障用药安全、有效维护人民健康起着十分重要的作用。药品标准是药品现代化生产和质量管理最重要的组成部分，是药品生产、供应、使用和监督管理部门共同遵循的法定依据。药品标准一般包括以下内容：法定名称、性状、鉴别、纯度检查、含量（效价或活性）测定、剂量、规格、贮藏、制备等。现在世界上主要药典有：《美国药典/国家处方集》《英国药典》《欧洲药典》《日本药局方》以及《中华人民共和国药典》或《中国药典》。

Text A
The United States Pharmacopoeia

The United States Pharmacopoeia-National Formulary (USP-NF) is published in continuing pursuit of the mission of United States Pharmacopoeia **Convention** (USPC) to improve the health of people around the world through public standards and related programs that help ensure the quality and safety of medicines and foods.

This text from USP-NF provides background information on USPC, as well as general information about the current version of USP-NF 2021 Issue 1 (formerly known as USP 44-NF 39).

1. History of USP-NF

On January 1, 1820, 11 physicians met in the **Senate Chamber** of the U.S. **Capitol** building to establish a pharmacopoeia for the United States. These practitioners sought to create a **compendium** of the best therapeutic products, gave them useful names, and provided **recipes** for their preparation. Nearly a year later, on December 15, 1820, the first edition of The Pharmacopoeia of the United States was published. Over time, the nature of the United States Pharmacopeia (USP) changed from being a compendium of recipes to a compendium of **documentary** standards that increasingly are allied with reference materials, which together establish the identity of an article through tests for strength, quality, and purity. The publishing schedule of the USP also changed over time. From 1820 to 1942, the USP was published at 10-year intervals; from 1942 to 2000, at 5-year intervals; and beginning in 2002, annually.

In 1888, the American Pharmaceutical Association published the first national formulary under the title *The National Formulary of Unofficial Preparations* (NF). Both the USP and the NF were recognized in the *Federal Food and Drugs Act* of 1906 and again in the *Federal Food, Drug, and Cosmetic Act* of 1938. In 1975, USP acquired the *National Formulary* (NF), which now contains **excipient** standards with references to allied reference materials. Today, USP continues to develop USP and NF through the work of the Council of Experts into compendia that provide standards for articles based on advances in analytical and **metrological** science. As these and allied sciences evolve, so do USP and NF.[1]

USP's governing, standards-setting, and advisory bodies include the USP Convention, the Board of **Trustees**, the Council of Experts and its Expert Committees, Advisory Panels, and staff. Additional volunteer bodies include **Stakeholder** Forums, Project Teams, and Advisory Groups, which act in an advisory capacity to provide input to USP's governing, standards-setting, and management bodies.[2]

2. Legal Recognition

USP-NF is recognized by law and custom in many countries throughout the world. In the United States, the *Federal Food, Drug, and Cosmetic Act* (FD&C Act) defines the term "official compendium" as the official USP, the official NF, the official *Homeopathic Pharmacopoeia of the United States*, or any supplement to them. The Food and Drug Administration (FDA) may enforce compliance with official standards in USP-NF under the adulteration and **misbranding** provisions of the FD&C Act. These provisions extend broad authority to the FDA to prevent entry or to remove **designated** products from the United States market on the basis of standards in the USP-NF.

The identity of an official article, as expressed by its name, is established if it conforms in all respects to the requirements of its **monograph** and other relevant portions of the compendia. The FD&C Act **stipulates** that an article may differ in strength, quality, or purity and still have the same name if the difference is stated on the article's label. The FDA requires that names for articles that are not official must be clearly distinguishing and differentiating from any name recognized in an official compendium. Official preparations (a drug product, a dietary supplement including nutritional supplements, or a finished device) may contain additional suitable ingredients.

Drugs USP's goal is to have substance and preparation (product) monographs in USP-NF for all FDA-approved drugs, including biologics, and their ingredients. USP also develops monographs for therapeutic products not approved by the FDA, e.g., pre-1938 drugs, dietary supplements, and compounded preparations. Although submission of information needed to develop a monograph by the Council of

Experts is voluntary, compliance with a USP-NF monograph, if available, is mandatory.

Biologics   In the United States, although some biologics are regulated under the provisions of the *Public Health Service Act* (PHSA), provisions of the FD&C Act also apply to these products. For this reason, products approved under the PHSA should comply with the adulteration and misbranding provisions of the FD&C Act at Section 501(b) and 502(g) and, thus, should conform to **applicable** official monographs in USP-NF.

Medical Devices   Section 201(h) of the FD&C Act defines a device as an instrument, apparatus, similar article, or component **thereof** recognized in USP-NF. There is no comparable recognition of USP's standards-setting authority and ability to define a medical device as exists for other FDA-regulated therapeutic products.

Dietary Supplements   *The Dietary Supplement Health and Education Act* of 1994 **amendments** to the FD&C Act name USP-NF as the official compendia for dietary supplements. The dietary supplement must be represented as conforming to a USP-NF dietary supplement monograph.

Compounded Preparations   Preparation monographs provide information or standards applicable in compounding. Standards in USP-NF for compounded preparations may be enforced at both the state and federal levels, e.g., if a practitioner writes a prescription for a compounded preparation that is named in a USP-NF monograph, the preparation, when tested, must conform to the stipulations of the monograph so named.

3. Pharmacopoeial Discussion Group's (PDG) Harmonious Activities

A pharmacopoeial monograph for an active ingredient or excipient, preparation, or other substance used in the manufacture or compounding of a medicinal product generally provides a name, definition, description, and sometimes packaging, labeling, and storage statements. Thereafter, the monograph provides tests, procedures, and acceptance criteria that constitute the specification. For frequently cited procedures, a monograph may refer to a general chapter for editorial convenience. The PDG works to harmonize excipient monographs and general chapters. This will reduce manufacturers' burden of performing analytical procedures in different ways, using different acceptance criteria. The PDG, which includes representatives from the European, Japanese, and United States pharmacopoeias, and WHO (as an observer), harmonizes pharmacopoeial excipient monographs and general chapters. At all times, the PDG works to maintain an optimal level of science consistent with protection of the public health.[3]

4. Revision of USP-NF

USP-NF is continuously revised. Revisions are presented annually in twice-yearly Supplements, and as monthly Accelerated Revisions on the USP website. USP uses its Accelerated Revision processes to **expedite** revisions to the USP-NF. Accelerated Revisions include Revision Bulletins, **Interim** Revision Announcements (IRAs), and **Errata**.

USP-NF Revision Processes Include:

Public Participation   Although USP's Council of Experts is the ultimate decision-making body for USP-NF standards, these standards are developed by an **exceptional** process of public involvement and **substantial** interaction between USP and its stakeholders, both domestically and internationally. Participation in the revision process results from the support of many individuals and groups and also from scientific, technical, and trade organizations.

USP monograph revisions can be requested by any stakeholder including industry and FDA to reflect the following: (1) New FDA approvals. Monographs are updated when FDA approves medicines with new or different quality specifications than those expressed in an existing monograph. (2) Changes requested by FDA or others based on safety data. A monograph may be revised to reflect new data or science, subsequent to FDA product approval or monograph publication. (3) Advances in technology. Monographs are revised to reflect new testing and manufacturing technologies.

Requests for revision of monographs, either new monographs or those needing updating, contain information submitted voluntarily by manufacturers and other interested parties. At times USP staff may develop information to support a monograph request for revision. USP has prepared a document titled *Guideline for Submitting Requests for Revision to USP-NF* available USP official website. Via pharmacopoeial forum (PF), USP **solicits** and encourages public comment on these monographs, general chapters, and other draft documents. USP scientific **liaisons** to Expert Committees review these responses and create draft proposals that are provided to the Council of Experts. These drafts become official when Expert Committees **ballot** to make them official in USP-NF. Thus, the USP standards-setting process gives those who manufacture, regulate, and use therapeutic products the opportunity to comment on the development and revision of USP-NF standards.

Working with the FDA As specified in U.S. law, USP works with the Secretary of the Department of Health and Human Services in many ways.[4] Principal agencies in the Department for this work are the Food and Drug Administration and the Centers for **Medicare** and **Medicaid** Services. The FDA liaison program allows FDA representatives to participate in Expert Committee meetings, enabling continuing interactions between the FDA scientific staff and Expert Committee activities. Staff in the FDA Centers who are responsible for review of **compendial** activities provide specific links and opportunities for exchange of comments.

5. USP-NF Publications

Before 2020, USP-NF publications were available in print form. In addition, USP-NF and its two annual Supplements were available in compact disc (CD) and online versions. The CD version made USP-NF accessible to users on their computer hard drives.[5] At the 200th anniversary of USP in 2020, the major milestone of USP's publication was the conclusion of USP-NF printed product and the future is digital. Therefore,the USP 43-NF 38 in 2020 is the last print edition.

Now, the *USP-NF Online* is the only source for all official USP-NF content. The online format allows individual registered users to access the online format through the Internet.[5] The online electronic format provides access to official USP-NF content, along with extensive search options. The electronic formats are **cumulatively** updated to integrate the content of Supplements. Frequent updates to online systems ensure access to the most current information. To search across multiple editions of the *USP-NF Online* instead of having to log out and then change editions is available. In addition, the USP-NF Mobile 1-Year **Subscription** provides mobile access to a simplified version of the *USP-NF Online*. The application is available for Apple and Android devices. Each subscription allows users to install and **activate** the application on up to two devices.

6. General Introduction of USP-NF 2021 Issue 1

Starting with the November 2020 USP-NF publication, the title of the publication is also changed to

USP-NF 2021, Issue 1 (formerly known as USP 44-NF 39). The USP-NF will make a **transition** to a new naming convention as follows:

USP-NF 2021 Issue 1 (previously USP 44-NF 39).

USP-NF 2021 Issue 2 (previously First Supplement to USP 44-NF 39).

USP-NF 2021 Issue 3 (previously Second Supplement to USP 44-NF 39).

Year-based naming convention better informs the end user of official dates of standards published on each scheduled revision date, with all newly published revisions generally becoming official in the same calendar year, responding directly to stakeholder input received through public survey, Stakeholder Forums, and Project Teams.

USP-NF 2021 Issue 1 is official on May 1, 2021. USP-NF contains official substance and preparation (product) monographs. The terms official substance and official preparation are defined in the General Notices of this Pharmacopeia. With few exceptions, all articles for which monographs are provided in USP-NF 2021 Issue 1 are legally marketed in the United States or are contained in legally marketed articles.

A USP-NF monograph for an official substance or preparation includes the article's definition; packaging, storage, and other requirements; and a specification. The specification consists of a series of universal (description, identification, impurities and assay) and specific tests, one or more analytical procedures for each test, and acceptance criteria. Ingredients are defined as either drug substances or excipients. An excipient is any component, other than the active substance(s), intentionally added to the formulation of a dosage form. Drug substances and excipients may be synthetic, **semisynthetic**, drawn from nature (natural source), or manufactured using recombinant technology. Larger molecules and mixtures requiring a potency test are usually referred to as **biologicals** or **biotechnological** articles.

USP-NF 2021 Issue 1 contains more than 4900 monographs and more than 350 general chapters providing clear, step-by-step guidance for assays, tests, and procedures. General Chapters provide frequently cited procedures, sometimes with acceptance criteria, in order to compile into one location repetitive information that appears in many monographs.

Word Study

1. activate ['æktɪveɪt] *v.* 激活
2. amendment [ə'mendmənt] *n.* (对法律或协议的) 修订，修正
3. applicable [ə'plɪkəbl] *adj.* 合适的，可用的
4. ballot ['bælət] *v.* 投票，抽签
5. biological [ˌbaɪə'lɒdʒɪkl] *n.* 生物制品，生物制剂
6. biotechnological [ˌbaɪəʊteknə'lɒdʒikl] *adj.* 生物技术的，生物工艺的
7. Capitol ['kæpɪtl] *n.* the Capitol (美国) 国会大厦
8. chamber ['tʃeɪmbə] *n.* 大厅，(尤指) 会议厅
9. compendial [kəm'pendiəl] *adj.* 与药典相关的
10. compendium [kəm'pendiəm] *n.* 手册，大全 (复数 compendia [kəm'pendiə])
11. convention [kən'venʃn] *n.* 惯例，习俗；(国际) 公约；大会，会议
12. cumulatively ['kjuːmjələtɪvli] *adj.* 累积地，渐增地
13. designated ['dezɪɡneɪtɪd] *adj.* 指定的，标出的
14. documentary [ˌdɒkju'mentri] *adj.* 文献的，书面的
15. errata [e'rɑːtə] *n.* (*pl*) 勘误表 (单数 erratum)

16. exceptional [ɪkˈsepʃənl] *adj.* 超常的，独特的

17. excipient [ɪkˈsɪpɪənt] *n.* [药学]赋形剂，辅料

18. expedite [ˈekspədaɪt] *v.* 促进，加快

19. guideline [ˈɡaɪdlaɪn] *n.* 指导方针，准则，指标

20. homeopathic [ˌhɒmɪəˈpæθɪk] *adj.* 顺势疗法的

21. interim [ˈɪntərɪm] *adj.* （只用在名字前面）临时的，过渡性的

22. liaison [liˈeɪzn] *n.* 通讯，联络

23. medicare [ˈmedɪkeə] *n.* （美国）医疗保健制

24. medicaid [ˈmedɪkeɪd] *n.* （美国）医疗补助制

25. metrological [ˌmetrəˈlɒdʒɪkl] *adj.* 计量的

26. misbrand [ˈmɪsˈbrænd] *v.* 标示不符，贴错标签

27. monograph [ˈmɒnəɡrɑːf] *n.* （药典中的）各论，专著

28. pharmacopoeia [ˌfɑːməkəˈpiːə] *n.* （同 pharmacopeia）药典

29. pharmacopoeial [ˌfɑːməkəˈpiːəl] *adj.* （pharmacopeial）药典的

30. recipe [ˈresəpi] *n.* 处方，食谱，烹调法

31. semisynthetic [ˈsemɪsɪnˈθetɪk] *adj.* 半合成的

32. senate [ˈsenət] *n.* the Senate（美国）参议院

33. solicit [səˈlɪsɪt] *v.* 恳求，征求

34. stakeholder [ˈsteɪkhəʊldə] *n.* 股东，利益相关者

35. stipulate [ˈstɪpjuleɪt] *v.* 约定，规定

36. subscription [səbˈskrɪpʃn] *n.* 订阅

37. substantial [səbˈstænʃl] *adj.* 大量的，多的；真实的，实际的

38. thereof [ˌðeərˈɒv] *adv.* (*formal*) 其，在其中，关于那

39. transition [trænˈzɪʃn] *n.* 过渡，转换

40. trustee [trʌˈstiː] *n.* 受托人，托管小组成员

Notes

1. As these and allied sciences evolve, so do USP and NF. 意思是 "有了这些工作和科学的进展，USP 和 NF 也得到发展。"这个句子是一个固定结构：As + 主语 + 动词，so + 倒装结构，意思是 "有了……，就有……"。如：As you sow, so will you reap. 种瓜得瓜，种豆得豆。

2. Additional volunteer bodies include Stakeholder Forums, Project Teams, and Advisory Groups, which act in an advisory capacity to provide input to USP's governing, standards-setting, and management bodies. 意思是 "其他志愿机构包括股东论坛、项目团队和顾问小组，他们以顾问身份给《美国药典》的管理、标准制定和经营机构提供信息。"in an advisory capacity：以顾问身份。相比较 as an advisor（作为一个顾问），这是一个比较正式的说法，又如：in professional/personal/advisory capacity (formal)：以专家/个人/顾问身份。

3. 在理解 "At all times, the PDG works to maintain an optimal level of science consistent with protection of the public health." 这个句子的时候，要注意它的结构，"consistent with protection of the public health" 是个形容词短语，做定语修饰前面的 "an optimal level of science"。这个句子的意思是："药典讨论小组的工作始终就是维持最理想的科学水平，以及保护公共健康"。"at all times" 的意思是 "总是，一直"；"be consistent with" 的意思是 "始终如一的，与……一致的"。

4. As specified in U.S. law, USP works with the Secretary of the Department of Health and Human

Services in many ways. 根据美国法律规定, 美国药典委员会在许多方面与卫生及公共服务部秘书处有工作关系。注意 "As specified in U.S. law" 这个结构, 在 "as" 后面省略了 "is/was"; 在意思理解上, as 就代表后面的句子。又如, As stated in the package insert: 正如药品说明书所说。

5. The CD version makes USP-NF accessible to users on their computer hard drives. The online format allows individual registered users to access the online format through the Internet. CD 版可让用户在电脑硬盘上使用 USP-NF。在线版允许个人注册用户通过网络使用。"make ...accessible to sb" 意思是 "使某人能够使用 / 得到……"; "allow sb to access" 意思是 "允许……使用 / 进入"; "registered users" 意思是 "注册用户"。

Exercises

1. Decide whether each of the following statements is true (T) or false (F) according to the passage.

1) In the United States, the *Federal Food, Drug, and Cosmetic Act* (FD&C Act) defines the term "official compendium" as the official USP, the official NF, the official *Homeopathic Pharmacopeia of the United States*, but the supplements to them are not included.

2) The FD&C Act stipulates that the article different in strength, quality, or purity may still have the same name if the difference is stated on the article's label.

3) If a practitioner writes a prescription for a compounded preparation that is named in a USP-NF monograph, the preparation, when tested, must conform to the stipulations of the monograph so named.

4) USP-NF is continuously revised. Revisions are presented annually, in twice-yearly Supplements, in IRAs, and in Revision Bulletins on the USP website.

5) USP-NF and its two annual Supplements are available in print form, and in compact disc (CD) and online versions.

6) An excipient is any component, including the active substance(s), intentionally added to the formulation of a dosage form, and excipients are the necessarily inert in USP. They may be synthetic, semisynthetic, drawn from nature (natural source), or manufactured using recombinant technology.

2. Questions for oral discussion.

1) What is the mission of USPC? Can you explain how it pursues it?

2) What is the legal status of USP in the United States and in the world? Why?

3) What do you think of USP's revision processes? Which process do you think is the most crucial one?

4) What is the relationship between USP-NF and Supplements? Are they both official?

3. Multiple Choice

1) The _____ designates the USP-NF as official compendia for drugs marketed in the United States.

    A. United States Pharmacopoeia Convention   B. *U.S. Federal Food, Drug, and Cosmetics Act*

    C. Pharmacopoeial Discussion Group   D. Food and Drug Administration

2) A drug product in the U.S. market must conform to the standards in _____ to avoid possible charges of adulteration and misbranding.

    A. USP-NF   B. *United States Pharmacopoeia*

    C. *National Formulary*   D. *International Pharmacopoeia*

3) USP-NF is a book of public pharmacopoeial standards for chemical and biological drug substances, dosage forms, and _____.

    A. compounded preparations   B. excipients

    C. medical devices   D. dietary supplements

4) _____ and the PDG, harmonizes pharmacopoeial excipient monographs and General Chapters.

    A. FDA   B. WHO

    C. The Federal Government   D. NMPA

5) Although _____ is the ultimate decision-making body for USP-NF standards, these standards are developed by an exceptional process of public involvement and substantial interaction between USP and its domestic stakeholders.

    A. Pharmacopoeial Forum   B. Pharmacopoeial Discussion Group

    C. USP's Council of Experts   D. United States Pharmacopoeia Convention

6) Tests and procedures referred to in multiple monographs are described in detail in the USP-NF _____.

    A. general notices   B. general chapters

    C. excipient   D. compendial notice

7) USP-NF contains official substance and preparation (product) monographs and all the texts in USP-NF 2022 are official as of _____.

    A. May 1, 2015   B. May 1, 2020

    C. May 1, 2021   D. May 1, 2022

8) An _____ is any component, other than the active substance(s), intentionally added to the formulation of a dosage form.

    A. excipient   B. placebo

    C. additive   D. ingredient

9) _____ in pharmacopoeia set forth the article's name, definition, specification and other requirements related to packaging, storage, and labelling.

    A. General Chapters   B. *National Formulary*

    C. Monographs   D. USP dictionary

10) The _____ is an official compendium containing drug standard and specifications in a country.

    A. General Chapters   B. *National Formulary*

    C. Monographs   D. Pharmacopoeia

4. Vocabulary work

Fill in the blanks of the following sentences with the words given in the box, and change the forms of the words if necessary.

> molecular weight, official name, molecular formula, chemical name, chemical abstract registry number, graphic structure, identification, test, assay, *British Pharmacopoeia*, *United States Pharmacopoeia/National Formulary*.

1)

Aspirin ①

$C_9H_8O_4$ ③   180.16 ④

Benzoic acid, 2-(acetyloxy)-Salicylic acid acetate ⑤   [*50-78-2*] ⑥

①_____   ②_____   ③_____
④_____   ⑤_____   ⑥_____

2) To control the quality of drugs, the monograph of a particular drug in pharmacopoeia must include _____ item to identify the quality, _____ item to know the purity, and _____ to determinate the quantity of the drug.

3) The _____ and the *European Pharmacopoeia* are two official compendia within the United Kingdom.

5. Translate the following sentences or paragraphs into Chinese.

1) The U.S. Pharmacopeial Convention (USPC) is a scientific nonprofit organization that sets standards for the identity, strength, quality, and purity of medicines, food ingredients, and dietary supplements manufactured, distributed and consumed worldwide.

2) USP-NF is published in continuing pursuit of the mission of U.S. Pharmacopeial Convention: To improve global health through public standards and related programs that help ensure the quality, safety, and benefit of medicines and foods.

3) USP-NF is a combination of two compendia, the *United States Pharmacopeia* (USP) and the *National Formulary* (NF). Monographs for drug substances, dosage forms, and compounded preparations are featured in the USP. Monographs for dietary supplements and ingredients appear in a separate section of the USP. Excipient monographs are in the NF.

4) Medicinal ingredients and products will have the stipulated strength, quality, and purity if they conform to the requirements of the monograph and relevant general chapters.

5) Drug substances and excipients may be synthetic, semisynthetic, drawn from nature (natural source), or manufactured using recombinant technology. Larger molecules and mixtures requiring a potency test are usually referred to as biological or biotechnological articles.

6) A USP-NF monograph for an official substance or preparation includes the article's definition; packaging, storage, and other requirements; and a specification. The specification consists of a series of universal (description, identification, impurities and assay) and specific tests, one or more analytical procedures for each test, and acceptance criteria.

7) Before 2020, all USP-NF publications were available in print form. In addition, USP-NF and its two annual Supplements were available in compact disc (CD) and online versions. The CD version made USP-NF accessible to users on their computer hard drives. The online format allows individual registered users to access the online format through the Internet.

Value-Oriented Reflective Reading

FDA Nods for Chinese Cancer Treatment

The United States Food and Drug Administration's approval for Chinese biomedicine company BeiGene Ltd's Brukinsa (zanubrutinib) capsules marked a breakthrough for Chinese drug developers. It is the first time an innovative therapy from a Chinese mainland drug developer will enter the US market, while the majority of new drugs, especially cancer therapies, from the Chinese market are imported, industry insiders said.

The FDA announced on Nov 15, 2019 Beijing time its Accelerated Approval of the drug for treatment of adult patients with mantle cell lymphoma who have received at least one prior therapy, based on the overall response rate or how many patients experience a complete or partial shrinkage of their tumors after treatment.

Accelerated Approval is designed for drugs that treat serious conditions to fill an unmet medical need based on results that are considered to be reasonably likely to offer clinical benefits to patients. The FDA accepted the application in August, granting it Priority Review.

Previously, the FDA had designated the drug a Breakthrough Therapy in January, a first for cancer therapies developed by Chinese companies as well as new drugs from Chinese mainland overall.

Shi Lichen, founder of medical consultancy Beijing Dingchen Consultancy, said the approval reflected Chinese pharmaceutical companies' increasing attention to innovation and new drug research and development.

"China has a population of 1.4 billion, with 4 million new cancer cases arising annually, but around 90 percent of innovative and patented cancer drugs in China are imported, and highly-priced," Wang Lai, BeiGene's senior vice-president said, "We already have world players in industries such as heavy equipment manufacturing, high-speed trains and IT, and now China's biomedicine is also gaining more presence in the world as it catches up with the top-tier leaders."

Since Brukinsa was granted Accelerated Approval, further clinical trials may be required to verify and describe the drug's clinical benefit, according to the FDA. By the way, the drug was also granted Fast Track designation by the FDA for the treatment of patients with WM in July 2018. And new drug applications to China's National Medical Products Administration for relapsed or refractory MCL in August 2018, and for relapsed or refractory chronic lymphocytic leukemia or small lymphocytic lymphoma, later in October 2018, have been accepted and granted priority review. The company said it believes approvals from NMPA will soon be granted.

The FDA approved zanubrutinib as the following contents:

HIGHLIGHTS OF PRESCRIBING INFORMATION
These highlights do not include all the information needed to use BRUKINSA safely and effectively. See full prescribing information for BRUKINSA.

BRUKINSA™(zanubrutinib) capsules, for oral use
Initial U.S. Approval: 2019

INDICATIONS AND USAGE
BRUKINSA is a kinase inhibitor indicated for the treatment of adult patients with mantle cell lymphoma (MCL) who have received at least one prior therapy. (1) This indication is approved under accelerated approval based on overall response rate. Continued approval for this indication may be contingent upon verification and description of clinical benefit in a confirmatory trial.

DOSAGE AND ADMINISTRATION
- Recommended dose: 160 mg orally twice daily or 320 mg orally once daily; swallow whole with water and with or without food. (2.1)
- Reduce BRUKINSA dose in patients with severe hepatic impairment. (2.2, 8.7)

- Advise patients not to open, break, or chew capsules. (2.1)
- Manage toxicity using treatment interruption, dose reduction, or discontinuation. (2.4)

DOSAGE FORMS AND STRENGTHS
Capsules: 80 mg. (3)

CONTRAINDICATIONS
None. (4)

WARNINGS AND PRECAUTIONS
Hemorrhage: Monitor for bleeding and manage appropriately. (5.1)

Infections: Monitor patients for signs and symptoms of infection, including opportunistic infections, and treat as needed. (5.2)

Cytopenias: Monitor complete blood counts during treatment. (5.3)

Second Primary Malignancies: Other malignancies have occurred in patients including skin cancers. Advise patients to use sun protection. (5.4)

Cardiac Arrhythmias: Monitor for atrial fibrillation and atrial flutter and manage appropriately. (5.5)

Embryo-Fetal Toxicity: Can cause fetal harm. Advise women of the potential risk to a fetus and to avoid pregnancy. (5.6)

ADVERSE REACTIONS

The most common adverse reactions (≥20%) included neutrophil count decreased, platelet count decreased, upper respiratory tract infection, white blood cell count decrcased, hemoglobin decreased, rash, bruising, diarrhea and cough.(6.1)

To report SUSPECTED ADVERSE REACTIONS, contact BeiGene at 1-877-828-5596 or FDA at 1-800-FDA-1088 or *www.fda.gov/medwatch.*

DRUG INTERACTIONS

- CYP3A Inhibitors: Modify BRUKINSA dose with moderate or strong CYP3A inhibitors as described. (2.3,7.1)
- CYP3A Inducers: Avoid co-administration with moderate or strong CYP3A inducers. (7.1)

USE IN SPECIFIC POPULATIONS

Lactation: Advise not to breastfeed.(8.2)

See 17 for PATIENT COUNSELING INFORMATION

Revised: 11/2019

Questions for discussion:

1. What is the approved indication of zanubrutinib?

2. Which government approved this anticancer drug first? China or the US?

3. Please discuss with your classmates and give your opinions on the research and development of anti-cancer drug in China.

Text B
The **Calcium Citrate** Monograph from USP 2021 Issue 1

Calcium Citrate[1]

$$Ca^{2+} \left[Ca^{2+} \begin{matrix} O^- & O \\ & \\ O^- & OH & O^- \\ O & O \end{matrix} \right]_2 \cdot 4H_2O$$

$C_{12}H_{10}Ca_3O_{14} \cdot 4H_2O$ 570.49

1,2,3-Propanetricarboxylic acid, 2-hydroxy-, calcium salt (2 : 3), tetrahydrate;

Calcium citrate (3 : 2), tetrahydrate [5785-44-4].

DEFINITION[2]

Calcium Citrate contains four molecules of water of **hydration**. When dried at 150 ℃ to constant weight, it contains not less than (NLT) 97.5% and not more than (NMT) 100.5% of $Ca_3(C_6H_5O_7)_2$.

IDENTIFICATION[3]

● **A.**

Analysis: **Dissolve** 0.5 g in a mixture of 10 mL of water and 2.5 mL of 2 N **nitric acid**. Add 1 mL of **mercuric sulfate** test solution (TS), heat to boiling, and add 1 mL of **potassium permanganate** TS.

Acceptance criteria: A white **precipitate** is formed.

● **B.**

Sample: 0.5 g of Calcium Citrate

Analysis: **Ignite** completely the sample at as low a temperature as possible, cool, and dissolve the **residue** in **dilute glacial acetic acid** (1 : 10). Filter, and add 10 mL of **ammonium oxalate** TS to the **filtrate**.

Acceptance criteria: A **voluminous** white precipitate that is soluble in **hydrochloric acid** is formed.

ASSAY[4]

● **PROCEDURE**

Sample solution: Dissolve 350 mg of Calcium Citrate, previously dried at 150 ℃ to constant weight, in 12 mL of 0.5 M hydrochloric acid, and <u>dilute with water to about 100 mL</u>.[5]

Analysis: While stirring the sample solution, add 30 ml of 0.05 mol/L **edetate disodium** VS from a 50-mL **buret**. Add 15 mL of 1 N **sodium hydroxide** and 300 mg of **hydroxy naphthol blue**, and continue the **titration** to a blue endpoint. Each mL of 0.05 M edetate disodium is equivalent to 8.307 mg of calcium citrate $Ca_3(C_6H_5O_7)_2$.

Acceptance criteria: 97.5%–100.5% on the dried basis

IMPURITIES[6]

● **ARSENIC**, Method I <211>

Test preparation: Dissolve 1 g of calcium citrate in 5 mL of 3 N hydrochloric acid, and dilute with water to 35 mL.

Acceptance criteria: NMT 3 **part per million (ppm)**

● **LEAD** <251>

Test preparation: Dissolve 0.5 g of calcium citrate in 20 mL of 3 N hydrochloric acid. **Evaporate**

this solution on a steam bath to 10 mL, dilute with water to 20 mL, and cool. Use 5 mL of diluted standard lead solution (5 μg of Pb) for the test.

Acceptance criteria: NMT 10 ppm

● **LIMIT OF** FLUORIDE

[NOTE—Prepare and store all solutions in plastic containers.]

Standard stock solution: 1,000 μg/mL of fluoride ion from *USP Sodium Fluoride Reference Standard* (RS) in water.

Standard solution: 5 μg/mL of fluoride ion from standard stock solution. [NOTE—Prepare on the day of use.]

Linearity solution A: Transfer 1.0 mL of the standard solution to a 250-mL plastic beaker. Add 50 mL of water, 5 mL of 1 N hydrochloric acid, 10 mL of 1.0 M sodium citrate, and 10 mL of 0.2 M edetate disodium. If necessary, adjust with 1 N sodium hydroxide or 1 N hydrochloric acid to a pH of 5.5. Transfer to a 100-mL volumetric flask, and dilute with water to volume. This solution contains 0.05 μg/mL of fluoride.

Linearity solution B: Transfer 5.0 mL of the standard solution to a 250-mL plastic beaker, and proceed as directed for Linearity solution A beginning with "add 50 mL of water". This solution contains 0.25 μg/mL of fluoride.

Linearity solution C: Transfer 10.0 mL of the standard solution to a 250-mL plastic beaker, and proceed as directed for Linearity solution A beginning with "add 50 mL of water". This solution contains 0.50 μg/mL of fluoride.

Sample solution: Transfer 1.0 g of calcium citrate to a 100-mL beaker. Add 10 mL of water and, while stirring, 10 mL of 1 N hydrochloric acid. When dissolved, boil rapidly for 1 min, transfer the solution to a 250-mL plastic beaker, and cool in ice water. Add 15 mL of 1.0 M sodium citrate and 10 mL of 0.2 M edetate disodium, and adjust with 1 N sodium hydroxide or 1 N hydrochloric acid to a pH of 5.5. Transfer this solution to a 100-mL volumetric flask, and dilute with water to volume.

Electrode system: Use a fluoride-specific, ion-indicating electrode and a silver-silver chloride reference electrode connected to a pH meter capable of measuring potentials with a minimum reproducibility of ± 0.2 mV (see pH<791>).

Analysis

Samples: Linearity solution A, Linearity solution B, Linearity solution C, and Sample solution.

Transfer 50 mL of each Linearity solution A, Linearity solution B, and Linearity solution C to separate 250-mL plastic beakers, and measure the potential of each solution with the Electrode system. Between each reading wash the electrodes with water, and absorb any residual water by blotting the electrodes dry. Plot the logarithms of the fluoride concentrations (0.05, 0.25, and 0.50 μg/mL, respectively) versus potential to obtain a standard response line.

Transfer 50 mL of the sample solution to a 250-mL plastic beaker, and measure the potential with the Electrode system. From the measured potential and the standard response line determine the concentration, C, in μg/mL, of fluoride ion in the sample solution. Calculate the percentage of fluoride in the specimen taken by multiplying C by 0.01.

Acceptance criteria: NMT 0.003%

● LIMIT OF ACID-INSOLUBLE SUBSTANCES

Sample solution:

Dissolve 5 g of calcium citrate by heating with a mixture of hydrochloric acid and water (10∶50) for 30 min.

Analysis: Filter, wash, and dry at 105℃ for 2 h the residue so obtained.

Acceptance criteria: The weight of the residue is NMT 10 mg (0.2%).

SPECIFIC TESTS

● LOSS ON DRYING <731>: Dry a sample at 150 ℃ for 4 h: it loses from 10.0% to 13.3% of its weight.

ADDITIONAL REQUIREMENTS

● PACKAGING AND STORAGE:

Preserve in well-closed containers.

● USP REFERENCE STANDARDS <11>

USP Sodium Fluoride RS

Word Study

1. ammonium oxalate [əˈmouniəm ˈɒksəˌleɪt] *n.* [化] 草酸铵

2. arsenic [ˈɑːsnɪk] *n.* 砷盐

3. assay [əˈsei] *n.* 含量测定

4. beaker [ˈbiːkə] *n.* 烧杯

5. blot [blɒt] *v.* (用软纸) 吸干

6. buret [bjuəˈret] *n.* [分化] 滴定管,玻璃量管

7. calcium citrate [ˈkælsiəm ˈsaɪtreɪt] *n.* 枸橼酸钙,柠檬酸钙

8. concentration [ˌkɒnsənˈtreɪʃən] *n.* 含量,浓度

9. dilute [daɪˈluːt] *v.* 稀释,冲淡

10. dissolve [dɪˈzɒlv] *v.* 溶解

11. edetate disodium [ˈiːdɪtət daɪˈsəʊdɪəm] *n.* 依地酸二钠,乙二胺四乙酸二钠

12. electrode [ɪˈlektrəʊd] *n.* [电] 电极

13. evaporate [ɪˈvæpəreɪt] *v.* (使) 蒸发,挥发

14. filtrate [ˈfɪltreɪt] *n.* 滤液

15. fluoride [ˈflɔːraɪd] *n.* 氟化物

16. glacial [ˈgleɪʃl] *adj.* 冰冷的,冰的

17. glacial acetic acid [ˈgleɪʃl əˈsiːtɪk ˈæsɪd] *n.* [有化] 冰醋酸,冰乙酸

18. hydration [haɪˈdreɪʃn] *n.* [化学] 水合作用

19. hydrochloric acid [ˈhaɪdrəˈklɒrɪk ˈæsɪd] *n.* [无化] 盐酸

20. hydroxide [haɪˈdrɒksaɪd] *n.* [无化] 氢氧化物,羟化物

21. hydroxy naphthol blue [haɪˈdrɒksɪ ˈnæfθəʊl bluː] *n.* 羟基萘酚蓝

22. identification [aɪˌdentɪfɪˈkeɪʃn] *n.* 鉴别

23. ignite [ɪgˈnaɪt] *v.* 炽灼

24. ion [ˈaɪən] *n.* [化学] 离子

25. lead [led] *n.* (一种重金属) 铅

26. linearity solution [ˌlɪniˈærəti səˈluːʃn] *n.* 线性 (标准) 溶液

27. logarithm [ˈlɒgərɪðəm] *n.* [数] 对数

28. mercuric sulfate [mɜːˈkjʊrɪk ˈsʌlfeit] *n.* [无化] 硫酸汞

29. nitric acid [ˈnaɪtrɪk ˈæsɪd] *n.* [无化] 硝酸

30. part per million (ppm) 百万分之一

31. plot [plɒt] v. 标出，标记，绘制（曲线、图表）

32. potassium permanganate [pə'tæsiəm pɜ:'mæŋɡəneɪt] n. ［无化］高锰酸钾

33. potential [pə'tenʃl] n. 电极电位

34. precipitate [prɪ'sɪpɪteɪt] n. 沉淀物；v.（使）沉淀，淀析

35. reproducibility [rɪprədju:sə'bɪlɪtɪ] n. 重现性，再现性

36. residual [rɪ'zɪdjuəl] adj. 剩余的

37. residue ['rezɪdju:] n. 残渣，滤渣

38. silver-silver chloride reference electrode ['sɪlvə 'sɪlvə 'klɔ:raɪd 'refrəns ɪ'lektrəʊd] n. 银 - 氯化银参比电极

39. sodium citrate ['səʊdiəm 'sɪtreɪt] n. ［有化］枸橼酸钠，柠檬酸钠

40. sodium hydroxide ['səʊdiəm haɪ'drɒksaɪd] n. ［无化］氢氧化钠

41. specimen ['spesɪmən] n. 样品，试样

42. titration [tɪ'treɪʃn] n. ［分化］滴定，滴定法

43. volumetric flask [ˌvɒljʊ'metrɪk flɑ:sk] n. ［分化］量瓶，容量瓶

44. voluminous [və'lu:mɪnəs] n. 大量的

Notes

1. 药典各论中所收载的原料药以法定名称（official name）开头，然后给出药物的描述性信息，包括结构式（graphic structure）、化学式（molecular formula）、分子量（molecular weight）、化学名称（chemical name）和化学文摘登记号（Chemical Abstract registry number）。

2. 各论中第一项是药物定义。定义项下的含量限度建立于含量测定项基础之上，以化学分子式的百分含量计，按干燥品或无水物计算。合成药物的含量通常在 98.0%~102.0%；发酵产物、天然药物或生物制品含量可以用每毫克中的微克数或单位数来表示；制剂的含量限度则是根据其生产过程精密度制定，以活性成分的化学分子式占标示量的百分含量来表示，一般范围是 90.0%~110.0%。

3. 鉴别试验提供帮助核实药物身份的方法。鉴别项首选的方法是红外吸收光谱法，也采用薄层色谱法和紫外吸收光谱等方法。对于以盐形式存在的药物（如本文中的枸橼酸钙），一般有酸、碱或盐的鉴别试验。

4. 原料药的含量测定多采用精密度较高的滴定分析法，如本文中的枸橼酸钙的含量测定采用了配位滴定法；制剂的含量测定多采用专属性较高的高效液相色谱法。抗生素的含量测定趋向于采用高效液相色谱法代替微生物效价测定法，对于含有多个活性成分的抗生素来说，微生物价测定法依然是最佳选择。

5. dilute with water to about 100 mL. 用水稀释到 100 mL。理解这句话时，"with water" 这个介词短语表示 "用某种溶剂（水）"，"to 100 mL" 这个介词短语表示 "到多少体积（到 100 mL）"。

6. 杂质检查是控制原料药纯度的必要途径。根据药物中可能存在的杂质来确定杂质检查项，采用限量检查法。药物合成或降解过程产生的毒性杂质称为特殊杂质。这些有害杂质必须通过合适的检查方法控制在用药安全的水平。特殊杂质限量检查通常采用色谱法或专属、灵敏的光谱分析法和化学法。

Supplementary Parts

1. Medical and Pharmaceutical Terminology (12): Morphemes from Latin and Greek in Medical and Pharmaceutical English Terms

在医药英语术语中,我们经常可以发现表达某一个含义的词素不止一个。这往往是由于它们分别来自希腊语、拉丁语等不同语言。一般来说,来自希腊语的词素往往出现在更为专业的术语中,来自拉丁语的词素往往出现在相对基础的专业术语中。在此,我们通过下表中列举的部分词根来加以提醒。

Latin	Greek	English Meaning	Chinese Meaning	Examples
ventro-	coelio-, laparo-	belly (abdomen)	腹	ventrodorsad 向腹背 coeliotomy 腹部切开术 laparoscope 腹腔镜
bili-	chole-	bile	胆	bilirubin 胆红素 cholecyst 胆囊
vesico-	cysto-	bladder	膀胱	vesicotomy 膀胱切开术 cystolith 膀胱结石
sangui-	em- hemo- hemato-	blood	血	sanguinopoietic 造血的 anemia 贫血 hemoperitoneum 腹腔积血 hematemesis 吐血,咯血
os(se)o-	osteo-	bone	骨	osseous 骨的,骨质的 osteomyelitis 骨髓炎
mammo-	masto-	breast	乳	mammography 乳房 X 线照相术 mastoid 乳头状的
auri-	oto-	ear	耳	auricular 耳状的 otitis 耳炎
oculo-	ophthalmo-	eye	眼	binocular 用两眼的 ophthalmology 眼科学
palpebro-	blepharo-	eyelid	睑	palpebral conjunctiva 睑结膜 blepharitis 睑缘炎
lip-	steato-	fat	脂肪	lipemia 脂血症 steatorrhea 脂肪泻
gingivo-	ulo-	gum	龈	gingivitis 牙龈炎 ulorrhagia 牙龈出血
cord-	cardi-	heart	心	cordiform 心形的 cardiology 心(脏)病学
reno-	nephro-	kidney	肾	renal 肾的 nephrectomy 肾切除术
labio	cheilo-	lip	唇	labionasal 唇鼻音,唇鼻音的 cheiloschisis 唇裂(畸形)
pulmo-	pneumo-	lung, air	肺,气	pulmonary 肺部的 pneumothorax 气胸
oro-	stomato	mouth	口	orolingual 口与舌的 stomatology 口腔医学
ungui-	onychi-	nail	甲	unguis 爪,蹄 onychia 甲床炎
nerv-	neuro-	nerve	神经	nervous 神经的 neuroblast 成神经细胞

续表

Latin	Greek	English Meaning	Chinese Meaning	Examples
naso-	rhino-	nose	鼻	nasopharynx　鼻咽 rhinology　鼻科学
palato-	urano-	palatine	腭	palatitis　腭炎 uranoschisis　腭裂
cutano-	derm(at)o-	skin	皮	cutaneous　皮肤的,影响皮肤的 dermoid　皮样的,皮状的
lieno-	spleno	spleen	脾	lienectomy　脾切除术 splenomegaly　脾大
lacrimo-	dacryo-	tear	泪	lacrimal　泪腺的,泪的 dacryocyst　泪囊
denti-	odonto-	tooth	牙齿	dentistry　牙科 odontodynia　牙痛
omphalo-	umbilico-	umbilicus	脐	omphalitis　（幼小动物患的）脐炎 umbilical hernia　脐疝
vagino-	colpo-	vagina	阴道	vaginorrhaphy　阴道缝合术 colposcope　阴道镜
veno-	phlebo-	vein	静脉	venograft　静脉移植 phlebitis　静脉炎
vaso-	angio-	vessel	血管	vasomotor　血管收缩的 angiography　血管造影术
utero-	hystero- metro-	womb, uterus	子宫	uterine　子宫的 hysteroscope　宫腔镜 endometrium　子宫内膜

(1) Fill in the blanks with certain Latin affix, Greek affix or its English meaning according to the given Chinese meaning.

Chinese meaning	Latin affix	Greek affix	English meaning
Sample: 腹	ventro-	coelio-, laparo-	belly (abdomen)
静脉	veno-		vein
神经	nerv-		
心		cardi-	heart
骨			bone
膀胱	vesico-		

(2) Fill in the blanks with the missing word root, prefix or suffix.

1) _____rubin　胆红素

2) _____nopoietic　造血的

3) _____cular　耳状的

4) bin_____　用两眼的

5) _____emia　脂血症

6) _____rrhagia　牙龈出血

7) _____ectomy　肾切除术

8) _____logy　口腔医学

9) _____pharynx　鼻咽

10) _____megaly　脾大

11) _____cyst　泪囊

12) _____graphy　血管造影术

2. English-Chinese Translation Skills: 药学英语翻译技巧 (8)：状语从句翻译

　　药学英语语篇较多使用状语从句,表示时间、原因、条件、让步、目的、结果等意义。状语从句通常可以直接翻译,但需要注意的是在翻译过程中如何正确处理状语从句与主句的位置。由于英汉两种语言的表达形式不同,翻译状语从句要根据汉语言表达习惯灵活处理。

　　状语从句翻译也要看句子具体情况而定,并非所有状语从句都要直接翻译出来,有时候状语从句也可以跟主句糅合在一起。如下。

　　例 1：There are two types of diabetes. Type 1 occurs when the body doesn't produce any insulin. People with type 2 diabetes don't produce enough insulin or their cells ignore the insulin.

　　参考译文：糖尿病分为两型。1 型是人体不能制造胰岛素。2 型是人体无法制造足够多的胰岛素或是人体细胞不识别胰岛素。

　　说明：译文很好地将时间状语从句 when the body doesn't produce any insulin 与主句 Type 1 occurs 糅合在一起,没有改变原句意思,汉语表述简洁流畅。

　　翻译状语从句时,要正确划分主句和从句,理清楚主句与从句之间的逻辑关系。例如在翻译原因状语从句时,要根据句子内容出发确定好哪个是"因",哪个是"果",如下。

　　例 2：Isolation of natural products differs from that of the more commonly occurring biological macromolecules because natural products are smaller and chemically more diverse than the relatively consistent proteins, nucleic acids and carbohydrates, and isolation methods must take this into account.

　　参考译文：天然产物的分离不同于通常出现的生物大分子,因为天然产物与常见的组成成分蛋白质、核酸和碳水化合物相比,分子量小且更具化学多样性,所以分离方法也要将这些因素考虑在内。

　　说明：例句原文由三个小句组成,结构并不复杂,正确理解和翻译的关键是判断 because 引导的原因状语从句到哪里结束,这是翻译药学英语状语从句较为重要的环节。根据原文意思并结合药学基础知识,译文通过增加连词"所以",很好地界定了原文三个小句之间的逻辑关系。

　　有时候,状语从句与主句之间的逻辑关系并不是十分明显,翻译时可以将主从句关系处理成并列关系。

　　例 3：A few antibiotics have such toxic effects that their usefulness is strictly limited.

　　参考译文：有些抗生素有毒性作用,其应用受到严格限制。

　　说明：例句中 such...that... 结构表示"如此……以至于……",是结果状语从句,译文将这种显然的"因果"关系处理成两个并列小句,没有改变原句意思。

　　有时候,不同逻辑关系状语从句也可以因为表达需要而进行转换,前提当然还是不能够改变原句意思。如下。

　　例 4：Drugs with such serious potential dangers as these should be used only if life is threatened and nothing else will work.

　　参考译文：这些有严重潜在危险的药物只有在生命受到威胁或其他药物无效时才使用。

　　说明：原例句中 only if 引导条件状语从句,译文在没有改变原句意思的情况下将这个从句处理成时间状语从句。如下。

　　例 5：All the possible troubles that can result from antibiotic treatment should not keep anyone from using one of these drugs when it is clearly indicated. Nor should they discourage certain preventive uses of antibiotics which have proved extremely valuable.

　　参考译文：由于有些抗生素疗效确切,使用抗生素所带来的所有可能的麻烦也不能阻止任何人用任何一种抗生素,对于被证明是有效的抗生素,人们不会不鼓励它们的使用。

说明:例句有两个小句。第一句中,主句是 All the possible troubles should not keep anyone from using one of these drugs,从句是 when 引导的时间状语从句。译文没有将 when 引导的从句翻译成时间状语从句,而是译成原因状语从句:"由于有些抗生素疗效确切",并没有改变原句的意思。第二句中没有状语从句,只有 which 引导的定语从句修饰 antibiotics,但是译文将这个定语从句处理成了状语:"对于被证明是有效的抗生素"。从整个句子来看,参考译文虽有将从句功能进行转译,但没有改变原文意思,而且符合汉语言表达习惯。

(龚长华　陈　芸　史志祥　陈　菁)

Unit Thirteen

International Pharmaceutical Registration

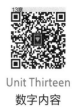

Unit Thirteen
数字内容

The role of therapeutic goods regulation is designed mainly to protect the health and safety of the population. Regulation is aimed at ensuring the safety, quality, and efficacy of the therapeutic goods. In most jurisdictions, therapeutic goods must be registered before they are allowed to be sold. There is usually some degree of restriction on the availability of certain therapeutic goods, depending on their risk to consumers.

Registration of drugs, also known as product licensing or marketing authorization, is an essential element of drug regulation. All drugs that are marketed, distributed and used in the country should be registered by the national competent regulatory authority.

Only the inspection of manufacturing plants and laboratory quality control analysis certainly does not guarantee product quality and safety. Drug regulation should therefore include the scientific evaluation of products before registration, to ensure that all marketed pharmaceutical products meet the criteria of safety, efficacy and quality. Although these criteria are applicable to all medicines including biological products (including vaccines, blood products, monoclonal antibodies, cell and tissue therapies) and herbal medicines (also other traditional and complementary medicines), there are substantial differences in the regulatory requirements for some groups of medicines.

Innovative medicines (originator products) are new medicines that have not been used in humans earlier and contain new active ingredients. Nowadays these medicines are usually first approved by regulators in well-resourced countries using regulatory requirements harmonized in the framework of International Conference on Harmonization of Technical Requirements for the Registration of Pharmaceuticals for Human Use (ICH).

治疗用品监管的作用主要是为了保护人民的健康和安全。监管的目的是确保治疗产品的安全性、质量和有效性。在大多数司法管辖区,治疗用品必须在被允许销售之前进行注册。由于某些治疗产品给消费者可能带来风险,通常对其上市有一定程度的限制。

药品注册也称为产品许可或上市许可,是药物监管的一个重要组成部分。所有在一个国家上市、流通和使用的药物都必须在该国职能监管机构进行注册。

只检查生产设施以及实验室质量控制分析,肯定不能保证产品的质量和安全性。因此,药物监管应包括在注册前对产品进行科学评价,以确保所有上市的药品符合安全、功效和质量标准。虽然这些标准适用于所有药物,包括生物制品(包括疫苗、血液产品、单克隆抗体、细胞和组织疗法)以及草药(以及其他传统和补充药物),但对于某些种类的药物来说,监管要求上会存在较大的差异。

创新药物(原研产品)是人类之前没有使用过的新药,它们包含新的活性成分。现在,这些药物通常首先被掌握资源较多的国家的监管机构首先批准,采用在国际人用药品注册技术协调会(ICH)框架下协调的监管要求。

A generic drug product is one that is comparable to a patented drug product in dosage form, strength, route of administration, quality, performance characteristics and intended use. Generic drug applications are generally not required to include preclinical (animal and *in vitro*) and clinical (human) trial data to establish safety and effectiveness. Instead, generic applicants must scientifically demonstrate that their product is bioequivalent (i.e., performs in the same manner as the innovator drug).

仿制药是指在剂型、剂量、给药途径、质量、性能特点和预期用途等方面与专利药品相媲美的药品。仿制药申请通常不需要包括临床前(动物和体外)和临床(人体)试验数据来建立其安全性和有效性。不过,仿制药申请人必须科学地证明其产品的生物等效性(即与原研药作用方式相同)。

As more than 95% of new medicines are worked out in the ICH "regions", the technical requirements for the safety, efficacy and quality of new medicines is determined at large by ICH technical guidelines. The application format for registration (marketing authorization) of new medicines in ICH and associated countries (such as Canada, Switzerland and Australia) has to follow *The Common Technical Document* (CTD), which provides harmonized structure and format for new product applications.

由于超过 95% 的新药是在 ICH "地区" 推出的,对新药安全性、功效和质量的技术要求普遍基于 ICH 技术指南。在 ICH 和相关国家(如加拿大、瑞士和澳大利亚)的新药注册(上市许可)的申请格式必须遵循通用技术文档(CTD)的要求,它为新产品的申请提供统一的结构和格式。

This Common Technical Document is divided into four separate sections and 5 modules. The four sections address the application organization (M4: Organization), the Quality section (M4Q), the Safety section (M4S) and the Efficacy section (M4E) of the harmonized application. Module 1 contains ICH region specific administrative data and prescribing information and is not part of CTD. Module 2 contains CTD summaries, Module 3 is dedicated to quality, Module 4 for non-clinical study reports and Module 5 on clinical study reports.

该通用技术文档分为 4 个单独部分和 5 个模块。这 4 个部分具体涉及一个协调申请项目的申请机构(M4:组织)、质量部分(M4Q)、安全性部分(M4S)和有效性部分(M4E)。模块 1 包含 ICH 区域具体行政数据和规定信息,这并不是 CTD 的必要部分。模块 2 包含 CTD 总结,模块 3 关注质量,模块 4 为非临床研究报告,模块 5 为临床研究报告。

Text A
The Electronic Common Technical Document

Electronic **submissions** have been part of the **regulatory** landscape since the first formats were developed in the early 1990s. The electronic Common Technical Document (eCTD) is an International Council on Harmonisation of Technical Requirements for the Registration of Pharmaceuticals for Human Use (ICH) created and maintained format for electronic submissions that aims to support the regional and international submission requirements of the Common Technical Document (CTD) in the three ICH regions and beyond.[1]

Since the desktop PC became a common part of the office working environment of the pharmaceutical industry and regulatory agencies, there have been efforts to use the technology to improve the efficiency of the review and approval process through the creation and use of electronic submissions. The fact that the data and documents that form part of the regulatory submission were being created using electronic systems led to efforts to find a way to submit these in an electronic format rather than printing them to paper and losing some of the opportunities to explore making review procedures more efficient.

The simplest definition of an electronic submission is any set of files submitted to aid the review of a **dossier**. The objective in submitting the content of a submission electronically is <u>to take advantage of the technology to provide a more efficient navigation around the content of the dossier</u>[2], to provide content that can be searched and queried, to provide content that can be more easily copied into assessment reports and other documents, to reduce the amount of paper submitted, and to allow the creation of different views of the submitted data.

Not all of the simplest electronic submissions will meet all of these objectives but all meet at least one of them. For example, the requests made by many agencies to receive copies of key summary and labeling documents in an electronic format are usually to aid in the review, preparing comments, and creation of assessment reports. The requests by some agencies to receive data files are usually to allow the reprocessing and analysis of the data and also <u>to reduce the amount of paper received</u>[3].

The FDA in the United States started one of the first electronic submission programs when they began the CANDA (Computer-Aided New Drug Application) project in the early 1990s. Applicants could work with the agency to deliver a complete new drug application (<u>NDA</u>[4]) submission in an electronic format to aid in the review of the dossier. Many companies who were making submissions in both the United States and Europe started to explore the way in which they could reuse this technology in Europe and European agencies started accepting electronic submissions in 1993 and 1994. Often, these early electronic submissions consisted not only of the set of submission files but also of the hardware and software necessary for the agency to be able to use and review the submission. The other main feature of these submissions was that the ways in which the data were presented, though conforming to the dossier standards of the region, would vary because of the different software applications used by the applicants in their creation.

The late 1990s saw the introduction of a number of standardized ways of presenting a dossier in an electronic format. The electronic NDA (eNDA) in the United States grew from initial efforts to standardize the presentation of the data submitted in items 11 and 12 of the NDA and resulted in a published standard employing the adobe portable document file (PDF) and <u>SAS</u>[5] formats, for documents and datasets respectively, for the entire content of the dossier. The FDA went further to develop the supporting processes to allow the electronic-only submission of the dossier without the need for any paper.

The growing use of electronic submissions on a global basis demonstrated that the concept and the objectives behind their use were all valid. However, for global companies there remained issues that the increased standardization of the electronic format was still taking place on a country or regional basis and that global companies could not get the greatest benefit of content reuse on an international basis.

Against this background, the <u>ICH</u>[6] Steering Committee approved the adoption of the global electronic submission standard as a project under the M2 (*Electronic Standards for the Transmission of Regulatory Information*, ESTRI) group. There was only one small problem—without a global standard for the presentation of regulatory content, there would be a significant issue in developing an electronic submission specification. The M4 topic to create the CTD was approved to create the structure for the submission of regulatory information, and as this was developed, M2 was able to start the work to define the electronic specification.

The main objectives of the ICH eCTD specification are the same as those of other electronic submission formats, to provide a global specification for the transport of a submission meeting the CTD structure from an applicant to the regulatory agency. The eCTD submission provides the specification to meet the basic requirements for the presentation of documents and the means to navigate within and between them in the dossier structure.

In addition to providing the specification to meet the structural and navigation requirements, the eCTD has sought to provide a standardized solution to the problem of relating submissions to each other. In the paper submission world, it has long been a desire of regulatory agencies to be able to see how each subsequent dossier relates to the previous ones. In some cases, it has been a requirement to submit the changed pages on different color paper so that they could be identified in an updated volume on the shelf. The possibilities offered by electronic submission technologies have long been seen as providing a more efficient way to resolve this problem. The FDA started a project known as the cumulative Table of Contents (c-TOC) in about 1998 to create an electronic submission solution to this problem. When the ICH adopted the eCTD project, the experience from c-TOC was brought to the project and it was decided that the specification should include a means to create and manage the relationships between documents and dossiers over the life of the drug product. Within the eCTD topic, this is known as life-cycle management.

Key to the resolution of the life-cycle management requirements is the ability to be able to submit submission content only once and to provide a means to refer to this from later submissions, without the need to resubmit the content. From this initial requirement, the specification must also be able to identify when content is submitted and what its relationship is to previously submitted data.

Another major part of the ICH eCTD business case would be the ability to design a specification that could also be extended to cover the regional aspects of the CTD. It is understood that the ICH CTD could only describe content that would be common to all three of the ICH regions, but that each region would have regional requirements that would need to be defined locally. The eCTD specification would need to accommodate the global and regional needs and attempt to do so in a way that would be **compatible** so that processes and the applications for creating the eCTD could be broadly similar between regions.

The ICH M2 group also wanted to learn from and reuse other parts of the existing regional and national specifications. Therefore, individual parts of these would be copied and reused wherever they could be as the new specification was developed.

Lastly, wherever possible, the eCTD specification should employ open standards and avoid using **proprietary** formats. There was a concern that if the standard was to be employed for submissions that would need to be readable and reusable over the potentially long lives of drug products, then one of the best ways to ensure this was by using formats less **susceptible** to a vendor's developmental **whims**.

The eCTD consists of four main components: files, folders, XML (eXtensible Markup Language) backbone files and utility files to manage the XML backbone files. The first two components, files and folders, are the common elements that the eCTD shares with other earlier electronic submission formats. The defining feature of the eCTD is the use of XML to manage the **metadata** about the documents and dossier that allows the relationships over the product life cycle to be managed.

The ability to establish and manage the relationships between documents and dossiers is the biggest functional difference between the eCTD and previous electronic submission formats. The relationships between individual documents are established primarily by the operation and modified-file attributes of the leaf elements[7] in the eCTD. The four allowed values of the operation attribute are reasonably self-explanatory, but experience has shown that the use of the operation attribute is dependent crucially on the business processes and document **granularity** adopted by the applicant.

A finer document granularity allows management of the content in smaller **chunks** and this may be advantageous when submitting **supplements** or variations as the scale of the change can be controlled more tightly. However, the finer granularity gives the applicant a bigger document management task and also means that there may be more external hyperlinks between files, something that is more difficult to create and manage.[8]

The concepts of dossier life-cycle management are probably not as well developed in the eCTD specifications as those of the document life cycle. The concept is managed mainly by the definition of the application and the use of the related-sequence metadata value to show the regulatory activity.

An element of dossier life-cycle management also comes from the decisions taken over the structure of the submission, particularly in Module 3. This will then define the way in which the applicant manages future supplements and variations within the overall life cycle.

The original eCTD design requirements suggested that the eCTD should be something that could be created without **recourse** to **sophisticated** tools and experience has shown that single eCTD submissions can be created using basic text editor tools. However, the complexity of managing document and dossier life cycles within the regulatory submission timelines means that some tools are almost certainly required to assist in the creation, **validation**, viewing, and reviewing of the eCTD.

eCTD creation tools come with a variety of functionalities. The simpler tools require the user to create the content files separately and will create the XML backbone and folder structure. More complex tools might introduce functionality to integrate with an electronic document management system, to manage the creation of the PDF files from source files and to better manage the document relationships over the life of the eCTD.

Validation of the eCTD is a key requirement and tools can assist in this task greatly. The DTD (document type definition) defines the rules to create a technically valid eCTD and a parsing XML editor can check that these rules are being followed. However, there are many additional business rules, such as the checking of the MD5 **checksums**, that also apply for an eCTD to be valid and tools are required to assist in these checks.

Viewing of a single eCTD sequence can be achieved using the stylesheets that accompany the eCTD specifications. However, to display the full life-cycle relationships between documents and dossiers, a tool is required. Reviewing tools will add functionality to annotate the content and assist in the creation of assessment reports at the agencies.

Only four regions/countries have fully implemented the eCTD since the ICH specification was first published in 2002 by publishing a regional specification to accompany the ICH one. These are Canada, the European Union, Japan, and the United States.

The European Union was the first region to publish its draft Module 1 specification in March 2002 with an initial statement to accept submissions in the eCTD format from June 2003. However, it was not until July 2004 that Version 1.0 of the European Union Module 1 specification was finally published. Since then, there have been three further updates to the European Union Module 1 specification. The driver for all of these changes has been changes to the European Union regulation requiring new sections in Module 1. At the same time, the opportunity has been used to review the technical specification of Module 1 and to implement other updates. Version 1.1 was released in January 2006, Version 1.2.1 in October 2006, and

Version 1.3 in May 2008.

In February 2005, the European Union Heads of Medicines Agencies resolved that by the end of 2009 all the European Union Member States would be able to accept submissions electronically without paper and that the format would be the eCTD. Since then, the individual National Competent Authorities (NCAs) and the European Medicines Agency (<u>EMEA</u>[9]) have worked to implement the eCTD. Individually, the Medicines Evaluation Board (MEB) in the Netherlands was the first NCA to publish guidance about electronic submissions and the acceptability of the eCTD, but they have been followed by at least 10 other NCAs who have also published guidance. The EMEA published a *Statement of Intent* about the acceptability of the eCTD in the *Centralized Procedure*[10] in January 2008, making the procedure fully electronic from January 1, 2009, and making eCTD the **mandatory** electronic submission format from January 1, 2010.

Despite the early adoption of the standard, the numbers of eCTDs have been relatively low. Gathering data has been difficult due to the problems of getting figures from all of the European Union Member States, but the best estimate is that about 5,000 eCTD sequences have been submitted. The EMEA *Statement of Intent* has led to eCTD numbers in the *Centralized Procedure* rising with 90% of products registered via this process having some submissions made using the format, although the overall percentage of eCTD is somewhere about 30% of all submissions. In the other procedures, the numbers are a lot smaller with a maximum estimate of 3% of submissions being made in the eCTD format. Work continues in Europe to increase the numbers of eCTDs through the transition to electronic working and then to the eCTD.

In the United States, the initial draft guidance for Module 1 and the use of the eCTD in Modules 2–5 were published in August 2003, but full implementation waited until the publishing of the ICH STF (*Study Tagging Files*) specification in November 2004. The STF specification describes how to organize study information and is vital in allowing the eCTD to be used in the United States during the <u>IND</u>[11] phase as well as the NDA phase. At the end of 2007, the FDA announced that the eCTD would become the only acceptable format for electronic submissions from January 1, 2008, although a waiver process was put in place so that the older eNDA could still be used under certain conditions.

As of the end of October 2008, the FDA had received just over 44,000 eCTD sequences associated with just over 4,000 applications. These numbers show the overall success of the eCTD implementation in the United States. However it is worth noting that an analysis by the FDA of all their 2007 submissions showed that of around 167,000 submissions, 11% were electronic only and 8% were mixed paper and electronic, meaning that 81% of submissions were still in paper only. Further analysis showed that the percentage of eCTD submissions for the various NDA types (original applications and various supplement types) varied between 24% and 71%. The greatest percentage of paper submissions remains in the IND where paper accounts for over 90% of all submissions.

The ICH eCTD specification has been around in pretty much the same form since Version 3.0 was published in 2002 (the update to Version 3.2 in February 2004 was a fairly minor change to the specification). The challenge for the ICH M2 group has been to support the eCTD specification's adoption by only making changes absolutely necessary to support the business needs, but not making so many changes that industry and the eCTD tool vendors are unable to implement because of the frequent changes.

In 2007, the ICH Steering Committee approved the ICH M2 group to begin the collection of the business requirements for the development of the *Next Major Version* of the eCTD. In October 2008, the ICH Steering Committee approved the development of the *Next Major Version* of the eCTD through a process involving Standards Development Organizations (SDOs). SDOs are accredited organizations that develop standards to meet the requirements of individual national or international standards bodies. Some of the better-known SDOs in the health-care industry are the International Standards Organisation[12] (ISO), the European Standards Organisation (CEN), and Health Level 7 (HL7), an SDO accredited by the American National Standards Institute[13] (ANSI). The processes used by these individual organizations are required to be followed by the mandates of some of the individual regions within the ICH if the resulting standard is to have a legal status and basis in the region.

Work in adopting the eCTD in other regions and countries is also continuing, though slowly. Although other countries are working on electronic submission formats, they will borrow ideas from the eCTD. It is hoped that the development of the eCTD through a process that involves international standards organizations may improve the chances of adoption of the standard outside the three ICH regions. As the eCTD becomes more widely adopted, national formats will be withdrawn and the eCTD can become a truly global standard.

Word Study

1. checksum [ˈtʃeksʌm] *n.* 检查和，校验和
2. chunk [tʃʌŋk] *n.* 厚块，大块
3. compatible [kəmˈpætəbl] *adj.* 一致的，兼容的
4. dossier [ˈdɒsieɪ] *n.* 档案材料，卷宗
5. granularity [grænjʊˈlærɪtɪ] *n.* 颗粒度，粒度
6. mandatory [ˈmændətəri] *adj.* 法定的，义务的，强制性的
7. metadata [ˈmetədeɪtə] *n.* 元数据
8. proprietary [prəˈpraɪətri] *adj.* 专利的，所有权的
9. recourse [rɪˈkɔːs] *n.* 依赖，求助
10. regulatory [ˈregjələtəri] *adj.* 管理的，控制的
11. sophisticated [səˈfɪstɪkeɪtɪd] *adj.* 复杂的
12. submission [səbˈmɪʃn] *n.* 提交，提交的文件
13. supplement [ˈsʌplɪmənt] *n.* 补充物
14. susceptible [səˈseptəb(ə)l] *adj.* 易受外界影响的，易受感染的，容许……的
15. validation [ˌvælɪˈdeɪʃn] *n.* 确认，批准，验证
16. whim [wɪm] *n.* 一时的兴致，奇想

Notes

1. The electronic Common Technical Document (eCTD) is an International Council on Harmonisation of Technical Requirements for the Registration of Pharmaceuticals for Human Use (ICH) created and maintained format for electronic submissions that aims to support the regional and international submission requirements of the Common Technical Document (CTD) in the three ICH regions and beyond. 译文：电子通用技术文档（eCTD）是人用药品技术要求国际协调理事会（ICH）创建和维护的电子文件提交格式，旨在规范通用技术文档（CTD）在ICH覆盖的三个地区以及其他地区和国际文件提交要求。注意，这里的 an International Council on Harmonisation of Technical Requirements for the Registration of Pharmaceuticals for Human Use (ICH) created and maintained

format 相当于 a format that is created and maintained by the International Council on Harmonisation of Technical Requirements for the Registration of Pharmaceuticals for Human Use (ICH).

2. ... to take advantage of the technology to provide a more efficient navigation around the content of the dossier 意思是：利用技术围绕文档内容进行更有效的导航。注意：这里的 navigation 指 "针对文档内容进行的定位、导航"。

3. ... to reduce the amount of paper received 意思是：减少所收到的纸质材料的数量。注意：这里的 paper 在文中出现多次，指 "纸质材料"，不要误解为 "论文、纸张" 等。

4. NDA 意思是新药申请。NDA 主要针对新分子实体（NME）；新化学实体（NCE）；原批准药品相同化学成分的新盐基、新酯基；原批准药品的新配方组成；原批准药品的新适应证（包括处方药转非处方药使用）；新剂型、新给药途径、新规格（单位含量）；两种以上原批准药品的新组合。

5. SAS 指 Statistical Analysis System，它是一个模块化、集成化的大型应用软件系统。

6. ICH 指 The International Council for Harmonisation of Technical Requirements for Pharmaceuticals for Human Use。ICH 为英文的首字母缩写，中文通常译为 "国际人用药品注册技术协调会"。

7. leaf elements 意思是 "叶子元素"，在档案中会被重复使用。

8. However, the finer granularity gives the applicant a bigger document management task and also means that there may be more external hyperlinks between files, something that is more difficult to create and manage. 译文：然而，更细的粒度给申请人带来更大的文档管理任务，也就意味着文件之间可能有更多的外部超链接，更难以创建和管理。

9. EMEA 指欧洲药物评审组织（The European Agency for the Evaluation of Medicinal Products）。

10. Centralized Procedure 指由 EMEA 负责的这个程序，称之为 "集中程序、集中审批程序、集中注册程序"。

11. IND 是 Investigational New Drug 的缩写，指新药临床研究审批。

12. International Standards Organisation 指国际标准化组织（International Organization for Standardization），简称 ISO。它是一个全球性的非政府组织，是国际标准化领域中一个十分重要的组织。

13. American National Standards Institute 指美国国家标准学会（American National Standard Institute），缩略为 ANSI。它是美国非营利性民间标准化团体，自愿性标准体系的协调中心，成立于 1918 年，总部设在纽约，有 250 多个专业学会、协会、消费者组织以及 1 000 多个公司（包括外国公司）参加。

Exercises

1. Decide whether each of the following statements is true (T) or false (F) according to the passage.

(1) The ways in which the data were presented in those early electronic submissions should be broadly similar.

(2) The FDA developed the supporting processes to allow the electronic submission of the dossier as well as paper filings.

(3) The resolution of the life-cycle management requirements is to submit submission content more than once.

(4) The eCTD specification should employ proprietary formats.

(5) The eCTD should be created with recourse to some other tools besides the basic text editor.

(6) Reviewing tools can check and edit the content and assist in the creation of assessment reports at the agencies.

2. Questions for oral discussion.

(1) What are the differences between electronic submissions and paper submissions?

(2) What do you think of the adoption of open standards rather than proprietary formats in the eCTD specification?

(3) Why have the numbers of eCTDs been relatively low in the European Union?

(4) Is it a complete success of the eCTD implementation in the United States?

3. Choose the best answer to each of the following questions.

(1) The creation of electronic submissions aims mainly to improve the _____.

 A. accuracy   B. stability

 C. efficiency   D. technicality

(2) Which of the following is not the objective in submitting the content of a submission electronically?

 A. To provide a more efficient navigation.

 B. To provide content that can be searched and queried.

 C. To abolish the requirement of paper submitted.

 D. To allow the creation of different views of the submitted data.

(3) These early electronic submissions consisted of all the following EXCEPT _____.

 A. a set of submission files   B. the hardware

 C. the software   D. a basic text editor

(4) What's the problem global companies faced along with the growing use of electronic submissions on a global basis?

 A. The standardization took place on a regional basis.

 B. They could not benefit greatly on an international basis.

 C. The data presented conformed to the local standards.

 D. Different software applications were used by the applicants.

(5) We should use formats less _____ to the vendors.

 A. alternative   B. susceptible

 C. adaptable   D. reusable

(6) A finer document granularity means _____.

 A. a bigger document management task

 B. more internal hyperlinks

 C. more light control

 D. easier creation and management

(7) The _____ of the submission will define the way in which the applicant manages future supplements and variations.

 A. validation   B. structure

 C. life cycle   D. decision

(8) The eCTD has been fully implemented except in _____.

 A. Canada   B. the European Union

 C. the United Nations   D. Japan

(9) The EMEA resolved that the eCTD would be the mandatory format from the year of _____.

 A. 2005   B. 2008

 C. 2009   D. 2010

(10) _____ of all the 2007 submissions the FDA received contains electronic format.

    A. 8%   B. 11%

    C. 19%   D. 81%

4. Match the words with the Chinese versions.

(1) ANSI	a.	标准开发组织
(2) CANDA	b.	国际标准组织
(3) CEN	c.	人用药品技术要求国际协调理事会
(4) CTD	d.	计算机辅助新药申请
(5) EMEA	e.	监管信息传输电子标准
(6) ESTRI	f.	美国国家标准协会
(7) ICH	g.	欧洲标准组织
(8) ISO	h.	欧洲药品管理局
(9) MEB	i.	通用技术文件
(10) SDO	j.	药物评估委员会

5. Translate the following sentences into Chinese.

(1) *The electronic Common Technical Document* (eCTD) is an International Council on Harmonisation of Technical Requirements for the Registration of Pharmaceuticals for Human Use (ICH) created and maintained format for electronic submissions.

(2) The fact that the data and documents that form part of the regulatory submission were being created using electronic systems led to efforts to find a way to submit these in an electronic format rather than printing them to paper.

(3) Not all of the simplest electronic submissions will meet all of these objectives but all meet at least one of them.

(4) The other main feature of these submissions was that the ways in which the data were presented, though conforming to the dossier standards of the region, would vary because of the different software applications used by the applicants in their creation.

(5) The growing use of electronic submissions on a global basis demonstrated that the concept and the objectives behind their use were all valid.

(6) In addition to providing the specification to meet the structural and navigation requirements, the eCTD has sought to provide a standardized solution to the problem of relating submissions to each other.

(7) The four allowed values of the operation attribute are reasonably self-explanatory, but experience has shown that the use of the operation attribute is dependent crucially on the business processes and document granularity adopted by the applicant.

Value-Oriented Reflective Reading

Everything Done for Patients Should be Done with Patients

Patient engagement into the entire drug life cycle, ranging from early research and clinical trials to review and approval of new drugs, is quite important. Global experience shows that patient engagement can promote drug research and development and objectively influence government decision-making, thereby improving drug accessibility. The earlier patients participate in the process, the more their views and demands will be considered in designing clinical studies. This will help improve the quality of life of patients and clinical researches, and eventually improve the success rate of drug development. A survey by *The Economist* magazine indicates that in the second or third phase of clinical trials of all diseases, the success rate of medicine eventually hitting the market is 18% higher in patient-centered clinical trials on average than in the ordinary clinical trials.

"As we see the need for patient centricity and involvement of patients in developing new and exciting therapies, the need for patient engagement is becoming greater and greater," said James Kissell, director of Rare Cancers Australia, an organization committed to bringing affordable and equitable cancer medicines to rare cancer patients in Australia.

According to a report published by Chinese Organization for Rare Disorders (CORD), which now serves more than 50,000 families nationwide and covers over 100 different types of rare diseases, currently 90% of rare diseases globally have no corresponding treatment plans yet. Chinese patients with rare disease, who mainly depend on imported medicines, especially suffer from drug shortages. Accelerating the drug research and development for the country's 16.8 million rare disease patients is an urgent task.

CORD has and manage a large number of patients, and cooperates with scientific researchers and clinicians to do research and makes its contributions in this regard. It can also help recruit patients for clinical research projects, and advocate the government to speed up approval of drugs. In the registration and approval stage, patient organizations can appeal from the perspective of patients rather than pharmaceutical companies, which may be more acceptable to the government and the society.

Different from clinical data of research institutions, real-world data collected by patient groups from patients on their treatment feelings, life quality and economic burdens, can reflect the real scenarios of drug use. These data, translated into real-world evidence, could become the "hard core competitiveness" of patient organizations. They can be used to assist research institutions for drug development more directly, and help regulators to better understand the effectiveness of drugs. By having patient organizations involved in data generation, especially to show in real clinical settings, as to what kind of effectiveness the drug can bring to patients, we can generate data much faster and bring more valuable data to the government for decision-making.

Pharmaceutical companies aim to provide communication platforms with patient organizations, whose involvement in drug development is believed to be vital for the companies to achieve the mission of providing personalized healthcare solution for patients. It can benefit both patients and pharmaceutical companies. Everything done for patients should be done with patients.

Questions for discussion:

1. Why is patient engagement into the entire drug life cycle important to the research and development of a new drug?

2. What can organizations for patients with rare diseases do to speed up approval of a new drug?

3. What do you think the government can do to help patients with rare diseases?

Text B
Review and Approval of Drugs in China

China is the second largest drug market in the world. Registering drugs in China is more accessible today than ever. That does not mean it is easy or straightforward. Before attempting to do so, international drug companies should research the **prevalence** of the disease their specific drug treats in China to make sure it will be welcomed by the Chinese government and people, and see whether your drug has real advantages over alternative existing treatments in China.

The process of getting a new drug approved in China can be complex and time-consuming. It involves multiple stages of testing and review by regulatory agencies to ensure the drug's safety and efficacy.

In this article, we'll provide a comprehensive guide to China's drug approval process, including an overview of the regulatory agency, preclinical studies, clinical trials, NMPA review, and post-market **surveillance**.

China's Drug Regulatory Agency

The National Medical Products Administration (NMPA)[1] is China's regulatory agency responsible for the approval of drugs, medical devices, and cosmetics. The NMPA was established in 2018, merging the China Food and Drug Administration (CFDA)[2] and other related agencies. The NMPA has a significant role in ensuring the safety, efficacy, and quality of drugs sold in China. Moreover, it implements strict regulations to ensure that all drugs meet the same standards as those set by the World Health Organization (WHO). The agency establishes **stringent** safety and efficacy requirements for drug approval.

NMPA's major responsibilities include:

(1) To supervise the safety of drugs (including traditional Chinese medicines (TCMs) and **ethno-medicines**), medical devices and cosmetics; to draw up regulatory policy plans, organize the drafting of laws and regulations, formulate **normative** documents, and supervise the implementation **thereof**; to research and formulate regulatory and supportive policies that encourage new technologies and new products for drugs, medical devices and cosmetics.

(2) To undertake standards management for drugs, medical devices and cosmetics; to organize the formulation and publication of the Chinese Pharmacopoeia[3] and other drug and medical device standards, organize the drafting of cosmetic standards, organize the formulation of the classification management system, and supervise the implementation thereof; to participate in formulating the National Essential Medicine List[4], and assist in the implementation of the national essential medicine system.

(3) To regulate the registration of drugs, medical devices and cosmetics; to develop the registration system, conduct strict review and approval for marketing, improve measures to facilitate the review and approval process, and organize the implementation thereof.

(4) To undertake quality management for drugs, medical devices and cosmetics; to develop Good Laboratory Practices (GLP) and Good Clinical Practices (GCP), and supervise the implementation thereof; to develop Good Manufacturing Practices (GMP) and supervise the implementation thereof in line with NMPA's responsibilities; to develop good practices on the distribution and use of medical products and guide the implementation thereof.

(5) To undertake post-market risk management for drugs, medical devices and cosmetics; to organize

the monitoring, evaluation, and handling of adverse drug reactions, medical device adverse events, and cosmetic adverse reactions; to undertake emergency response management for drugs, medical devices and cosmetics in accordance with law.

(6) To undertake management of qualifications for <u>licensed</u> pharmacists[5]; to formulate regulations of qualifications for licensed pharmacists, and guide and supervise the registration of licensed pharmacists.

(7) To organize and guide the supervision and inspection of drugs, medical devices and cosmetics; to develop the inspection system, investigate and punish illegal activities during the registration process for drugs, medical devices and cosmetics in accordance with law, and organize and guide the investigation and punishment of illegal activities during the manufacturing process in line with NMPA's responsibilities.

(8) To engage in international exchange and cooperation in the regulation of drugs, medical devices and cosmetics, and participate in developing relevant international regulatory rules and standards.

China Drug Registration

China's National Medical Products Administration (NMPA) is the overarching government agency that approves drugs. Under the NMPA, the <u>Center for Drug Evaluation (CDE)</u>[6] does the initial review. CDE plays a critical role in the approval process for clinical trials and pharmaceuticals. A key legal framework that governs various aspects of drug-related activities is the <u>Drug Administration Law of the People's Republic of China</u>[7], which encompasses drug development, registration, manufacturing, and the marketing of drugs.

Drugs are classified in China as-1. Small molecule drugs, 2. Traditional Chinese Medicine, or 3.Therapeutic Biologics. Each class has sub-categories to further designate classification and registration paths.

To submit a drug application in China, you need a <u>Marketing Authorization Holder (MAH)</u>[8]. For drugs made overseas, the Chinese MAH is usually the foreign drug manufacturer; for drugs made in China, the MAH is normally a domestic Chinese drug company.

Preclinical Studies

Before a new drug can be tested in humans, it must undergo preclinical studies to evaluate its safety and efficacy. In China, preclinical studies must be conducted in compliance with Good Laboratory Practice (GLP) guidelines. These studies include pharmacological and toxicological testing and are required for the new drug application process in China.

Pharmacological testing involves studying the drug's mechanism of action and its effects on biological systems. Toxicological testing involves evaluating the drug's potential toxicity to living organisms. The results of these studies are included in the new drug application package submitted to the NMPA.

Clinical Trials

Clinical trials are conducted to evaluate the safety and efficacy of the new drug in humans. In China, the clinical trial process consists of three phases.

(1) Phase 1 involves a small group of healthy volunteers to evaluate the drug's safety and dosing.

(2) Phase 2 includes a larger group of patients to evaluate the drug's efficacy and side effects.

(3) Phase 3 involves a larger patient population to confirm the drug's efficacy and monitor any adverse events.

The clinical trial data must be submitted to the NMPA in the new drug application (NDA) package. The data must follow Good Clinical Practice (GCP) guidelines and include detailed information on the trial design, patient **demographics**, adverse events, and efficacy outcomes.

Foreign drug companies can utilize three main strategies when doing clinical trials for China drug registration. First, you can do China trials simultaneously with your other global clinical trials. This is the fastest and cheapest way to proceed in China since you will be able to **leverage** overseas clinical data and reduce the number of patients in your local China clinical study. Second, foreign drug companies that have already completed their clinical trials in the West, can do an Asian multi-regional clinical study including about 50% of the patients from China. While this is more expensive than the first option above, more and more companies are choosing this strategy for their China/Asian drug development. Finally, as has been the main strategy in the past, foreign drug companies that have already completed their clinical trials in the West and received drug approval, can do a **standalone** Phase 3 study in China. This will be the most expensive way to proceed and delay the **submittal** of a registration application in China.

China has improved its clinical trial requirements in a number of ways over the last five years. First, it only takes 60 days to get a clinical trial application (CTA) approved. Second, imported drugs do not need to be approved overseas or complete Phase 2 studies, in advance of starting their China clinical trial. Third, more foreign clinical data is being accepted in China, especially if ethnic differences can be accounted for. There are also other changes that have made the clinical trial process easier for foreign drug companies.

NMPA Review

The NMPA review process is a critical step in the drug approval process in China. The process consists of three stages, each of which plays an important role in ensuring the safety and efficacy of drugs sold in China. Here are the three stages of the NMPA review process:

1. Technical Review

The technical review is the first stage of the NMPA review process.

In this process, they evaluate the new drug application package submitted by the drug manufacturer to ensure it meets all regulatory requirements. This can be checking that the preclinical data and clinical trial data meet the required standards, and that the drug's manufacturing process meets Good Manufacturing Practice (GMP) guidelines.

If the application package meets all regulatory requirements, the NMPA will proceed to the next stage of the review process. If there are any issues with the application package, the NMPA will request additional information or clarification from the drug manufacturer.

2. Onsite Inspection

During this stage, the NMPA conducts an inspection of the drug manufacturing facility to ensure compliance with GMP guidelines. The inspection involves a review of the manufacturing process, quality control systems, and documentation procedures.

The NMPA may also inspect the clinical trial sites to ensure compliance with Good Clinical Practice (GCP) guidelines.

If the onsite inspection identifies any issues, the NMPA will request **corrective** action from the drug manufacturer. The drug manufacturer must address any issues identified during the onsite inspection before the NMPA can proceed to the final stage of the review process.

3. Expert Review

Next, a panel of experts evaluates the data submitted in the new drug application package. The panel includes experts in pharmacology, toxicology, clinical medicine, statistics, and drug regulatory affairs.

The expert review evaluates the safety, efficacy, and quality of the drug, as well as the manufacturing process. The experts may request additional information or clarification from the drug manufacturer before making a final decision on the drug's approval.

If the expert review identifies any issues, the drug manufacturer must address them before the drug can be approved for sale in China.

The NMPA considers multiple factors in its review process, including the drug's safety, efficacy, quality, and manufacturing process. The length of the NMPA review process can vary, but it typically takes around 1–2 years for a new drug to be approved in China.

Post-Market Surveillance[9]

Once a drug is approved for sale in China, the NMPA requires post-market surveillance to monitor the drug's safety and efficacy. The drug manufacturer is required to submit **periodic** safety reports and conduct ongoing monitoring of adverse events. The NMPA may also conduct inspections of the drug manufacturing facility to ensure compliance with GMP guidelines.

China's drug approval can be a challenging but necessary process for pharmaceutical companies seeking to develop and market drugs in China. The NMPA plays a crucial role in ensuring the safety and efficacy of drugs sold in China, and pharmaceutical companies must adhere to strict regulatory guidelines throughout the drug development and post-approval processes.

As China continues to develop its healthcare system, we can expect to see further developments in the drug approval process aimed at improving the efficiency of drug approval while maintaining high safety and efficacy standards.

Word Study

1. corrective [kəˈrektɪv] *adj.* 纠正的，矫正的
2. demographics [ˌdeməˈɡræfɪks] *n.* 人口统计资料，人口统计学
3. ethno-medicine [ˈeθnə ˈmedɪsn] *n.* 民族药
4. leverage [ˈliːvərɪdʒ] *v.* 充分利用
5. license [ˈlaɪs(ə)ns] *v.* 许可，特许
6. normative [ˈnɔːmətɪv] *adj.* 规范的，标准的
7. periodic [ˌpɪəriˈɒdɪk] *adj.* 周期的，定期的
8. prevalence [ˈprevələns] *n.* 流行，盛行
9. standalone [ˈstændəˌləʊn] *n.* 独立运行
10. stringent [ˈstrɪndʒənt] *adj.* 严格的，严厉的
11. submittal [səbˈmɪtl] *n.* 提交，服从
12. surveillance [sɜːˈveɪləns] *n.* 监测，监视
13. thereof [ˌðeərˈɒv] *adv.* 在其中，由此

Notes

1. National Medical Products Administration (NMPA)：（中国）国家药品监督管理局（https://www.

nmpa.gov.cn/）

2. China Food and Drug Administration (CFDA)：（中国）国家食品药品监督管理总局（2018 年更名为 National Medical Products Administration，NMPA，国家药品监督管理局）。

3. Chinese Pharmacopoeia：全称为 Pharmacopoeia of the People's Republic of China（《中华人民共和国药典》），简称 Chinese Pharmacopoeia（ChP）。最新版为 2020 年版，由一部、二部、三部和四部构成，收载品种共计 5 911 种。一部中药收载 2 711 种；二部化学药收载 2 712 种；三部生物制品收载 153 种；四部收载通用技术要求 361 个，其中制剂通则 38 个、检测方法及其他通则 281 个、指导原则 42 个；药用辅料收载 335 种。

4. National Essential Medicine List：（中国）国家基本药物目录（是医疗机构配备使用药品的依据，包括两部分：基层医疗卫生机构配备使用部分和其他医疗机构配备使用部分。基本药物目录中的药品是适应基本医疗卫生需求，剂型适宜，价格合理，能够保障供应，公众可公平获得的药品，中国自 2009 年 9 月 21 日起施行国家基本药物目录。）

5. licensed pharmacist：执业药师（指经全国统一考试合格，取得《中华人民共和国执业药师职业资格证书》并经注册，在药品生产、经营、使用和其他需要提供药学服务的单位中执业的药学技术人员。）

6. Center for Drug Evaluation (CDE)：（中国）国家药品审评中心，为 NMPA 直属单位，完整名称为 Center for Drug Evaluation，NMPA（国家药品监督管理局药品审评中心）。

7. Drug Administration Law of the People's Republic of China：中华人民共和国药品管理法（是为了加强药品管理，保证药品质量，保障公众用药安全和合法权益，保护和促进公众健康而制定的法律。1984 年 9 月 20 日第六届全国人民代表大会常务委员会第七次会议通过，自 1985 年 7 月 1 日起施行。2019 年 8 月 26 日，新修订的《中华人民共和国药品管理法》经十三届全国人大常委会第十二次会议表决通过，于 2019 年 12 月 1 日起施行。）

8. Marketing Authorization Holder (MAH)：药品上市许可人制度（是指将上市许可与生产许可分离的管理模式。这种机制下，上市许可和生产许可相互独立，上市许可持有人可以将产品委托给不同的生产商生产，药品的安全性、有效性和质量可控性均由上市许可人对公众负责。）

9. post-market surveillance：药品上市后监测。

Supplementary Parts

1. Medical and Pharmaceutical Terminology (13): Common Morphemes in English Terms for Chemistry

Morpheme	Meaning	Example
chem	化学	biochemistry　生物化学
chrom	铬	chromic　铬的
bar	钡	barium　钡
arg	银	argentaffin　嗜银的
kal	钾	hyperkalemia　高钾血症
natr	钠	hypernatremia　高钠血症
magnes	镁	magnesium　镁
sider	铁	sideropenia　铁（质）缺乏
ferr	铁	ferrated　含铁的
ferro	（二价）铁	ferrous　亚铁的，二价铁的
ferri	（三价）铁	ferric　高铁的，三价铁的
calc	钙	calcium　钙

续表

Morpheme	Meaning	Example
mercur	汞	mercury 汞,水银
bor	硼	borax 硼砂,硼酸钠
silic	硅	silicon 硅
thi	硫	thiacetazone 氨硫脲
sulf	硫	sulfur 硫
carb	碳	carbon 碳
arsen	砷	arsenic 砷
iod	碘	iodide 碘化物
bromo	溴	bromide 溴化物
hal	卤素	halide 卤化物
fluor	氟	fluorine 氟
hydr	氢	hydrogen 氢
oxy	氧	oxygen 氧
oxid	氧	oxidant 氧化剂
deoxy	脱氧	deoxycytidylic acid 脱氧胞苷酸
desoxy	脱氧	desoxymorphine 脱氧吗啡
chlor	氯	chlorine 氯
nitr	氮,硝基	nitrogen 氮
amin	氨	amine 胺
ammon	氨	ammonia 氨
cyan	氰	cyanide 氰化物
anthrac	炭	anthracosis 炭末沉着病,炭肺
hydr	水	hydragogue 水泻剂
meth	甲基	methane 甲烷,沼气
methyl	甲基	methyl 甲基
ethyl	乙基	ethyl 乙基,乙烷基
acet	乙基	acetaldehyde 乙醛
acyl	酰基	acylase 酰化酶
acetyl	乙酰基	acetylcholine 乙酰胆碱
amyl	戊基	amyl 戊基
phen	苯基	phenacetin 乙酰对氨苯乙醚(非那西汀)
phenyl	苯基	phenylalanine 苯丙氨酸
benzyl	苯甲基,苄基	benzyl 苄基,苯甲基
alkyl	烷基	alkylation 烷化
keto	酮基	ketogenesis 生酮作用
aceton	丙酮基	acetonuria 丙酮尿
phenol	酚基	phentolamine 酚妥拉明
hydroxy	羟基	hydroxyamphetamine 羟苯丙胺
carboxyl	羧基	carboxylase 羧化酶
prote	蛋白质	protease 蛋白酶
globulin	球蛋白	globulinuria 球蛋白尿
hemoglobin	血红蛋白	hemoglobinopathy 血红蛋白病
fibrin	纤维蛋白	fibrinogen 纤维蛋白原
pept	肽	dipeptide 二肽

续表

Morpheme	Meaning	Example
zym	酶	zymogen 酶原
glyc	糖	glycogen 糖原
sacchar	糖	saccharide 糖类,糖化物
carbohydro	糖	carbohydrate 碳水化合物,糖类
gluc	葡萄糖	glucagon （胰）高血糖素
fruct	果糖	fructosuria 果糖尿
rib	核糖	ribosome 核糖体
amyl	淀粉	amyloid 淀粉样的
lip	脂肪	lipid 脂类,油脂
adip	脂肪	adipose 脂肪的
glycer	甘油	glycerin 甘油,丙三醇
salicyl	水杨酸	salicylic acid 水杨酸
phosph	磷酸	phosphagen 磷酸肌酸
chlorhydr	盐酸	chlorhydric acid 盐酸,氢氯酸
hydrochlor	盐酸	hydrochloric acid 盐酸,氢氯酸
glycin	甘氨酸	glycinate 甘氨酸盐
uric	尿酸	uricacidemia 尿酸血症
bas	碱	basophil 嗜碱性粒细胞
alkal	碱	alkali 碱,强碱
ald	醛	aldehyde 醛
formal	甲醛	formalin 甲醛,福尔马林
sorb	山梨醇	sorbitol 山梨醇
sulf	磺胺	sulfonamide 磺胺
cyt	胞苷	cytidine 胞苷
quin	喹啉	quinine 奎宁
quinon	醌	quinone 醌,苯醌
erg	麦角	ergometrine 麦角新碱
pyrazin	吡嗪	pyrazinamide 吡嗪酰胺
pyrazon	唑酮	sulfinpyrazone 磺吡酮
pyrim	嘧啶	pyrimidine 嘧啶
uracil	尿嘧啶	fluorouracil 氟尿嘧啶
uridine	尿苷	floxuridine 氟尿苷
lys	分解	lysin 溶素,溶解素
solv,solut	分解,溶解	solution 解决,溶液,溶解
tox	毒	toxemia 毒血症
coll	胶体	colloid 胶体,胶质
gel	凝胶	gelatin 明胶

(1) Fill in the blanks with the missing word root, prefix or suffix.

1) hyper_____mia 高钠血症

2) _____ated 含铁的

3) _____ium 钙

4) _____ide 碘化物

5) _____ant 氧化剂

6) _____osis 炭末沉着病

7) _____agogue 水泻剂

8) _____ation 烷化

9) _____genesis 生酮作用

10) _____acidemia 尿酸血症

11) _____ophil 嗜碱性粒细胞

12) _____metrine 麦角新碱

(2) Word-matching.

1) chromic	A. 嘧啶
2) silicon	B. 奎宁
3) mercury	C. 苄基
4) methyl	D. 蛋白酶
5) pyrimidine	E. 甲醛
6) formalin	F. 铬的
7) quinine	G. 汞,水银
8) magnesium	H. 甲基
9) protease	I. 戊基
10) benzyl	J. 甲烷,沼气
11) methane	K. 镁
12) amyl	L. 硅

2. English-Chinese Translation Skills: 药学英语翻译技巧 (9): 名词性从句翻译

英语中名词性从句包括主语从句、表语从句、宾语从句、同位语从句等,由于汉语句子结构相对松散,这类名词性从句在汉语中一般没有固定格式。名词性从句大量使用在药学英语语篇中。翻译名词性从句本身没有什么特别之处,最重要的是要考虑这类从句在复合句中的位置。在英译汉过程中,大多数语序可以不变,即可按原文顺序翻译,但有时也需要一些其他处理方法。

例 1: The FD&C Act stipulates that an article may differ in strength, quality, or purity and still have the same name if the difference is stated on the article's label.

参考译文:《食品、药品及化妆品法案》规定品种在规格、质量或者纯度方面可以有不同,而且只要在品种标签上注明可以用同样的名称。

说明:例句中谓语动词 stipulate 后面有一个 that 引导的宾语从句,翻译这类句子时,只需要按照正常顺序表述即可。

例 2: What was stated above obviously indicates that pharmacy service quality is in urgent need of improving.

参考译文:上述内容明显地表明了药学监护质量亟待提高。

说明:例句中 what stated above 是一个主语从句,译文没有调整原句子顺序,采用顺译法翻译,很好地表达了英语原句意思,也符合汉语表达习惯。但有时候名词性从句在翻译过程中需要调整顺序。如下。

例 3: This is supported by the fact that secondary metabolites are often unique to a particular species or group of organisms and, while many act as antifeedants, sex attractants, or antibiotic agents, many have no apparent biological role. It is likely that all these concepts can play some part in understanding the production of the broad group of compounds that come under the heading of secondary metabolite.

参考译文：事实表明次级代谢产物通常对特殊物种或某些有机体是独一无二的，有一些常用作拒食剂、性引诱剂、抗生素等，还有很多并没有明显的生物作用。这些概念很有可能在理解次级代谢旺盛期大量各种化合物的产生方面起重要作用。

说明：上面例句有两个名词性从句。一个是在 fact 后面 that 引导的同位语从句，另一个构成英语中的特殊结构：It is likely that+ 从句。译文在处理这两个名词性从句时没有简单教条地按照英语结构形式来表达，而是跳出英语原来的结构，将原句意思用流畅得体的汉语结构表述出来。第一句的主要结构是 This is supported by the fact that...，为了意义表达需要译文将主句 This is supported by the fact 省略，直接将名词性从句独立成句，语言简洁流畅。第二句是英语中特有的句子结构，汉语中没有。译文直接按照汉语表达结构译成："很有可能……"，通顺自然。翻译这类套用英语固定结构的名词性从句时，可以直接使用对应的汉语表达结构，再如下。

例 4：It is worth bearing in mind that the relationship between the degrees of purity achieved in a natural product extraction, and the amount of work required to achieve this, is very approximately exponential.

参考译文：值得记住的是，天然产物提取过程中要达到的纯度和所需要工作量之间接近于指数关系。

说明：例句也是英语中一个句型：It is worth *v*-ing that+ 名词性从句，翻译这样句子可以直接采用汉语表达结构："值得……是……"。同样是类似句型，在翻译过程中有时候需要适当添加一些成分，如下。

例 5：It is also probably true to say that this exponential relationship also often holds for the degree of purity achieved versus the yield of natural product.

参考译文：我们或许真的可以说所得到的纯度与天然产物的产量之间也是指数关系。

翻译名词性从句本身没有特别技巧，只要正确理解并表述从句意义即可，但是名词性从句往往都跟英语特定句型连在一起使用，故处理好名词性从句与句型之间的位置关系显得更加重要。

（史志祥　张朝慧　赵　岩　龚长华　陈　菁）

Unit Fourteen

Drug Instructions

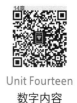

If you don't feel well, probably you will go to a hospital. When you get the prescription filled in the pharmacy, the pharmacist usually gives you some additional written information, or you may receive a very detailed "package insert" filled with information provided by the drug manufacturer and approved by the National Medical Products Administration (NMPA). Such package inserts are available for all prescription medications approved by the NMPA. Similar information is available for nonprescription medicines and for some herbal medicines and dietary supplements as well. The package insert is a good source of information to be used in addition to instructions your doctor or nurse may have given you. It's a good idea to review the package insert for any new medicine and to look at it again if anything about your health changes after taking the medicine. If it raises any questions in your mind, contact your doctor or nurse for an explanation.

The package insert follows a standard format for every medication, and written in technical language. After the brand name, chemical name and molecular formula of the product, the following sections appear: Description, Microbiology and Clinical Pharmacology, Indications and Usage, Contraindications, Warnings, Precautions, Adverse Reactions, Overdosage, Dosage and Administration, Pregnancy and Lactation, Interaction with other Drugs, Pharmacological and Toxicological Properties, Storage, Package, and Shelf Life etc.

如果你不舒服,你可能就会去医院看病。在药房用处方取药的时候,药师一般也会给你一些书面的用药信息,或者你会拿到一个详细的"药品说明书",上面有药厂提供的经过国家药品监督管理局(NMPA)批准的内容。NMPA批准的所有处方药都附有药品说明书。非处方药、一些草药和膳食补充剂也有类似的说明书。除了医生或者护士给你的用药指导以外,药品说明书也是一个很好的用药信息来源。使用任何新药都要仔细阅读说明书,如果用药后身体状况发生了变化要及时再看看说明书。如果有什么疑惑,要询问医生或者护士。

药品说明书都遵循一个标准格式,并且用专业术语撰写。在介绍商品名、化学名和分子式之后,说明书还包括其他信息,如:性状、微生物学和临床药理、适应证和用法、禁忌证、警告、注意事项、不良反应、药物过量、用法用量、孕妇及哺乳期妇女用药、药物相互作用、药理毒理、贮藏、包装和有效期等。

Text A
The New Drug Package Insert—Implications for Patient Safety

The package insert contains detailed drug information compiled and distributed by the drug manufacturer after the FDA's review and approval. The purpose of the package insert is to provide complete and **unbiased** prescribing and safety information to health professionals. In 1968, a two line warning placed on the **isoproterenol inhaler** package is considered as the first patient package insert. Although in 1970 the FDA **mandated** that a separate patient package insert detailing risks and benefits accompany each package of birth control pills, it was not until 1979 that the FDA **promulgated** the content and format of physician prescribing information inserts (also known as the package insert).[1] Within the "Warnings" section of this document, the term "boxed warning" (black box warning) was used for the first time in the FDA labeling requirements. Since then, the volume and detail of the package insert had increased significantly. In the 1980s, the FDA acknowledged that the information included in the package insert had become so lengthy, detailed, and complex that it was difficult for health practitioners to find specific information and to distinguish critical information from less important issues.

To address the problem, the FDA conducted a research to assess how prescription drug labeling was used by health care practitioners, and to determine which labeling information was considered the most important. The studies documented that many practitioners usually find the information they need, but that the process was often time-intensive and clinically inefficient. In addition, the package insert format **disproportionately** stressed the occurrence of extremely rare clinical events. As a result, the FDA developed a new package insert format that had three major sections: ①"The Highlights of Prescribing Information"; ②"Full Prescribing Information Table of Contents"; and ③"The Full Prescribing Information" (FPI). This new organization of information improved access to critical information and made the label more user-friendly. The new label format proposal was issued in December 2000 and, after public meetings and comment by practitioners, a final version became official in June 2006. A transition to the new format will not be mandatory for drugs that received the FDA's approval more than 5 years before the final ruling in June 2006. However, pharmaceutical companies may elect to **reformat** the package insert for these older drugs. Drugs approved within the 5-year window must resubmit the package insert in the revised label format during a 3-7-year phase-in period to comply with the new FDA standards. Here list some sections selected in the new drug package insert.

1. Highlights of Prescribing Information

Most of the information included in the "Highlights of Prescribing Information" section communicates risks or warning information. A **succinct** summary of critical clinical information is presented in a bulleted format that is **cross-referenced** to the FPI section for more in-depth explanation. The organization of the section reflects the priorities and most common patterns of product insert usage as expressed by practitioners during the FDA reformatting studies.

2. Black Box Warning

The black box warning is set apart as the most prominent information included in a product insert. Any warning **elevated** to the status of a black box warning must be bolded (only the heading must be in all capitals, not the text of the warning) and "boxed" by a solid black line on all four sides. A black box warning is indicated in the following three situations, but may be used in other situations to **highlight** warning information that is particularly important to the prescriber:

(1) There is an adverse reaction so serious in proportion to the potential benefit from the drug that it is essential that it be considered in assessing the risks and benefits of using the drug.[2] This includes potentially life threatening or permanently disabling adverse reactions.

(2) There is a serious reaction that can be prevented or reduced in frequency or **severity** by patient

selection, careful monitoring, avoiding certain concomitant therapy, addition of another drug or managing patient in a specific manner, or avoiding use in a specific clinical situation.

(3) The FDA has approved the drug with restrictions on use and distribution to assure safe use.

A black box warning has implications for the manufacturer, health care provider, and patients. Manufacturer implications include a restriction on the degree of advertising, a potentially negative impact on sales, a decreased use of the drug, and an increased risk of litigation. From the provider's and patients' perspective, the substitution of a drug without a black box warning may actually entail greater expense and exposure to another set of side effects than the use of the drug with a black box warning. Further, in the absence of patients' awareness of the potential dangers of a drug, when untoward events are precipitated by the drug, there is also an increased risk of litigation.

3. Recent Major Changes, Indications and Usage, Dosage and Administration, Dosage Forms and Strengths

The "Recent Major Changes" section lists only major changes in the boxed warning, indications and usage, dosage and administration, contraindications and warnings, and precautions sections. The three sections following Recent Major Changes are practical information giving indications and usage, dosage and administration, and dosage forms and strengths. These informational sections placed after the most serious warning issues have been identified to facilitate practical use of the label, whose major purpose is to provide dosage information for routine use.

The sections following the routine use information are warning or risk information of high importance. These sections include contraindications, warnings and precautions, adverse reactions, drug interactions, and use in specific populations.

4. Contraindications

A drug is classified as contraindicated in the clinical situation for which the risks outweigh any possible therapeutic benefit of the drug. Only known hazards, and not theoretical possibilities, can be listed. If there are no known contraindications for a drug, "none" must be designated in this section. The order in which the contraindications are presented in the text reflects the relative public health risk. The significance of the contraindications is based on the likelihood of occurrence and the size of the population potentially affected.

5. Warnings and Precautions

When an adverse reaction is considered clinically significant, or when the reaction risk is serious, it will be included in the "Warning and Precautions" section. There must be reasonable evidence of a causal relationship between the drug and the reaction. The order of the list of adverse reactions (ADRs) reflects their relative public health significance. The relative seriousness of the reaction and the ability to prevent or mitigate its occurrence are prioritized in this section. A description of the reaction and outcome, including time to resolution, significant sequelae, estimated risk of ADRs, and discussion of any known risk factors for the reaction, are required. Treatment or management strategies for the ADRs and discussion of any possible steps to reduce the risk, shorten the duration, or minimize the severity of a reaction are included in this section.

Observed ADRs and expected ADRs are included in the Warnings and Precautions section. Observed

ADRs are those events that have been observed in association with the use of the drug and that are serious or are otherwise clinically significant. "Clinically significant" means that the ADRs may require:

- adjustment of the drug dosage or **regimen**.
- discontinuation of the drug.
- supplement treatment with an additional drug.
- appropriate patient selection to avoid the ADRs.
- avoidance of **concomitant** therapy which triggers the ADRs.
- evaluation of the patient for medication compliance.
- use of alternative laboratory tests.

Expected ADRs are events that can be anticipated to occur with a drug, based on observations from other members of the drug class or animal studies. Expected ADRs are appropriate for warnings and precautions if the reaction is clinically serious, indicating that it could have an outcome of death, life-threatening illness, or require hospitalization to treat.

6. Drug Interactions

The "Drug Interactions" section includes concise information about the potential for interaction with other drugs or foods. These include both **pharmacokinetic** (e.g., food effects, **enzyme** induction and **inhibition**) and **pharmacodynamic** effects (e.g., **meperidine** with **monoamine oxidase** inhibitors).

7. Use in Specific Populations

This section on "Use in Specific Populations" lists clinically significant or important differences in patient response or the use of a drug in specific populations of patients.

8. FPI Contents

The purpose of the table of contents is to reference all the sections and subsections included in the FPI, some of which will not be cross-referenced in the Highlights. The Highlights contains cross-references to the FPI, which contains the full explanatory text for the bulleted summaries and is easily accessed by practitioners to encourage its use and discourage use of the Highlights section as the sole source of information. The sections of the FPI coincide with the order of the sections covered in the Highlights section. Also, similar to the Highlights, the most crucial dosing and warning sections are at the beginning of the FPI text. The sections dealing with risk information are grouped together. The informational sections not dealing with risk are grouped collectively. Additional sections in this part of the package insert include drug abuse and dependence, over-dosage, description, clinical pharmacology, non-clinical toxicology, clinical studies, references, how supplied/storage and handling, and patient counseling information.

Hospital-based medication errors and preventable adverse drug reactions occur at a rate of 400,000 per year according to a recent Institute of Medicine (IOM) study. These errors are reported to translate into an annual cost of $3.5 billion in extra hospital expense. The new format changes the landscape of drug information, and the FDA has expressed the hope that these changes would increase effective use of prescription of drugs and decrease medication errors.

Word Study

1.　concomitant [kən'kɒmɪtənt] *adj.* (*formal*) 相伴的，相随的

2. contraindication [ˌkɒntrəˌɪndəˈkeɪʃn] *n.*（医）禁忌证，禁忌证候

3. cross-referenced [ˈkrɔːsˈrefrənst] *adj.* 互相参照的，交叉引用的

4. designate [ˈdezɪgneɪt] *v.* 指定，标明，表示

5. disproportionately [ˌdɪsprəˈpɔːʃənətli] *adv.* 不成比例地

6. elevate [ˈelɪveɪt] *v.* 提高，提升

7. entail [ɪnˈteɪl] *v.* (*formal*) 使成为必要，导致

8. enzyme [ˈenzaɪm] *n.* 酶

9. highlight [ˈhaɪlaɪt] *n.* 最重要的细节或事件；*v.* 强调，使……突出

10. indication [ˌɪndɪˈkeɪʃn] *n.* 适应证

11. inhaler [ɪnˈheɪlə(r)] *n.* 吸入器

12. inhibition [ˌɪnhɪˈbɪʃn] *n.* 抑制，阻止

13. isoproterenol [aɪsoʊprəˈterənɒl] *n.* 异丙肾上腺素

14. litigation [ˌlɪtɪˈgeɪʃn] *n.* 诉讼，起诉

15. mandate [ˈmændeɪt] *v.* (*formal*) 命令，规定，颁布（法律）

16. meperidine [meˈperədiːn] *n.* 哌替啶，杜冷丁

17. mitigate [ˈmɪtɪgeɪt] *v.* (*formal*) 减轻，缓和

18. monoamine [ˌmɒnoʊˈeimiːn] *n.* 单胺

19. oxidase [ˈɒksɪdeɪs] *n.* 氧化酶

20. pharmacodynamic [fɑːməkoʊdaɪˈnæmɪk] *adj.* 药物效应动力学的，药效学的

21. pharmacokinetic [ˌfɑːməkoʊkɪˈnetɪk] *adj.* 药物代谢动力学的，药动学的

22. precipitate [prɪˈsɪpɪteɪt] *v.* (*formal*) 使（尤指坏事）发生，促成

23. promulgate [ˈprɒm(ə)lgeɪt] *v.* (*formal*) 发布，颁布，传播（观点等）

24. reformat [ˌriːˈfɔːmæt] *v.* 重新制定格式

25. regimen [ˈredʒɪmən] *n.* 养身之道，疗程，方案

26. sequelae [sɪˈkwiːliː] (*pl.*) *n.* 后遗症 (*sig.*) sequela [sɪˈkwiːlə]

27. severity [sɪˈverəti] *n.* 严重，严重性

28. succinct [səkˈsɪŋkt] *adj.* (*formal*) 言简意赅的，简明的

29. unbiased [ʌnˈbaɪəst] *adj.* 公正的

Notes

1. 在 "Although in 1970 the FDA mandated that a separate patient package insert detailing risk and benefits accompany each package of birth control pills, it was not until 1979 that the FDA promulgated the content and format of physician prescribing information inserts (also known as the package insert)." 句中，"although" 引导让步状语从句，动词 "mandate" 表示命令，后续从句中动词 "accompany" 前面省略了 "should"。

2. 在理解 "There is an adverse reaction so serious in proportion to the potential benefit from the drug that it is essential that it be considered in assessing the risks and benefits of using the drug." 这个句子的结构时，首先要知道，这个句子的主要结构是：There is an adverse reaction. 后面的 "so serious in proportion to the potential benefit from the drug that it is..." 都是做定语修饰 "an adverse reaction"。另外，在理解这个很长的定语部分时，要注意 3 个问题：①构成 "so...that..." 结构的是第一个 "that"，表示 "如此……以至于……"；②这个 "that" 引导的结果状语从句是一个句型：it is essential that it be considered in assessing the risks and benefits of using the drug，在这个句型中，第一个 "it"

是形式主语,真正的主语是后面 "that it be considered in assessing the risks and benefits of using the drug." 在这个主语中, "it" 代表的是前面的 "an adverse reaction"; ③在 "...that it be considered..." 的 "be" 前面,省略了 "should"。

Exercises

1. Decide whether each of the following statements is true (T) or false (F) according to the passage.

(1) In the 1980s, health practitioners found it easy to get specific information and to distinguish critical information from less important issues in the package insert.

(2) As far as the function of the package insert is concerned, the FDA finds that it is usually time-intensive and clinically inefficient for many practitioners to get the information they need, because the package insert format disproportionately stressed the occurrence of extremely rare clinical events.

(3) For the drugs that received the FDA's approval more than 5 years before the final ruling in June 2006, the pharmaceutical companies may elect either to continue the old format of the package insert or to reformat it.

(4) The "Recent Major Changes" section lists only major changes in the boxed warning, indications and usage, dosage and administration, contraindications and warnings, and precautions sections.

(5) The FPI contains cross-references to the Highlights, which contains the full explanatory text for the bulleted summaries and is easily accessed by practitioners to encourage its use and discourage use of the Highlights section as the sole source of information.

(6) In the FPI text, both the sections dealing with risk information and the sections not dealing with risk are grouped, but separately. But clinical pharmacology and patient counseling information are not included in this section.

2. Questions for oral discussion.

(1) What is "Black Box Warning"? In what situation should it be indicated?

(2) Are length, detail and complexity the criteria to judge a package insert? How do you comment on a package insert?

(3) What is included in "Highlights of Prescribing Information"?

(4) What are observed ADRs and expected ADRs in a package insert?

3. Choose the best answer to each of the following questions.

(1) Which of the following statements is true according to the passage?

A. The first package insert appeared in 1968, with a detailed warning placed on the isoproterenol inhaler package.

B. Since a separated package insert is required by the FDA, the package insert has become more lengthy and detailed.

C. "Boxed warning" is a summary of "Warnings" section, providing concise information about adverse reactions.

D. The package insert is compiled and distributed by drug manufacturers, providing detailed drug information to health practitioners.

(2) Why did FDA decide to reformat package insert in the 1980s?

A. Because the information the health professionals need in package insert is not accessible.

B. Because "Boxed warning" was not included in the package insert.

C. Because the occurrence of rare clinical events is not given enough stress in the package insert.

D. None of the above.

(3) According to the passage, the new format of a package insert issued by the FDA in 2000 _____.

　　A. was mandatory for all previously approved drugs

　　B. was more convenient for the users to get access to the critical information

　　C. excluded the information of less important clinical events

　　D. became less lengthy, detailed and complex

(4) Which of the following statements is true according to the passage?

　　A. The Highlights of Prescribing Information section contains the most prominent risk and warning information in detail.

　　B. Warning information can be found in both Black Box Warning section and Highlights of Prescribing Information section.

　　C. Some prescribers find that Black Box Warning can help them to avoid the risk of being accused.

　　D. The information in Black Box Warning is the most important in a package insert.

(5) Which of the following is NOT a possible influence of Black Box Warning?

　　A. The drug sale is negatively affected.

　　B. The degree of drug advertising is restricted.

　　C. Health practitioners may face less lawsuits.

　　D. A drug without a black box warning should be used as a substitution.

(6) Which of the following statements is right according to the passage?

　　A. Both known dangers and theoretical possibilities should be listed in "Contraindications".

　　B. Adverse reaction is usually included in Highlights of Prescribing Information section.

　　C. There is a relationship between the significance of the contraindications and the likelihood of occurrence and the size of population affected.

　　D. That there are no known contraindications for a drug means therapeutic benefits outweigh risks.

(7) In a drug insert, pharmacokinetic effects are included in _____ section.

　　A. Drug Interaction　　　　　　　　B. FPI Contents

　　C. Contraindications　　　　　　　　D. Recent Major Changes

(8) Some information in FPI Contents section is cross-referenced in _____ section.

　　A. Black Box Warning　　　　　　　B. Highlights of Prescribing Information

　　C. Contraindications　　　　　　　　D. Warnings and Precautions

(9) When an ADR requires adjusting drug dosage or regimen, discontinuing the drug and evaluating the patient for medication compliance, it means that the ADR associated with the drug use is _____.

　　A. clinically insignificant　　　　　　B. clinically insufficient

　　C. clinically significant　　　　　　　D. clinically sufficient

(10) Which of the following statements is right according to the passage?

　　A. Most hospital-based medication errors are due to the insufficient information in package insert.

　　B. The new package insert format has decreased $3.5 billion in hospital expenses.

　　C. Expected ADRs refer to the events that are anticipated to occur since they have been observed previously with a drug of similar class.

　　D. The FDA's purpose of developing a new package insert format is to provide more information to health care professionals.

4.　Fill in the blanks of the following incomplete sentences with the words given.

(1) _____ (Concomitant/Sequential) therapy involves the use of two or more drugs at the same time for

therapeutic purposes.

(2) In some countries or regions, the local pharmacy is the most common place for a patient to _____ (order/fill) a prescription.

(3) Many viral infections _____ (relieve /resolve) on their own without treatment.

(4) Ibuprofen tablet is _____ (indicated/labeled) for relief of the signs and symptoms of rheumatoid arthritis and osteoarthritis.

(5) Poor patient _____ (compliance/conformity) with drug dosing regimens can be a major problem to effective treatments.

(6) But infection with H. pylori alone does not lead to stomach cancer; other factors, like genetic _____ (susceptibility/sensibility) of the stomach, are also necessary for the condition to develop.

(7) Annual worldwide deaths from asthma have been estimated at 250,000, but the _____ (mortality/morbidity)does not appear to correlate well with prevalence.

(8) The SARS did great harm to them physically and mentally. Most of them have kinds of _____ (consequence/sequelae), like lung disease, especially the mental maladjustment, caused by people's discrimination

(9) Although this diet is not physically harmful, and can be helpful in reducing the weight in some instances, it's generally not wise to adopt this _____ (regimen/recipe).

(10) Pharmaceutical _____ (excess/excipient) is the important part of pharmaceutical preparations. It plays a key role in the improvements of the performance of drug form, bioavailability and reducing the side effect.

5. Translate the following sentences and paragraphs into Chinese.

(1) In 1968, a two line warning placed on the isoproterenol inhaler package is considered as the first patient package insert.

(2) There is an adverse reaction so serious in proportion to the potential benefit from the drug that it is essential that it be considered in assessing the risks and benefits of using the drug.

(3) The studies conducted by the FDA documented that many practitioners usually find the information they need, but that the process was often time-intensive and clinically inefficient.

(4) A drug is classified as contraindicated in the clinical situation for which the risks outweigh any possible therapeutic benefit of the drug.

(5) Hospital-based medication errors and preventable ADR occur at a rate of 400,000 per year according to a recent Institute of Medicine study. These errors are reported to translate into an annual cost of $3.5 billion in extra hospital expense.

(6) A black box warning has implications for the manufacturer, health care provider, and patients. From the provider's and patients' perspective, the substitution of a drug without a black box warning may actually entail greater expense and exposure to another set of side effects than the use of the drug with a black box warning. Further, in the absence of patients' awareness of the potential dangers of a drug, when untoward events are precipitated by the drug, there is also an increased risk of litigation.

(7) Observed ADRs are those events that have been observed in association with use of the drug and are serious or are otherwise clinically significant. Expected ADRs are events that can be anticipated to occur with a drug, based on observations from other members of the drug class or animal studies. Expected ADRs are appropriate for warnings and precautions if the reaction is clinically serious, indicating it could have an outcome of death, life-threatening illness, or require hospitalization to treat.

Value-Oriented Reflective Reading

Elixir Sulfanilamide, A Deadly Mistake That Led to Safer Medicine

In January 1937, the world-changing use of penicillin to treat infections was still five years away. When an article in the *Journal of the American Medical Association* suggested the antimicrobial drug sulfanilamide might fight strep infections, several companies rushed to develop capsules and tablets and get them to market.

Among those entering the fray was Tennessee's S.E. Massengill Company, which whipped up a raspberry-flavored liquid "elixir" to meet demand. The solution included 10 percent sulfanilamide, 16 percent water, small amounts of raspberry extract, saccharin（糖精）, amaranth and caramel—and 72 percent diethylene glycol. The company shipped its miracle drug to hundreds of pharmacies all over the country. But soon people were dying— 105 by the end of the crisis. Diethylene glycol, it turned out, was a poison and the elixir was toxic.

Diethylene glycol is a condensation product of ethylene glycol（乙二醇）production. It proved to be an excellent solvent and was used as a glycerine（甘油）substitute, as a moistening agent（润湿剂）, and in the production of resins and explosives. Its use in food products, however, was not permitted because of the paucity（少量）of scientific data proving it safe for oral administration. Back then, there were one or two scientific studies about its toxicity, but they weren't widely known. In 1931, Von Oettingen and Jirouch determined that the minimum lethal dose of diethylene glycol in mice was 5 mL/kg body weight of a 50% solution given subcutaneously. Histologic analysis showed marked hydropic degeneration（水样变性）of the kidney. In early 1937, Haag and Ambrose reported that ingestion of a 3% diethylene glycol solution was rapidly fatal in a rat model. Massengill's control lab tested the mixture for flavor, appearance, and fragrance and found it satisfactory. However, they failed to note the toxicity of this highly nephrotoxic agent to humans.

Before 1938, the United States FDA only had the power to prevent adulteration and mislabeling. Pharmaceutical companies couldn't, for example, sell tablets of flour and say it was medicine. That was against the law. But they could sell something that was poison with zero safety testing beforehand—as long as it was what was said on the label. The Massengill company's elixir contained exactly what they said it did: sulfonamides and diethylene glycol, with some water and flavoring. So they didn't technically break the law. They called the stuff an elixir, but that word was only supposed to be used for products that contained ethyl alcohol. Massengill's syrup had none. The FDA seized on this technicality. They used it to track down the tainted medicine and slap Massengill with an unprecedented fine under the charge of mislabeling.

There was an enormous public outcry from the sulfanilamide disaster. In November 1937, both Houses of the U.S. Congress passed resolutions requesting a full investigation into the tragedy. Finally, Congress passed the *Food, Drug and Cosmetic Act* (1938). It required that pharmaceutical companies submit a new drug application report to the FDA showing drug safety before the interstate shipment of any new pharmaceutical agent. The new statute also banned dangerous drugs (for example, radium water) and false and misleading labeling. Formula disclosures of all active ingredients were now required. Directions for use and warnings about possible misuse were also required unless the drug was sold by prescription.

Penalties for infractions（违反）of any of these regulations were also stiffened.

The sulfanilamide disaster remains a seminal moment in US pharmaceutical history. The tragedy ushered in standards that placed the highest responsibility on the drug manufacturer to establish whether their medicines were fit– and safe– for purpose. It remains one of the key turning points in drug development history, whose consequences reverberate to this day.

Questions for discussion:

1. What do you think are the causes of the Elixir Sulfanilamide disaster?
2. Why is drug safety important?
3. What can be done by the pharmaceutical industry and the government to ensure drug safety?

Text B
The Package Insert and Prescription

In 1937, **sulfanilamide**, the first **sulfa** antimicrobial drug, was marketed. The **diluent** for this sulfa preparation was **diethylene glycol**, a chemical **analog** of **antifreeze**. More than 100 people, many of whom were children, died after receiving the drug. As a result, the US Congress **enacted** the 1938 *Federal Food, Drug and Cosmetic Act*, which required proof of safety before the introduction of a new drug into clinical practice. This act also changed the focus of the FDA from a policing agency, with an emphasis on **confiscation** of adulterated drugs, to a regulatory agency supervising the evaluation of new drugs.

In the practice of pediatrics, drugs which are not approved by the Food and Drug Administration (FDA) as safe and effective in children are prescribed daily. This is due in part to the fact that many drugs released since 1962 carry an "orphaning clause" in the package insert such as, "not to be used in children, since clinical studies have been insufficient to establish recommendations for its use." What is the status of the package insert? Is it a legal directive to the physician, or is it intended as a guide for the physician in prescribing a drug?[1]

The package insert, by legal definition of the *Federal Food, Drug and Cosmetic Act*, is the official information piece for a drug. The information it contains is derived from data supplied by investigators and submitted by the pharmaceutical firm to the FDA. The insert is written and printed by the drug manufacturer, but its contents must be approved by the FDA. The *Food, Drug and Cosmetic Act*, as **amended** in 1962, requires full **disclosure** of all known facts **pertaining to** the use of the drug. Therefore, a great deal of information is included in the insert, including the chemical structure of the drug, a summary of its pharmacological and toxicological action, its clinical indications and contraindications, precautions, reported adverse reactions, dosage recommendations, and available dosage forms.

Many drugs have package inserts approved by the FDA before the *Drug Amendments* of 1962 when manufacturers were required to show the safety but not the effectiveness of their products. On the basis of evaluations of the efficacy of these older drugs by **panels** of experts selected by the National Academy of Sciences-National Research Council, the FDA is now requiring revision of these package inserts to eliminate unsupported claims and thus to make them more useful to the practitioner.

Is the pediatrician breaking the law when he prescribes drugs for his patients which carry the "orphaning clause?" No, he is not. The physician may exercise his professional judgment in the use of any drug. However, if he **deviates** from the instructions in the package insert and adverse reactions occur, he must be prepared to defend his position in court if there is a malpractice suit.

Many drugs are used by clinicians in the treatment of conditions not listed in the package insert. The FDA cannot require a pharmaceutical firm to include a new use for the drug product in the insert even if it has been clinically tested and found useful for a given problem. Economic considerations are among a number of factors that may influence such a policy on the part of the company. If a new use for a drug is not yet included in the package insert, the manufacturer cannot advertise his product for that particular use. The package insert is legally binding on the manufacturer in limiting the conditions under which he can promote the use of the drug.

Another fact not generally recognized is that a physician's failure to use a drug approved as effective treatment for a specific disease might be **construed** as **malpractice**. In regard to this, it is important that the physician be informed about the availability of the drug and bases his decision to use it or not to use it on rational grounds. It would be unlikely that information taken from the package insert could be used successfully as evidence against the physician in a **liability** suit.

The dilemma facing the physician is illustrated by **imipramine** (Tofranil) when used in the treatment of **enuresis**. In 1965, a controlled study was published showing that this drug was useful in "training enuretic children to be dry." Its mechanism of action was not defined, but it appeared to be effective when given to children between the age of 5 and 12 years in a dosage up to 50 mg at bedtime. Following publication of this paper, imipramine became widely used for the treatment of enuresis. A straw poll of 15 pediatricians in the Cleveland area showed that 12 had prescribed imipramine for this condition. When one examines the package insert supplied with imipramine, two points are clear: ①the treatment of enuresis is not listed under conditions for the use of this drug; and ②there is a clear statement that the drug is not recommended for use in patients under 12 years of age. If a severe reaction occurred and litigation followed, how would a court react if a physician admitted to the use of this drug for the treatment of enuresis in view of the prohibitions in the package insert? Possibly, if other physicians made themselves available to give expert medical **testimony** and if other physicians in the community used the drug for this purpose, would the published clinical study, plus the physician's judgment in prescribing the drug, **suffice**?

The purpose of the FDA control of the package insert is not to **legislate** for the practice of medicine. As in the past, the physician is the individual prescribing the drug. The fact that he followed the recommendations in the package insert does not absolve him from responsibility for harm resulting to his patient, nor does failure to follow the recommendations in the package insert necessarily render him legally **culpable**.

The statements made in the package insert and approved by the FDA are not in themselves legally binding on the physician in his practice of medicine. Furthermore, no physician should rely on the package insert as his sole source of drug information. Drug dosages, as given in the insert, are guides for instituting therapy. The dose may have to be increased or decreased, depending on the patient's response. And, each time a drug is used, the question of benefit versus risk to the patient must be considered.

American Academy of **Pediatrics** Committee on Drugs has taken the view that the insert should be viewed as a useful guide to the physician; its recommendations should be judged on an equal **footing** with other publications and research reports. The package insert contains useful information, but the physician's decision on therapy should be based on cumulative knowledge derived from many sources. When sound scientific data exist which have shown that a drug is reasonably safe and effective in the treatment of a specific disease in adults, it should not necessarily be **withheld** from a sick child with the same disease just because its use has not been studied in children.[2] However, if used under these circumstances the physician should be cautious and the use of the drug should be reported to the manufacturer, the FDA, or in the medical literature to add to the knowledge concerning such use. The **foregoing** situation must be distinguished from use of the drug when the package insert states that the drug is contraindicated in infants or children on the basis of studies showing it to be unsafe or ineffective in these age groups.

The Committee feels that the pediatrician is likely to ignore the "orphaning clause" in the insert if, in his judgment, his patient requires a particular medication for **optimal** treatment. Whether or not this places him in unusual legal **jeopardy** is a question not yet resolved by the courts. It is the opinion of the Committee that this practice should not be a problem if the physician is well informed on the pharmacology and toxicology of the drugs he uses and closely follows his patient's response to treatment.

Changing the directives in the package insert, except to disclose **pertinent** new data, will not solve the problem of "therapeutic orphans." Early in 1968, Harry Shirkey, a **pediatrician** and pediatric pharmacologist, criticized the prevailing climate "created by present regulations of human experimentation [that] makes drug testing difficult" and urged all pediatricians and pediatric **subspecialists** to take on the "responsibility for developing active programs of clinical pharmacology and drug testing in infants and children" lest children become "therapeutic orphans". Echoing Dr. Harry Shirkey's stand, the Committee believes that the ultimate solution requires the development of programs in pediatric clinical pharmacology to ensure that all drugs used in infants and children are adequately tested for safety and efficacy.

In 1994, the National **Institutes** of Health created the Pediatric Pharmacology Research Unit Network to support pharmaceutical testing of children. At that time, nearly 80% of drugs lacked a pediatric label. Between 1997 and 2002, new federal laws and regulations "increased both the number of medications in pediatric clinical trials and the number that are labeled for use in children." The new drug testing was encouraged by both a carrot and a stick. The carrot was the "Pediatric Exclusivity Provision", which granted an additional 6 months of patent protection or market **exclusivity** for new molecular entities **voluntarily** tested in children. The stick was the "*Pediatric Rule*," a requirement by the FDA that, in some circumstances, pharmaceutical companies would be required to test their molecular entities to get approval from the FDA. Although this regulation was struck down, Congress passed other legislation. By 2002, new policies from the National Institutes of Health and Congressional regulations promoting pediatric research led to the public recognition that the "'Therapeutic Orphan' has finally been adopted". The adoption was further **solidified** by the enactment of the *Food and Drug Administration Safety and **Innovation** Act* in 2012[3], which made these mandates permanent.

Word Study

1. amend [əˈmend] *v.* 修正, 改进
2. analog [ˈænəlɔːg] *adj.* 模拟的, 类比的 *n.* 类似物
3. antifreeze [ˈæntifriːz] *n.* 防冻剂, 防冻液
4. confiscation [ˌkɒnfɪsˈkeɪʃən] *n.* 没收, 把……充公
5. construe [kənˈstruː] *v.* (formal) 理解, 解释, 识解
6. culpable [ˈkʌlpəbl] *adj.* (formal) 该负责任的, 应受处罚的, 有罪的
7. deviate [ˈdiːvɪeɪt] *v.* 背离, 偏离
8. diethylene [dɪəˈθɪliːn] *n.* 二次乙基, ~ glycol [ˈglaɪkɒl] *n.* 二甘醇
9. diluent [ˈdɪljʊənt] *adj.* 稀释的 (=diluting) *n.* 稀释剂

10. disclosure [dɪsˈkləʊʒə(r)] *n.* 揭发,透露,公开(秘密等)

11. enact [ɪˈnækt] *v.* 制定(法律),通过(法案),颁布

12. enuresis [ˌenjʊəˈriːsɪs] *n.* 遗尿症

13. exclusivity [ˌekskluːˈsɪvəti] *n.* 独占权,独占期

14. footing [ˈfʊtɪŋ] *n.* 立场,基础

15. foregoing [ˈfɔːgoʊɪŋ] *adj.* 前面的,上述的

16. glycol [ˈglaɪkɒl] *n.* 二醇,乙二醇

17. imipramine [ɪˈmɪprəˌmiːn] *n.* 丙米嗪(一种抗抑郁药)

18. institute [ˈɪnstɪtjuːt] *v.* 创立,制定;开始,着手

19. jeopardy [ˈdʒepədɪ] *n.* 危险

20. legislate [ˈledʒɪsleɪt] *v.* 立法,制定法律

21. liability [ˌlaɪəˈbɪlətɪ] *n.* (赔偿等)责任,义务

22. malpractice [ˌmælˈpræktɪs] *n.* 医疗失当,医疗差错,行为不当

23. optimal [ˈɒptɪməl] *adj.* 最理想的,最佳的

24. panel [ˈpænl] *n.* 座谈小组,全体陪审员

25. pediatrician [ˌpiːdɪəˈtrɪʃn] *n.* 儿科医生

26. pediatrics [ˌpiːdɪˈætrɪks] *n.* 儿科学

27. pertain [pəˈteɪn] *v. (formal)* 从属,pertaining to 与……有关系,关于,固有的

28. pertinent [ˈpɜːtnənt] *adj. (formal)* 相关的,有关的

29. subspecialist [sʌbˈspeʃəlɪst] *n.* 亚专科专家

30. suffice [səˈfaɪs] *v. (formal)* 足够,使满足

31. sulfa [ˈsʌlfə] *adj.* 磺胺的, sulfa drug 磺胺药物

32. sulfanilamide [ˌsʌlfəˈnɪləmaɪd] *n.* 磺胺

33. testimony [ˈtestɪmənɪ] *n.* (法庭上的)证词

34. voluntarily [ˈvɒləntrəlɪ] *adv.* 主动地,自愿地

35. withhold [wɪðˈhəʊld] *v.* (...from...) 把……扣着,压住,隐瞒

Notes

1. 在 "Is it a legal directive to the physician, or is it intended as a guide for the physician in prescribing a drug?" 中, be intended for 意为:"打算供……用""是为……而准备的"。

2. 在理解 "When sound scientific data exist which have shown that a drug is reasonably safe and effective in the treatment of a specific disease in adults, it should not necessarily be withheld from a sick child with the same disease just because its use has not been studied in children." 这个句子时,要注意两点:① "which have shown that a drug is reasonably safe and effective in the treatment of a specific disease in adults" 是一个定语从句修饰前面的 "data",放在动词 "exist" 后面是为了平衡;② "a sick child with the same disease" 意思是 "患有同样疾病的儿童",这里 "with 结构" 做定语,修饰 "a sick child"。

3. 美国对于儿童用药的重要监管法案包括:1994 年, FDA 通过《儿科标签规范》(*Pediatric Labeling Rule*),要求企业提供已上市处方药的儿科安全性和有效性信息,或在说明书说标识无儿童用药经验;1997 年, FDA 出台《FDA 现代化法案》(*Food and Drug Administration Modernization Act*, FDAMA),设立了儿童用药的 "儿科独占权条款" (The Pediatric Exclusivity Provision),对儿科标签进行政策性鼓励;2002 年,国会通过了《最佳儿童药品法案》(*Best Pharmaceuticals for Children*

Act, BPCA），设立"儿科优先目录"，继续"自愿"但"经济刺激"鼓励企业进行儿科用药研究；2003 年国会又颁布了《儿科研究平等法》(*Pediatric Research Equity Act*, PREA)，除非准予豁免，强制规定企业在新药和仿制药申报中提供成人适应证的儿科临床评价信息。2012 年，国会将 PREA 和 BPCA 两部法案定为永久性法律，再次明确除非 FDA 同意豁免或延迟，所有新药申请均需在成人临床二期结束会议后 60 天内提交"儿科研究计划"（pediatric study plan, PSP）。

Supplementary Parts

1. Medical and Pharmaceutical Terminology (14): Common Morphemes in English Terms for Human Anatomy

Morpheme	Meaning	Example
spir/o	呼吸	respiration 呼吸
nas/o	鼻	oronasal 口鼻的
rhin/o	鼻	rhinitis 鼻炎
pharyng/o	咽	pharyngotomy 咽切开术
laryng/o	喉	laryngophony 喉听诊音
trache/o	气管	tracheostomy 气管造口术
bronch/o	支气管	bronchogenic 支气管源的
pulm/o	肺	pulmometry 肺容量测定法
pulmon/o	肺	pulmonary 肺的
pneum/o	气,肺	pneumococci 肺炎球菌
pneumon/o	气,肺	pneumonia 肺炎
pleur/o	胸膜	pleural 胸膜的
muc/o	黏液	mucosal 黏膜的
diaphragm/o	膈	diaphragmitis 膈炎
phren/o,phrenic/o	膈神经	phrenicectomy 膈神经切除术
-pnea	呼吸	eupnea 平静呼吸
atel/o	不完全的,有缺陷的	atelectasis 肺不张
myc/o	真菌	mycoplasmas 支原体
or/o	口,嘴	oral 口的
stomat/o	口,嘴	stomatopathy 口（腔）病
labi/o	唇	labial 唇的
cheil/o	唇	cheilostomatoplasty 唇口成形术
dent/i	牙齿	dentalgia 牙痛
odont/o	牙齿	periodontal 牙周的
lingu/o	舌	sublingual 舌下的
gloss/o	舌	glossitis 舌炎
aden/o	腺	adenoid 腺样的
saliv/a	涎,吐液	salivation 流涎
sial/o	涎,吐液	sialoangitis 涎管炎
pharyng/o	咽	pharyngolaryngitis 咽喉炎
esophag/o	食管	esophageal 食管的
gastr/o	胃	gastric 胃的
pylor/o	幽门	pylorospasm 幽门痉挛
lapar/o	腹壁	laparotomy 剖腹术

续表

Morpheme	Meaning	Example
enter/o	小肠	parenteral 胃肠外的
duoden/o	十二指肠	duodenostomy 十二指肠造口术
jejun/o	空肠	jejunitis 空肠炎
ile/o	回肠	ileal 回肠的
col/o	结肠	colitis 结肠炎
append/o	阑尾	appendectomy 阑尾切除术
rect/o	直肠	rectal 直肠的
an/o	肛门	anal 肛门的
proct/o	肛门和直肠	proctalgia 肛部痛
hepat/o	肝	hepatitis 肝炎
cholecyst/o	胆囊	cholecystotomy 胆囊切开术
bil/i	胆	bilirubin 胆红素
chol/e	胆	cholemia 胆血症
pancreat/o	胰	pancreatic 胰的
peritone/o	腹膜	intraperitoneal 腹膜内的
succ/o	汁,分泌,分泌物	succagogue 促分泌的
pept/i	消化	peptic 消化(性)的
peps/i	消化	dyspepsia 消化不良
chlorhydr/o	盐酸	achlorhydria 胃酸缺乏
gluc/o	糖	glucatonia 血糖极度降低
glyc/o	糖	glycemia 糖血
sacchar/o	糖	polysaccharide 多糖
amyl/o	淀粉	amyloid 淀粉样的
lip/o	油,脂肪	lipemia 脂血(症)
steat/o	油,脂肪	steatolysis 脂肪分解
fec/a	粪便	fecal 粪便的
-lithiasis	结石	cholelithiasis 胆石症
-helcosis	溃疡形成	gastrohelcosis 胃溃疡
herni/o	疝	herniorrhaphy 疝修补术
gingiv/o	齿龈	gingivitis [牙]龈炎
dentin/o	牙本质	dentinoma 牙本质瘤
cement/o	牙骨质	cementoblast 成牙骨质细胞
orth/o	直的	orthodontics 畸齿矫正术,口腔正畸学
py/o	脓	pyorrhea 脓溢
ren/o	肾	renal 肾的
nephr/o	肾	nephromegaly 肾肥大
pyel/o	肾盂	pyelolithotomy 肾盂切开取石术
ureter/o	输尿管	ureterolith 输尿管结石
vesic/jo	膀胱	vesicotomy 膀胱切开术
cyst/o	囊、膀胱	cystitis 膀胱炎
urethr/o	尿道	urethropexy 尿道固定术
ur/o	尿,尿道	diuretic 利尿剂
hydr/o	水	hydronephrosis 肾盂积水
lith/o	石,结石	lithonephrotomy 肾石切除术

续表

Morpheme	Meaning	Example
staphyl/o	一束	staphylococcus 葡萄球菌
cocc/o	球菌	micrococcus 微球菌
retro-	向隔,在后	retroperitoneal 腹膜后的
test/o	睾丸	testosterone 睾酮
orchi/o	睾丸	orchiocele 睾丸突出,睾丸瘤
andr/o	男性,雄性的	androgen 雄激素
epididym/o	附睾	epididymovasostomy 输精管附睾吻合术
prostat/o	前列腺	prostatectomy 前列腺切除术
pen/o	阴茎	penile 阴茎的
genit/o	生殖器	genital 生殖的,生殖器的
gon/o,gonad/o	性腺,生殖腺	gonorrhea 淋病
sperm/o	精子	spermicide 杀精子剂
zo/o	生物	spermatozoon 精子
gamet/o	配子	gametogenesis 配子发生
ov/o	卵,卵子	ovulation 排卵
oo/o	卵,卵子	oophoritis 卵巢炎
uter/o	子宫	uteritis 子宫炎
hystcr/o	子宫	hysterectomy 子宫切除术
cervic/o	颈,宫颈	cervicectomy 子宫颈切除术
vagin/o	阴道	intravaginal 阴道内的
men/o	月经	menorrhagia 月经过多
gynec/o	妇女,女性	gynecologist 妇科专家
embry/o	胎儿,胚胎	embryonic 胚胎的
par(t)/o	娩出	postpartum 产后的
umbilic/o	脐	umbilical 脐的
mamm/o	乳房	mammography 乳房 X 线照相术
mast/o	乳房	mastectomy 乳房切除术
pseud/o	假的,伪的	pseudohermaphrodite 假两性体
crypt/o	隐藏的	cryptorchidism 隐睾
-plasia	形成	hyperplasia 增生
cardi/o	心	electrocardiogram 心电图
coron/o	冠,心脏	coronary 冠状的
aort/o	主动脉	aortic 主动脉的
angi/o	血管	angiogram 血管造影照片
vas/o	血管	vasoconstrictor 血管收缩药
arteri/o	动脉	arteriostenosis 动脉狭窄
ven/o	静脉	venous 静脉的
phleb/o	静脉	phlebitis 静脉炎
capill/o	非常小的血管	capillary 毛细血管
steth/o	胸	stethoscope 听诊器
sphygm/o	脉搏	sphygmomanometer 血压计
hemat/o	血	hematuria 血尿
granul/o	小结节,颗粒	agranulocyte 无粒细胞
plasm/o	血浆	plasmapheresis 血浆去除术

续表

Morpheme	Meaning	Example
thromb/o	凝块,血块	thrombosis 血栓形成
-poiesis	产生	hemopoiesis 造血,血细胞生成
fibr/o	纤维,纤维组织	fibrous 纤维性的
reticul/o	网	reticular 网状的
agglutin/o	凝块,凝集	agglutinogen 凝集原
glob/o	圆的,球	globin 球蛋白
ser/o	血清	serous 血清的,血浆的
nucle/o	核	mononuclear 单核的
kary/o	核	megakaryocyte 巨核细胞
phag/o	吃,吞噬	phagocyte 吞噬细胞
immun/o	安全,免疫	immunology 免疫学
lymph/o	淋巴	lymphadenitis 淋巴结炎
nod/o	结	nodal 结的,节点的
splen/o	脾	splenocyte 脾细胞
thym/o	胸腺	thymic 胸腺的
tonsill/o	扁桃体	tonsillectomy 扁桃体切除术
ather/o	脂肪堆积	atherosclerosis 动脉粥样硬化
necr/o	死亡	necrosis 坏死
angin/o	阻塞	anginal （心）绞痛的
tach/o	快速	tachycardia 心动过速
brachy	短的	brachycardia 心动过缓
ster/o	固体	cholesterol 胆固醇
coll/o	胶	colloid 胶质
somat/o	身体	somatotropin 生长激素
thyr/o	甲状腺	thyrocele 甲状腺肿
adren/o	肾上腺	adrenal 肾上腺
neur/o	神经	neuroblast 成神经细胞
myelin/o	髓磷脂	myelinic 髓磷脂的
myel/o	脊髓	myelocele 脊髓突出
gangli/o	神经节	ganglionic 神经节的
cerebr/o	大脑	cerebral 大脑的
encephal/o	脑	encephalomeningocele 脑膜脑膨出
ventricul/o	室	ventricular 脑室的,心室的
thalam/o	丘脑	thalamic 丘脑的
menin/o, meningi/o	脑膜	meningitis 脑膜炎 meningioma 脑（脊）膜瘤
spin/o	脊髓	spinocerebellar 脊髓小脑的
sympath/o	自主神经系统交感部分	sympathoblast 成交感神经细胞
cut/i	皮肤	subcutaneous 皮下的
derm/o	皮肤	epidermis 表皮
kerat/o	角质的,硬的	keratonosis 皮肤角质层病
trich/o	毛发	trichosis 毛发病
pil/o	毛发	pilous 毛的

续表

Morpheme	Meaning	Example
hidr/o	汗	hidropoiesis　汗生成
hol/o	整个,全部	holocrine　全分泌的
mer/o	部分	merocrine　部分分泌的
oste/o	骨	osteoblast　成骨细胞
chondr/o	软骨	chondral　软骨的
cran/o	颅骨	craniotome　开颅器
cervic/o	颈	cervical　颈的,子宫颈的
thorac/o	胸	thoracic　胸的
lumb/o	腰、背下部	lumbar　腰的
spondyl/o	椎骨	spondylosyndesis　脊柱制动术
vertebr/o	椎骨	intervertebral　椎间的
myel	脊髓,骨髓	myelitis　脊髓炎,骨髓炎
pelv/o	骨盆	pelvic　骨盆的
my/o,myos/o	肌肉	myitis (myositis)　肌炎
muscul/o	肌肉	muscular　肌肉的
sarc/o	肉	sarcolemma　肌膜
arthr/o	关节	arthritis　关节炎
articul/o	关节	articulation　关节
synovi/o	滑液	synovial　滑液的
fibr/o	纤维组织	fibroblast　成纤维细胞
tend/o	腱	tendotome　腱刀
ophthalm/o	眼	ophthalmologist　眼科专家
ocul/o	眼	ocular　眼的
phac/o	晶体	phacomalacia　晶状体软化
pupill/o	瞳孔	pupillary　瞳孔的
core/o	瞳孔,虹膜	corectopia　瞳孔异位
corne/o	角性的,角膜	corneal　角膜的
kerat/o	角膜	keratomalacia　角膜软化
scler/o	巩膜	sclerectasia　巩膜膨胀
retin/o	视网膜	retinoscopy　视网膜检影法
lacrim/o	眼泪,泪小管	lacrimal　泪的,泪管的
dacry/o	眼泪	dacryoadenitis　泪腺炎
conjunctiv/o	结膜	conjunctivitis　结膜炎
audi/o	听觉	audiometer　听力计
acou/o	听觉	acoustic　听觉的
aur/o	耳	aural　耳的
ot/o	耳	otitis　耳炎

(1) Write down the Latin or Greek affixes according to the same Chinese meaning.

1) 鼻　　_____　　_____

2) 口,嘴　_____　　_____

3) 牙齿　_____　　_____

4) 胆　_____　　_____

5) 肾　_____　　_____

6) 子宫 ＿＿＿＿＿＿＿＿   ＿＿＿＿＿＿＿＿

7) 血管 ＿＿＿＿＿＿＿＿   ＿＿＿＿＿＿＿＿

8) 核 ＿＿＿＿＿＿＿＿   ＿＿＿＿＿＿＿＿

9) 皮肤 ＿＿＿＿＿＿＿＿   ＿＿＿＿＿＿＿＿

10) 毛发 ＿＿＿＿＿＿＿＿   ＿＿＿＿＿＿＿＿

11) 眼 ＿＿＿＿＿＿＿＿   ＿＿＿＿＿＿＿＿

12) 听觉 ＿＿＿＿＿＿＿＿   ＿＿＿＿＿＿＿＿

(2) Word-matching 1.

1) eupnea		A. 食管的	
2) esophageal		B. 气管造口术	
3) succagogue		C. 输尿管结石	
4) intraperitoneal		D. 平静呼吸	
5) laparotomy		E. 胸膜的	
6) tracheostomy		F. 咽切开术	
7) pleural		G. 口腔正畸学	
8) ovulation		H. 排卵	
9) pharyngotomy		I. 促分泌的	
10) ureterolith		J. 肺炎球菌	
11) orthodontics		K. 腹膜内的	
12) pneumococci		L. 剖腹术	

(3) Word-matching 2.

1) coronary		A. 神经节的	
2) atherosclerosis		B. 结膜炎	
3) thrombosis		C. 淋巴结炎	
4) brachycardia		D. 毛细血管	
5) ganglionic		E. 血栓形成	
6) lymphadenitis		F. 软骨的	
7) chondral		G. 冠状的	
8) conjunctivitis		H. 动脉粥样硬化	
9) capillary		I. 检影法	
10) retinoscopy		J. 胸的	
11) corectopia		K. 瞳孔异位	
12) thoracic		L. 心动过缓	

(4) Complete the following expression according to its Chinese meaning in the brackets.

1) （不良）＿＿＿＿＿＿＿reactions

2) （分子）＿＿＿＿＿＿＿weight

3) （肝）＿＿＿＿＿＿＿function

4) （过敏）＿＿＿＿＿＿＿reaction

5) （缓解）＿＿＿＿＿＿＿effect

6) （降压）＿＿＿＿＿＿＿action

7) （尿常规）＿＿＿＿＿＿＿examination

8) （失效）＿＿＿＿＿＿＿date

9)（胃肠道）_____ disorder

10) significant _____ effect（疗效）

11) cardiac _____（不全）

12)（兴奋）_____ effect

(5) Translate the following passage into Chinese.

Dosage & Administration:

Usual dosage:

Adult: two capsule to be taken three times daily or as directed by the physician. Children 6 to 12 years of age; one capsule to be taken three times daily or as directed by the physician.

Complete the whole treatment course even if the condition seems to be improved.

Acute urethritis: 3 grams daily in 2 divided doses.

Gonorrhoea: 3 grams in a single dose.

Side effects:

As with other penicillin, AMOXYCILLIN may cause occasionally gastrointestinal disturbances, urticaria, rash and hypersensitivity reactions which may occur in patients with history of asthma, hay fever and urticaria. However, such side effect may disappear after cease of the treatment.

Precaution: Caution use in penicillin–sensitive patients.

2. English-Chinese Translation Skills: 药学英语翻译中的语篇意识

药学英语翻译的直接目标是篇章翻译,单个句子翻译是很少的。系统功能语法认为语篇是由一组相互连贯的句子所体现的意义单位,或称为语言运用单位。根据语言学理论,判断一系列句子是否构成了一个篇章取决于句内与句间的连贯关系。判断语篇的完整性有七个标准,包括"衔接性"(cohesion)、"连贯性"(coherence)、"意图性"(intentionality)、"可接受性"(acceptability)、"信息性"(informativity)、"情境性"(situationality) 和 "互文性"(intertextuality)。在这七个标准中,衔接性和连贯性最为重要,语篇没有衔接性和连贯性,其他几个标准在一定程度上很难实现。药学英语翻译中的语篇意识可以从衔接手段和主位结构来分析。

功能语法将衔接分为五种:指称、替代、省略、连接和词汇衔接,词汇衔接包括重复、同义词 / 反义词以及上下义词等。衔接是语篇表层结构上的有形网络,当语篇中一个成分的含义依赖于另一个成分的解释时,便产生了衔接与连贯关系。由于英语和汉语语言结构存在差异,在翻译语篇时,要注意两种语言中衔接表达方式上的差异。如下。

例 1: Traditional Chinese herbal medicine draws on ancient practice. Herbal medicine is as old as humanity itself. Early human beings were hunter-gatherers whose survival depended on their knowledge of their environment. Direct experience taught them which plants were toxic, which ones imparted strength and sustained life, and which had special healing qualities.

Thousands of medicinal substances are used in China today. Indeed, more than a million tons of herbs are used each year in China. Thirty herbs, mostly tonics, account for more than 50 percent of this figure, with *Gancao* topping the list at 86,000 tons.

参考译文:中药源于古代社会实践,和人类历史一样久远。古人靠狩猎和采集为生,生存与否取决于他们对环境的了解。直接的经验教会他们哪些植物有毒,哪些可以助长力气、延年益寿,哪些有特殊的治疗作用。

今天中国有数千种中药仍在使用。实际上,中国每年消耗的中药材超过百万吨。其中 30 种中药,主要是补益药,使用量超过总量的 50%。甘草消耗量最大,每年用量 8.6 万吨。

说明:在第一小段中,前两个小句主语分别是 traditional Chinese herbal medicine 和 herbal medicine,两个意义重复的主语表明这两个句子之间的衔接。但是在翻译成汉语时,如果按照原文将两个重复主语翻译出来就显得啰嗦,汉语译文省略一个主语,符合汉语表达习惯也保留了两个小句的意义衔接。第二小段第一句中主语 "thousands of medicinal substances" 与第一段中的 "traditional Chinese herbal medicine" 以及本段中下面两句中的 "herbs" 形成重复,构成意义上的衔接,但是如果按照字面翻译将 "thousands of medicinal substances" 译成 "数千种药物",则明显破坏了整个语篇意义上的衔接。

例 2:[1] Another form of transmucosal delivery takes advantage of the superior absorptive properties of (the respiratory tract, nose, and bronchial tree). [2] Drugs can be delivered to (these tissues) via sprays. [3] The level at which the drug acts in (the respiratory system) can be controlled by the particle size. [4] Smaller particles penetrate further into (the lung) before they are filtered out.

[5] Spray delivery has already been used to deliver two peptides, gonadotrophin-releasing factor, a potential male contraceptive, and vasopressin, a pituitary hormone being tested for memory enhancement. [6] Spray delivery is now being tested with insulin. [7] Sprays are preferred for peptides because peptides, like proteins, are hydrolyzed in the stomach. [8] Respiratory delivery would also be advantageous for antibiotics used to treat pneumonia and for anticancer drugs for (lung) cancer. [9] Vaccines might ideally be administered this way. [10] And cardiovascular drugs should be more effective by this route since delivery to the highly vascular (lung) is equivalent to an intra-arterial injection.

参考译文:[1] 另一种经黏膜给药法利用了呼吸道、鼻子和支气管卓越的吸收特性。[2] 药物可以通过喷射进入这些组织。[3] 颗粒的大小可控制作用于呼吸道的药物水平。[4] 小颗粒在被滤出之前就可渗入肺的深处。

[5] 喷剂已用于两种肽给药,一种是潜在的男性避孕药,促性腺激素释放因子,另一种是正在测试其增强记忆功能的脑垂体激素加压素。[6] 喷剂也在试用于胰岛素的给药。[7] 喷剂更适用于肽,因为肽和蛋白质一样,可在胃中水解。[8] 呼吸道给药法对治疗肺炎的抗生素和治疗肺癌的抗癌药都有其优越性。[9] 也是服用疫苗的最佳途径。[10] 心血管药物通过这一途径服用会更有效,因为心血管密布的肺部送药与动脉内注射是一样的。

说明:该句是关于药物给药系统中的 "呼吸道给药法",共有两个小段,10 个小句,为了便于说明分别给每个小句标上 [1] 到 [10] 的编号。在第 [1] 句中 another form 与其前文中一定存在的 one form 构成连接,形成语篇上下文整体连贯。其他衔接关系如下。

(1) 第 [1]、[2]、[5]、[6]、[7]、[8] 句中的 delivery、spray deliver、spray 等构成重复关系。

(2) 第 [1]、[2]、[3]、[4]、[8]、[10] 句中的 the respiratory tract, nose, and bronchial tree、these tissues、the respiratory system、lung 等构成上下义词关系,其中 tissues, respiratory system 是上义词,其他名词则是下义词。

(3) 第 [9]、[10] 句中的 this way, this route 与前文中的 delivery 等构成指代关系。

(4) 第 [2]、[3]、[5]、[6]、[7]、[8]、[9]、[10] 中的 drug、peptides、insulin、antibiotics、anticancer drugs、vaccines、cardiovascular drugs 等构成重复和上下义词关系。

(5) 第 [3]、[4] 句中的 the particle size 和 smaller particles、they 等构成重复和指代关系。

从这些衔接关系分析中可见,(1)、(2) 和 (4) 表示的关系是本语篇的主要衔接关系,说明此语篇的主要内容是关于 "给(药)"(delivery)、"呼吸"(respiratory) 和 "(给)药"(drug)。

语法衔接关系构成语篇意义上的连贯,但是英汉两种语言差异要求在翻译时要注意不同语言在衔接与连贯关系表达上的差别,在翻译过程中不能够将源语言的衔接关系完全移植到目的语中。分析参考译文,第 [4] 句中的指代词 they 和第 [9] 句中的指导词 this way 都省略了,翻译过程中通过英汉语不同的衔接手段实现译文的语篇连贯。

功能语法将小句分为主位和述位两个部分,主位就是句子谓语动词前面的部分,除了主位,句子的其他成分就是述位。主位是话题,小句信息的出发点;述位是目标,小句信息传递的核心内容。英语和汉语主位结构相似,都是主位在前,述位在后;主位往往都是已知信息,述位都是新信息。英汉两种语言在主位结构上的相似性应用在翻译中可以采取顺着原句顺序保留原文的主位结构的直译方式,实现源语语篇和目的语语篇的结构对应。

在上面例 2 中的第一段,源语语篇有 4 个小句,其中小句 [3] 和小句 [4] 是复合小句,因此第一段中共有 6 个主位,它们分别是:[1] another form of transmucosal delivery, [2] drugs, [3] the level (...) 和定语从句中的 the drug, [4] smaller particles 和时间状语从句中的 they。分析这第一段的译文可见,小句 [1] 和小句 [2] 的翻译中保留了英语小句的主位结构;小句 [3] 的译文将原英语小句中的述位 "the particle size" 变成了主位,这里就值得商榷。按照语言学的理论,主位是已知信息,是小句信息的出发点,而译文中的主位 "颗粒大小" 却是前文中没有出现的,是 "新信息",这样处理破坏了原英语小句的信息结构。如果将小句 [3] 翻译成:"药物作用于呼吸道的水平可由颗粒大小控制",则可以较好地表述原句的信息,虽然原小句的主位 the level 和 drug 的位置发生了变化,但这是由英汉两种语言的结构差异所致。在小句 [4] 中,原英语小句中的一个主位 they 被省略了,但是原句的信息结构没有改变,这些语言上的变化属于必要性转变(obligatory shifts)。

在完整语篇中,连续小句的主位构成 "主位 - 述位" 推进。英语中 "主位 - 述位" 按照一定规律推进,小句间主位、述位交替,环环相扣,构成衔接有序的语篇。

再看例 2:

第一段中:小句 [2] 的述位中的 delivered 是小句 [1] 中的主位,小句 [3] 中的主位 drug 对应小句 [2] 的主位,小句 [4] 的主位是小句 [3] 的述位。在第二段中:小句 [5]、[6]、[7]、[8] 主位相同,而小句 [9]、[10] 的主位则是前面 4 个小句的述位(上下义关系或同义、并列关系)。再将第一段和第二段联合分析可见这段语篇中 10 个小句的主位推进模式构成了意义连贯的语篇。

药学英语属于科技英语语篇,语言结构严谨,内容丰富,专业性强。在药学英语翻译过程中,除了必须掌握基本的翻译技巧之外,更要注重英汉两种语言在构成语篇衔接性与连贯性上的异同性,使译文能够更好地传递原文的语篇信息。

(龚长华　易　玲　陈　菁　史志祥)